MYOCARDIAL ISCHEMIA AND LIPID METABOLISM

MYOCARDIAL ISCHEMIA AND LIPID METABOLISM

Edited by

R. Ferrari
University of Brescia
Brescia, Italy

A. M. Katz
University of Connecticut Health Center
School of Medicine
Farmington, Connecticut

A. Shug
William S. Middleton Memorial Veteran
  Hospital
Madison, Wisconsin

and

O. Visioli
University of Brescia
Brescia, Italy

PLENUM PRESS • NEW YORK AND LONDON

Library of Congress Cataloging in Publication Data

Main entry under title:

Myocardial ischemia and lipid metabolism.

"Proceedings of the International Society for Heart Research on Myocar-
dial Ischemia and Lipid Metabolism, held July 4–6, 1983, in Rome, Italy"
    Includes bibliographies and index.
    1. Coronary heart disease—Congresses. 2. Blood Lipids—Metabolism—
Congresses. I. Ferrari, R. (Roberto) II. International Society for Heart
Research. [DNLM: 1. Coronary Disease—etiology—congresses. 2. Lipids—
metabolism—congresses. 3. Lipids—adverse effects—congresses. WG
300 M9976 1983]
RC685.C6M956   1984   616.1′23   84-18103
ISBN 0-306-41832-0

Proceedings of the International Society for Heart Research on
Myocardial Ischemia and Lipid Metabolism,
held July 4–6, 1983, in Rome, Italy

©1984 Plenum Press, New York
A Division of Plenum Publishing Corporation
233 Spring Street, New York, N.Y. 10013

Printed in the United States of America

PREFACE

Over the past years, the thrust of research in cardiology has
been toward an understanding of the engineering of the heart as a
pump that transports blood to the various organs of the body. More
recently, the fields of biochemistry and biophysics have come to
influence heart research. The modern cardiologist can no longer
pretend to understand, for example, what is happening to the patient
with myocardial infarction or ischemia without understanding the
principles of molecular biology. The structure and function of the
heart are therefore central themes of cardiological research and
practice, which incorporate knowledge and discoveries from diverse
disciplines.

The importance of lipid metabolism in the myocardium has become
clearly understood. In the well-oxygenated heart, fatty acids are
the preferred substrates. The fact that the heart derives most of
its energy from the oxidation of lipids, which represent the largest energy store of the body, is logical for an organ that must
work throughout our lifetime. There are, however, several lines
of evidence that during ischemia, lipids may be harmful to the heart.
High levels of free fatty acids in the serum have been suggested to
play a role in causing life-threatening arryhthmias and damage in
the ischemic heart. The molecular basis for these effects remains
poorly understood, and several possible mechanisms for these harmful effects have been suggested.

Recognition of these important questions was the stimulus that
led to the organization of the meeting which served as the basis for
the present text. This book, therefore, is concerned with the intimate activities of lipids within the heart muscle cell; their distribution; their specific effects on heart membranes; the pathological effects of their abnormal accumulation during ischemia; the
possibility of reducing these toxic effects; and the clinical relevance of this rapidly growing body of knowledge. We believe that
bringing together these various aspects of lipid metabolism will be
of help not only to those working on these subjects, but all phy-
siologists, biochemists and clinicians to whom the myocardium is
important.

This book is, of course, not comprehensive, but contains selected highlights in the areas covered. The present work is intended to provide a basis for the continuing study of lipid metabolism during myocardial ischemia, to lead to a greater understanding of its complexity, and to help generate ideas for further research.

                              Odoardo Visioli, Chairman

ACKNOWLEDGMENTS

The Editors thank the International Society for Heart Research, for sponsoring the satellite meeting "MYOCARDIAL ISCHEMIA AND LIPID METABOLISM" in conjunction with its XI International Congress. This satellite meeting, held in Rome July 4-6, 1983, together with the interactions and exchange of ideas that it made possible, provided the stimulus for the development of the present text.

Our gratitude is also extended to the University of Brescia, the University of Bologna, and the Italian Society of Cardiology for their support and cooperation in arranging the meeting. We are especially grateful to Dr. Claudio Cavazza, President of Sigma Tau Pharmaceutical Company, for having made this meeting possible. We also thank Signora Vania Mainardi and Signora Nunzia Gaetani for many forms of administrative and secretarial assistance, and Mrs. Priscilla Adler who transferred all of the manuscripts to a computer so as to provide uniformity of style in this text.

Roberto Ferrari
Brescia, Italy

Arnold M. Katz
Farmington, U.S.A.

Austin L. Shug
Madison, U.S.A.

Odoardo Visioli
Brescia, Italy

CONTENTS

ISCHEMIA AND LIPID-INDUCED CHANGES
IN MYOCARDIAL FUNCTION

INTERVENTIONS USED TO MODIFY LIPID-INDUCED
ABNORMALITIES IN THE HEART

IMPORTANCE OF LIPID METABOLISM IN MAN

OVERVIEW OF LIPID METABOLISM

N. Siliprandi, F. Di Lisa,
C.R. Rossi and A. Toninello

Istituto di Chimica Biologica, Universita di Padova and
Centro Studio Fisiologia Mitocondriale C.N.R., 35131
Padova, Italy

Cardiac muscle is a typical aerobic tissue; its metabolism
is closely dependent on oxygen, so that oxygen restriction leads
to more or less profound functional and structural damages.
Myocardial cells are extremely rich in mitochondria, which
occupy ~ 40 per cent of the cellular volume, in myoglobin, and
in carnitine (1.3 μmoles/g wet wt of tissue). More than 95 per
cent of the ATP utilized in contraction is produced by oxidative
phosphorylation.

In the well oxygenated heart, fatty acids and ketone bodies
have been identified as the preferential substrates by both in
vitro and in vivo studies (for review see 1). The fact that the
heart derives most of its energy (approximately 80%) from
lipids, by far the largest energy stores in the body, is
appropriate for an organ that must work for a life-time without
stopping. The pattern of lipid metabolism in the heart does not
differ significantly from that of other tissues with the only
exception of lipogenesis, which is practically absent. This
means that, unlike other tissues, the heart is unable to convert
glucose into fatty acids.

In the present report, two aspects of cardiac lipid
metabolism will be considered briefly: i) the transport of
fatty acids across sarcolemma and within the cytoplasm; and ii)
the activation of fatty acids and their compartmentation.

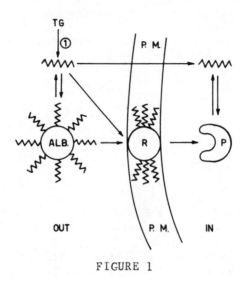

FIGURE 1

Proposed pathway for fatty acid transport across the
sarcolemma. P.M.: plasma membrane; ALB.: albumin; R: fatty acid
receptor; P:.fatty acid binding protein; TG: triglycerides; ① :
lipoprotein lipase; ⋀⋀⋀ : unbound fatty acids.

Transport of Fatty Acids in the Cardiac Cell

Despite extensive investigations into cellular uptake of
fatty acids, there is still no precise answer as to how these
compounds enter the cell. Both simple diffusion (2) and a
facilitated transport dependent on binding of fatty acids to a
receptor in the sarcolemma (3) have been demonstrated. In
either case, Ca^{2+} seems to be an important regulator of fatty
acid transfer across cell membrane (4). As illustrated in
Figure 1, a portion of the fatty acids taken up by the heart are
albumin-bound, in which form they are transported from adipose
tissue. Albumin-bound fatty acids are in equilibrium with
unbound fatty acids present in the blood at very low
concentration; this small pool is free to bind to the surface of
the myocardial cell (5). However, direct transfer of fatty
acids from albumin to a more or less specific receptor present
in the sarcolemma cannot be excluded. A dual mechanism for the
fatty acid entry into the cell was proposed by Stein and Stein
(6), who proposed that fatty acids enter the cell through
selective anatomical channels by means of two non-energy

dependent mechanisms, one resembling passive diffusion down a
concentration gradient and the other being a saturable fatty
acid binding process between proteins in the blood and on the
myocardial sarcolemma. A second portion of fatty acids is
derived from plasma triglycerides by the action of lipoprotein
lipase located int he capillary endothelium. The relative
contributions of these two sources is dependent on the
nutritional state and hormonal equilibrium of the subject.

    Once in the cytosol, free fatty acids bind to a cytoplasmic
protein that assists in the fatty acid distribution to various
pools and pathways. Fournier et al. have recently isolated a
soluble myocardial protein, molecular weight 12,000, considered
to be the specific transcytoplasmic fatty acid carrier (7, 8).
This protein, which is also able to bind acyl CoA and acyl
carnitine, may self-aggregate in at least four distinct
molecular species, each having a different fatty acid binding
capacity. As illustrated in Figure 2, the monomer has little,

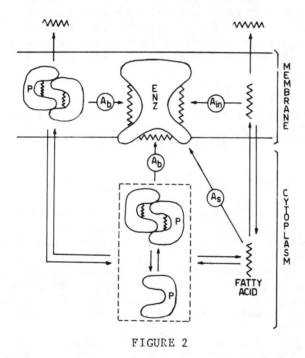

FIGURE 2

Interaction of fatty acid or acyl CoA with cytoplasmic binding
protein. ENZ.: membrane enzymes (acyl CoA synthetase or acyl
transferases). Fatty acids free in cytoplasm (A_s), bound to
the protein (A_b) and free in the membrane (A_{in}). P: fatty
acid binding protein. Reproduced from Biochemistry 22: 1863
(1983) with the author's permission.

if any, binding capacity for fatty acids or their derivatives. According to Fournier et al. (7), the self-aggregating properties of the cardiac fatty acid carrier have important metabolic implications. For instance, the activity of acyl CoA synthetases and carnitine or α-glycerophosphate acyl transferase might be strongly regulated by the concentration and the status of the carrier. Two types of regulation by this carrier protein are possible: a long-term and a short-term regulation. The former is likely occur in vivo, since the protein is inducible by a fat-rich diet (9). A short-term regulation can be predicted on the basis of the uneven distribution of the protein in the cytosol and the equilibrium among the multiaggregated states of the protein. Fournier et al. (8) assume that the short-term regulation might occur, for instance, during each cardiac cycle. It can also be postulated that a deficiency of the fatty acid binding protein, or abnormalities of its structure or a self-aggregation capability might be responsible for the damage induced by free fatty acids or their derivatives. According to Gloster and Harris (10), myoglobin, rather than specific fatty acid binding proteins, may transport fatty acids as well as oxygen. Indeed, the myocardium is very rich in myoglobin and it is very likely that myoglobin may act, if not primarily as a transporter, as a buffer for fatty acids in the cytoplasm.

Regarding the existence of cytoplasmic fatty acid-binding proteins having a high affinity for acyl CoA (11), the possible role of long-chain fatty acids as regulators of mitochondrial ATP-ADP exchanger (12) seems to be rather doubtful, at least in vivo (13).

Fatty Acid Activation

Oxidation, as well as any other metabolic utilization of fatty acids, requires an initial investment of energy (in the form of ATP or GTP) for the activation step leading to acyl CoA formation. For this reason, a critical concentration of nucleotide triphosphates is required in order to initiate fatty acid oxidation. The activation process consists of two reactions catalyzed by the ATP-dependent acyl CoA synthetase (acid:CoA ligase (AMP), E.C.6.2.1.2) respectively:

$$1) \quad R-C\overset{O}{\underset{OH}{\diagup}} + CoASH + ATP \rightleftharpoons R-C\overset{O}{\underset{SCoA}{\diagup}} + \boxed{AMP} + PPi \longrightarrow 2Pi$$

ATP-dependent acyl CoA synthetase

2) $\quad R-C\!\!\begin{smallmatrix}\nearrow O\\\searrow OH\end{smallmatrix} + \text{CoASH} + \text{GTP} \rightleftharpoons R-C\!\!\begin{smallmatrix}\nearrow O\\\searrow \text{SCoA}\end{smallmatrix} + \quad \text{GDP} \quad + \quad \boxed{\text{Pi}}$

GTP-dependent acyl CoA synthetase.

The ATP-dependent enzymes are present both in the extramitochondrial space (outer mitochondrial membrane and sarcoplasmic reticulum) and in the "inner membrane-matrix" space; the GTP-dependent acyl CoA synthetase is uniquely present in the intramitochondrial space.

It is important to note that the ATP-dependent synthetases are inhibited by AMP, whereas the GTP-dependent synthetase is inhibited by inorganic phosphate (14); note that both AMP and inorganic phosphate are products of the reactions.

"External" fatty acid activation

Fatty acids, when activated by the extramitochondrial ATP-dependent acyl CoA synthetase, require carnitine as a "carrier" in order to reach the oxidation site, located within the "inner membrane-matrix" space: carnitine dependent oxidation (15). Figure 3 shows the conditions under which the oxidation of fatty acids activated at the external site takes place and illustrates the mechanism involved. Under the conditions of a typical experiment, represented by the oxygen trace in Figure 3, mitochondrial synthesis of ATP is prevented by an uncoupler (DNP) and the entry of extramitochondrial ATP is prevented by atractyloside; consequently, the intramitochondrial activation of fatty acid is abolished. Note that oleate is not oxidized unless ATP and carnitine are added: ATP is necessary for the "external" activation of oleate, while carnitine is necessary for the translocation of activated acyl into the inner compartment.

The carnitine-dependent acyl translocation allows controlled access of the acyls to the oxidation site. However, in the heart the mechanism of this regulation is much less clear than in the liver, where malonyl CoA, the presence of which in the heart is doubtful, has a predominant role (16).

"Internal" ATP-dependent fatty acid activation

Intramitochondrial ATP-dependent activation, preliminary to the so-called "carnitine-independent" oxidation, involves fatty acids that diffuse freely into the mitochondrion or are

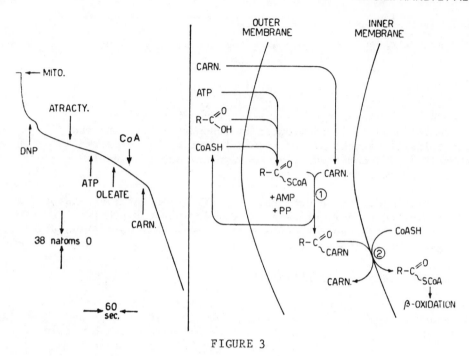

FIGURE 3

Fatty acid "carnitine dependent oxidation". Left: oleate
oxidation by rat heart mitochondria. The incubation system
contained 16 mM phosphate buffer (pH 7.2), 0.2 M sucrose, 10 mM
HEPES, 2 mM $MgCl_2$ and 10 mM malonate. At the points indicated
by arrows, 5 mg of mitochondrial protein (MITO), 0.1 µmole of
2,4-dinitrophenol (DNP), 50 µmoles of atractyloside (ATRACTY), 2
µmoles of ATP, 0.2 µmole of oleate (OLE), 0.3 µmole of CoA and 1
µmole of L-carnitine (CARN) were added. Total volume was 2.0
ml. Right: scheme of the mechanism involved in the fatty acid
oxidation supported by "external" activation. ① external
acyl-carnitine transferase. ② carnitine translocase.

generated in situ by the activity of phospholipases. It occurs
at expense of endogenous ATP, produced either by respiratory
chain-coupled phosphorylation or substrate-linked
phosphorylation. Unlike external activation, the internal
ATP-dependent activation does not require added ATP and
carnitine (Figure 4). The presence of two ATP-dependent acyl
CoA synthetases, external and internal to the inner membrane,

has been confirmed by their identification in submitochondrial fractions (17).

The dual localization of the ATP-dependent acyl CoA synthetase can be reasonably interpreted as a device for the synthesis of acyl CoA, impermeable to the inner membrane, in the same site as its metabolic utilization. Acyl CoA formed in the inner compartment is utilized in the oxidation processes occurring within this compartment, while acyl CoA synthesized in the outer compartment is directly available for glyceride

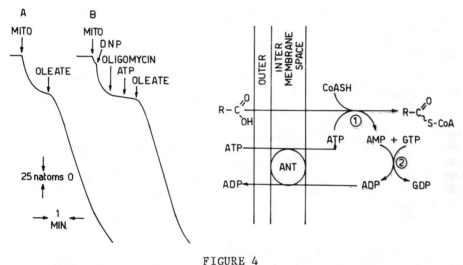

FIGURE 4

"Internal ATP dependent and carnitine independent oleate oxidation. Left: (A) coupled and (B) uncoupled rat heart mitochondria. Experimental conditions as in Fig. 3 except that no malonate was present. At the points indicated by arrows 5 mg of mitochondrial protein (MITO), 0.2 μmole of oleate, 0.1 μmole of DNP, 2 μg/ml protein of oligomycin, 2 μmoles of ATP were added. Right: scheme of the mechanism involved in the fatty acid oxidation supported by internal activation. ① ATP dependent acyl CoA synthetase. ② GTP-AMP phosphotransferase. ANT: adenine nucleotide translocase.

and phospholipid synthesis. However, when the acyl production
in one or the other compartment exceeds its utilization in situ,
translocation mediated by the carnitine-dependent system ensures
a redistribution according to the physiological demand.

The extent to which long chain fatty acids are oxidized in
vivo by the carnitine-independent process is unknown. To our
knowledge a condition of absolute carnitine deficiency in the
heart, which might resolve this question, has not been described
so far. However, the concept that the carnitine-dependent
process is by far the most important for fatty acid oxidation in
the heart can be inferred from many experimental and clinical
observations. For instance, the finding by Bressler and Wittels
(18) that triglyceride accumulation in diphtheritic myocarditis

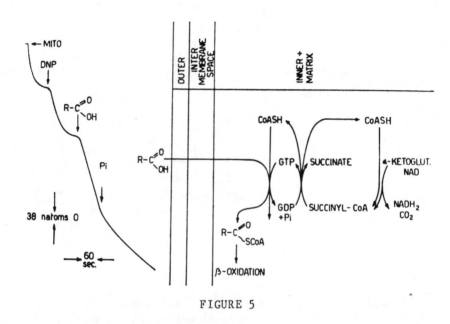

FIGURE 5

GTP-dependent fatty acid oxidation. Left: oleate oxidation by
rat heart mitochondria in the absence of inorganic phosphate.
Experimental conditions as in Fig. 3 except that inorganic
phosphate and malonate were omitted. At the points indicated by
arrows 5 mg of mitochondrial protein (MITO), 0.1 μmole of DNP,
0.2 μmole of oleate (OLE), 30 μmoles of inorganic phosphate were
added. Right: scheme of the reactions involved in the
GTP-dependent fatty acid oxidation.

is associated with a depressed rate of oxidation of fatty acids and a decreased content of carnitine, and oxidation and acyl carnitine synthesis to normal (19) underlines a clearcut relation between the carnitine system and fatty acid oxidation. Similarly, other conditions of triglyceride accumulation in myocardium (for review see 20) might be referred to an impairment of the carnitine-dependent process for fatty acid translocation into the mitochondrial inner space.

GTP-dependent fatty acid activation

This process is located in the "inner membrane matrix" space and is dependent on GTP produced in the same compartment at the α-ketoglutarate oxidation step in the Krebs cycle. As shown in Figure 5 the GTP activation is insensitive to uncouplers and sensitive to both phosphate and arsenate. The responsible synthetase, isolated and purified by Rossi et al. (20), has a molecular weight of about 20,000 and contains a cofactor identified as 4´-phosphopantotheine. This process, which is very active in liver mitochondria (22), has very low activity in myocardium (23). The existence of the three fatty acid activation processes (carnitine-dependent, carnitine-independent and GTP-dependent) in the heart is shown in Figure 6.

Significance of fatty acid activation in the heart

The ATP-dependent activation (intra- and extra-mitochondrial), the most important if not the only system for fatty acid activation in the heart, produces one mole of AMP per mole of acyl CoA formed. It is well known that AMP, unlike ATP and ADP, is unable to cross the inner mitochondrial membrane and, if not phosphorylated to ADP, remains sequestered in the same compartment where it is formed. When AMP accumulates above a critical value, the activity of ATP-dependent synthetase is inhibited. Furthermore, accumulation of AMP in the cytosolic space leads to a stimulation of fructose-6-phosphate kinase. Therefore, oscillations in the extra-mitochondrial ATP/AMP ratio represent a regulatory mechanism whereby the rates of carbohydrate and lipid utilization are integrated. On the other hand, accumulation of AMP within the matrix space (Figure 7) stimulates α-ketoglutarate oxidation by promoting a continuous supply of GDP, which is necessary for α-ketoglutarate oxidation in the reaction catalyzed by the GTP-AMP phosphotransferase:

$$GTP + AMP \rightleftharpoons GDP + ADP$$

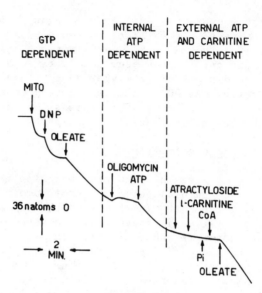

FIGURE 6

Evidence for the existence of the three fatty acid activation
processes in rat heart mitochondria: GTP-dependent, internal
ATP-dependent, external ATP- and carnitine-dependent.
Experimental conditions as in Fig. 3 except that inorganic
phosphate and malonate were omitted. At the points indicated by
arrows 5 mg of mitochondrial protein (MITO), 0.1 μmole of DNP,
0.2 μmole of oleate, 2 μg/mg protein of oligomycin, 2 μmoles of
ATP, 50 nmoles of atractyloside, 1 μmole of L-carnitine, 0.3
μmole of CoA, 30 μmoles of inorganic phosphate were added.

At the same time AMP is converted into ADP and the inhibition of
the ATP-dependent acyl CoA synthetase is progressively removed.
Therefore, changes of the intramitochondrial ATP/AMP ratio
impose a mutual control to α-ketoglutarate and fatty acid
oxidations. A high ATP/AMP ratio stimulates fatty acid
oxidation, whereas a low ATP/AMP ratio stimulates
α-ketoglutarate oxidation and substrate level phosphorylation.
Furthermore, fatty acid activation promotes and sustains
α-ketoglutarate oxidation and vice versa. Therefore, it is
likely that fatty acid activation, rather than oxidation (24),
might control the metabolic flux in the Krebs cycle.

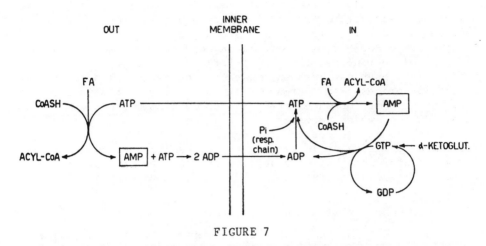

FIGURE 7

Scheme for adenine nucleotide changes consequent to fatty acid
activation in the extra- and intra-mitochondrial space. It is
shown that accumulated AMP is removed by the adenylate kinase
reaction in the extramitochondrial space, and by GTP-AMP
phosphotransferase in the intramitochondrial space. Since GTP
is produced by α-ketoglutarate oxidation, this reaction is
critical for the internal fatty acid activation process.

     Another important condition involved in this regulation is
the availability of free CoA within the "inner membrane matrix"
space. Free CoA is necessary for the oxidation of both fatty
acids and α-ketoglutarate. Overproduction of acyl CoA causes a
shortage of free CoA which, in turn, induces an inhibition of
α-ketoglutarate oxidation. This inhibition can be relieved by
carnitine which, through the transacylation reactions, makes
more CoA available (25). This sparing action of carnitine,
together with its role in redistributing acyls between cellular
compartments is important in the regulation of mitochondrial
oxidation. The acyl buffering action of carnitine and the
consequent improvement of the metabolic flux in the Krebs cycle
might be relevant to hypoxic conditions, in which fatty acids
and their metabolites accumulate in the cardiac cell.

It is generally accepted that the accumulation of fatty acids and their derivatives in hypoxic conditions aggravate the functional and structural lesions induced by oxygen restriction. However, in the scrutiny of the underlying biochemical mechanisms, fatty acid activation and its implications have not been extensively considered. Indeed, the activation process may continue even when fatty acid oxidation is blocked. For instance, the deacylation of membrane phospholipids, which seems to be accelerated in ischemic tissue as the result of activation of phospholipase A_2 (26), represents a futile cycle leading to progressive accumulation of AMP and contributing signficantly to the degeneration of the ischemic tissue.

REFERENCES

1. Neely, J.R. & Morgan, H.E. (1974): Ann. Rev. Physiol. 36: 413.
2. DeGrelle, R.T. & Light, R.J. (1980): J. Biol. Chem. 255: 9739.
3. Samuel, D., Paris, S., & Aihaud, G. (1976): Eur. J. Biochem. 64: 583.
4. Schroeder, F. & Soler-Argilaga, C. (1983): Eur. J. Biochem. 132: 517.
5. Harris, P., Gloster, J.A., & Ward, B.J. (1980): Arch. Mal. Coeur 73: 593.
6. Stein, O. & Stein, Y. (1968): J. Cell Biol. 36: 62.
7. Fournier, N.C., Geoffroy, M., & Deshusses, J. (1978): Biochim. Biophys. Acta 533: 457.
8. Fournier, N.C., Zuker, M., Williams, R.E., & Smith, I.C.P. (1983): Biochemistry 22: 1863.
9. Ockner, R.K. & Manning, J.A. (1974): J. Clin. Invest. 54: 326.
10. Gloster, J. & Harris, P. (1977): Biochem. Biophys. Res. Commun. 74: 506.
11. Lunzer, M.A., Manning, J.A., & Ockner, R.K. (1977): J. Biol. Chem. 252: 5483.
12. Shug, A., Lerner, E., Elson, C., & Shrago, E. (1971): Biochem. Biophys. Res. Commun. 43: 557.
13. Barbour, R.L. & Chan, S.H.P. (1979): Biochem. Biophys. Res. Commun. 89: 1168.
14. Alexandre, A., Rossi, C.R., Sartorelli, L., & Siliprandi, N. (1969): FEBS Letters 3: 279.
15. Rossi, C.R., Galzigna, L., Alexandre, A., & Gibson, D.M. (1967): J. Biol. Chem. 242: 2102.
16. McGarry, J.D. & Foster, D.W. (1979): J. Biol. Chem. 254: 8163.
17. deLong, J.W. & Hulsmann, W.C. (1970): Biochim. Biophys. Acta 197: 127.

18. Wittels, B. & Bressler, R. (1964): J. Clin. Invest. 43: 630.
19. Bressler, R. & Wittels, B. (1965): Biochim. Biophys. Acta 104: 30.
20. Opie, L.H. (1968): Am. Heart J. 76: 685.
21. Rossi, C.R., Alexandre, A., Galzigna, L., Sartorelli, L., & Gibson, D.M. (1970): J. Biol. Chem. 245: 414.
22. Rossi, C.R., Alexandre, A., Carignani, G., & Siliprandi, N. (1972): Adv. Enzyme Reg. 10: 171.
23. Di Lisa, F., Siliprandi, N., & Toninello, A. Unpublished results.
24. Garland, P.B. & Randle, P.J. (1964): Biochem. J. 93: 678.
25. Hulsmann, W.C., Siliprandi, D., Ciman, M., & Siliprandi, N. (1964): Biochim. Biophys. Acta 93: 166.
26. Liedtke, A.J. (1981): Prog. Cardiovasc. Dis. 23: 321.

FACTORS INFLUENCING THE CARNITINE-DEPENDENT OXIDATION OF FATTY ACIDS IN THE HEART

J. Bremer, E.J. Davis* and B. Borrebaek

Institute of Medical Biochemistry, University of Oslo
Norway, *Department of Biochemistry, Indiana University
School of Medicine, Indianapolis, Indiana, U.S.A.

The availability of fatty acids is a dominating factor in
the regulation of the rate of fatty acid oxidation in the
heart. When the heart is offered both fatty acids and glucose,
fatty acids are the preferred substrate, even in the presence of
insulin. Uptake and oxidation increase with the concentration
of free fatty acids in the perfusion fluid. With high
concentrations of fatty acids (0.75 mM on 2% albumin) 80-90% of
the total CO_2 produced in the normal heart will be derived
from the fatty acids (1-3).

However, the rate of oxidation is not regulated by the
availability of fatty acids alone. An increased work load
accelerates fatty acid uptake and oxidation (4). Glucose can
inhibit fatty acid oxidation (2), and ketone bodies have a
strong inhibitory effect (5). Free acetate, which inhibits
glucose oxidation, has almost no effect on fatty acid oxidation
(6). Thus, the heart exhibits hierarchy in its substrate
preferences. Fatty acid oxidation in the heart is also
influenced by the endocrine state of the animal. Thus, glucose
plus insulin inhibits fatty acid oxidation less in hearts from
alloxan diabetic rats than in normal hearts (2).

The oxidation of long chain fatty acids is
carnitine-dependent, and the rate of oxidation varies with the
level of long chain acyl-CoA and acylcarnitines (7, 8). The
endocrine state of the animal seems to influence the formation
of long-chain acyl-CoA and acyl-carnitines from endogenous

substrates. Thus, perfused hearts from diabetic rats release
more glycerol, showing a more active lipolysis of endogenous
triglyceride (2), and contain higher levels of acyl-CoA and
acylcarnitines than normal hearts (9).

In the following discussion the difference between heart and
liver in their regulation of fatty acid oxidation will be
examined. This comparison is useful for our understanding of
the regulation of fatty acid oxidation in both organs.

Uptake and Activation

In both the heart and liver the uptake and activation of
fatty acids seem to depend mainly on the concentration of free
fatty acids in the blood. Acyl-CoA causes product inhibition of
the activation (10). Thus, accelerated removal of acyl-CoA,
e.g. by increased oxidation, will increase fatty acid uptake
even at an unchanged concentration of fatty acids. No other
regulatory mechanism for the synthesis of long-chain acyl-CoA
has been established.

Does Esterification Compete with Oxidation in the Heart?

Esterification and oxidation are the main alternatives for
fatty acids in the body. In the liver the activity of the
glycerophosphate acyltransferase, which catalyses the initial
step in the synthesis of triacylglycerol, is relatively high in
both the endoplasmic reticulum and mitochondria, while it is
relatively low in the heart (11, 12). Accordingly it has been
demonstrated in liver mitochondria and in isolated hepatocytes
that glycerophosphate can inhibit fatty acid oxidation by
directing the fatty acids towards esterification (12-15).

At a fixed low concentration of palmityl-CoA,
glycerophosphate inhibits the carnitine dependent oxidation of
palmityl-CoA in liver mitochondria (Table 1). It should be
noted that under the conditions of these experiments (state 3,
ADP added) glycerophosphate does not act as a competing
oxidizable substrate (16). Presumably the glycerophosphate
acyltransferase in the outer membrane of the mitochondria
prevents the acyl-CoA from reaching the carnitine
acyltransferase in the inner membrane.

However, glycerophosphate had no effect on the oxidation of
palmityl-CoA in heart mitochondria. This is in agreement with
the low activity of glycerophosphate acyltransferase (12), and
with relatively slow esterification and rapid oxidation of fatty
acids observed in the normal heart (17). It is therefore
unlikely that variable triacylglycerol synthesis has any

TABLE 1: The effect of free CoA and of α-glycerophosphate on the carnitine-dependent oxidation of palmityl-CoA in liver and heart mitochondria.

	[1-^{14}C]palmityl-CoA recovered as acid soluble products: (nmol x min^{-1} x mg protein^{-1})			
Additions	Liver		Heart	
None	0.52	0.54	0.55	0.52
Glycerophosphate	0.33	0.32	0.54	0.52
CoA	0.25	0.24	0.42	0.39
CoA + gl.P.	0.11	0.11	0.42	0.39

[1-^{14}C]Palmityl-CoA, 11 μM; (-)carnitine, 0.25 mM (liver) or 1 mM (heart); and mitochondria, 1.1 mg protein (liver) or 0.7 mg protein (heart), were incubated with Tris, pH 7.4, 20 mM; potassium phosphate, 5 mM; malate, 5 mM; ADP, 2.5 mM; mannitol, 60 mM; and KCL, 40-50 mM; and, where noted, free CoA, 50 μM; and DL-α-glycerophosphate, 2 mM.

significant influence on the rate of fatty acid oxidation in the heart. However, the rate of esterification seems to increase when oxidation is inhibited. Thus, loss of carnitine from the heart caused by diphtheria toxin leads to triacylglycerol accumulation (18). A similar phenomenon is seen in skeletal muscle and heart low in carnitine because of an inborn error of carnitine metabolism and transport (19).

Other mechanisms that impair fatty acid oxidation also lead to accumulation of triacylglycerol. Diets high in erucic acid or other C_{22} fatty acids lead to a temporary lipidosis in the heart, presumably because these long chain fatty acids are poor substrates for the mitochondria, and may also inhibit the oxidation of other fatty acids (17, 20).

Decreased oxidation in hypoxia also leads to increased esterification and accumulation of triacylglycerol in the heart (21).

Carnitine-Dependent Transport of Fatty Acids into the Mitochondria

In the heart, 85-90% of the CoA is found in the mitochondria, whereas 90% of the carnitine is outside the mitochondria (10). Since carnitine and acylcarnitines can

penetrate the inner mitochondrial membrane, while CoA and
acyl-CoA cannot, fatty acid oxidation in the heart is carnitine
dependent. The distribution of carnitine and CoA suggests that
fatty acids are automatically directed toward oxidation in the
mitochondria. Only a relatively small fraction of the fatty
acids is normally esterified as triacylglycerol in the heart
(17).

In both the liver and heart of the newborn, the outer
carnitine palmityltransferases have a low activity, but their
activities increase rapidly after birth (22, 23). It seems
likely that the carnitine palmityltransferase and the ability to
oxidize fatty acids is turned on immediately after birth. It is
not known how the apparently latent enzyme is activated in the
newborn animal, but in isolated mitochondria it can be activated
by preincubation of the mitochondria under different conditions
(24, 25) or by treatment with phospholipase (26).

A low activity of the outer carnitine palmityltransferase is
also found in mitochondria from hearts exposed to chronic
ischemia (27). The mechanism of this inactivation is not known.

Several differences between the heart and liver carnitine
systems have been reported. The concentration of carnitine in
the heart is normally higher (about 1 mM in the rat) than in the
liver (0.3 mM). In the heart, carnitine concentration is
relatively invariable, while in the liver it increases
signficantly in fasted and in diabetic animals. Especially
marked variations are found in the livers of sheep (28).

TABLE 2: The effect of malonyl-CoA and of free CoA on the carnitine-
dependent oxidation of palmityl-CoA in heart mitochondria.

Additions	$[1-^{14}C]$Palmityl-CoA recovered as acid soluble products (nmol $\times$ min^{-1} $\times$ mg protein^{-1})	
None	1.70	1.65
CoA	1.32	1.24
Malonyl-CoA	1.24	1.21
CoA + malonyl-CoA	1.01	1.00

$[1-^{14}C]$Palmityl-CoA, 2 μM; (-)carnitine, 1 mM; and
mitochondria, 0.65 mg protein, were incubated with HEPES, pH
7.4, 25 mM; potassium phosphate, 5 mM; malate, 2 mM; ADP, 2 mM;
KCl, 50-60 mM; mannitol, 30 mM; albumin, 1%; and, where noted,
malonyl-CoA, 20 μM; and CoA, 50 μM.

TABLE 3. The effect of malonyl-CoA and of free CoA on the
         carnitine dependent oxidation of palmityl-CoA in liver
         mitochondria.

Additions	[1-^{14}C]Palmityl-CoA recovered as acid soluble products (nmol x min^{-1} x mg protein^{-1})	
None	1.88	1.81
CoA	1.16	1.19
Malonyl-CoA	0.49	0.57
CoA + malonyl-CoA	0.23	0.27

[1-^{14}C]Palmityl-CoA, 45 μM; (-)carnitine, 0.25 mM; and
mitochondria, 3 mg protein; were incubated with Tris, 33 mM, pH
7.4; potassium phosphate, 5 mM; malate, 5 mM; KCl, 100 mM; and
ADP, 5 mM; albumin, 1%; and where noted, malonyl-CoA, 20 μM; and
CoA, 100 μM.

In the liver the activity of the outer carnitine
palmityltransferase is increased by fasting (12, 13, 29) and by
triiodothyronin (30), but no such changes have been found in the
heart.

Malonyl-CoA

The outer carnitine palmityltransferase is inhibited by
malonyl-CoA (31, 32). In liver mitochondria this inhibition is
increased by a low pH (33), and decreased when the animal is
fasted (29, 34, 35). These effects have not been found in heart
mitochondria.

The oxidation of palmityl-CoA is inhibited by free CoA to
about the same extent in heart and liver (Tables 1, 2, and 3).
However, we found malonyl-CoA relatively less inhibitory on
palmityl-CoA oxidation in heart mitochondria (Tables 2 and 3).
This was unexpected since the heart carnitine palmityltransferase has been found to be more sensitive to malonyl-CoA
than the liver enzyme (32). It is still not established that
malonyl-CoA takes part in the regulation of fatty acid oxidation
in the heart. We have measured malonyl-CoA in the hearts of fed
and fasted rats, and malonyl-CoA indeed is found in the heart in
similar concentrations as in the liver (Table 4). Its
concentration is decreased in fasted animals, although to a
smaller extent than in the liver. Since the heart enzyme
apparently is very sensitive to malonyl-CoA (32), it is possible

TABLE 4. Malonyl-CoA content of tissues of fed and fasted rats
         according to Singh et al. (39).

| | Malonyl-CoA (nmol/g fresh tissue) | | |
	Liver	Heart	Kidney
Fed	4.1 ± 0.12	3.7 ± 0.3	0.7 ± 0.05
Fasted	1.4 ± 0.09	2.8 ± 0.22	0.6 ± 0.05

that malonyl-CoA participates in the regulation of fatty acid
oxidation in the heart.

The carnitine acetyltransferase of the heart is not
inhibited by malonyl-CoA, while the liver enzyme is (36). It
appears that fatty acid oxidation can be inhibited by
malonyl-CoA without interfering with the formation of
acetylcarnitine.

Interaction of Fatty Acid Oxidation with the Citric Acid Cycle

In liver the formation of ketone bodies permits β-oxidation
to proceed independently of the citric acid cycle, while in
heart fatty acid oxidation depends on the citric acid cycle for
the oxidation of the acetyl-CoA. This difference in the
dependence on the citric acid cycle in heart and liver is
demonstrated by the effect of fluoroacetyl-carnitine on the
oxidation of palmitylcarnitine in heart and liver mitochondria.
In both types of mitochondria formation of fluorocitrate is
followed by an accumulation of citrate which inhibits its own
synthesis by feedback inhibition of citrate synthetase (37,
38). In liver mitochondria the increased acetyl-CoA is disposed
of by acetoacetate formation, and fatty acid oxidation continues
almost abated.

In heart mitochondria, which have no ketogenesis to consume
the acetyl-CoA, palmitylcarnitine oxidation is strongly
inhibited. However, the inhibition is not total. In the
inhibited mitochondria free acetate is formed by acetyl-CoA
hydrolase which becomes active when the acetyl-CoA/CoA ratio
increases (37). This illustrates the function of acyl-CoA
hydrolases as a "safety valve" securing some regeneration of
free CoA under conditions where the mitochondria or the cell is
"flooded" by acetyl- or fatty acyl groups. However, the

TABLE 5. The effect of malate, glutamate and ADP on the
carnitine dependent oxidation of palmityl-CoA in rat
heart mitochondria.

| | $[1-^{14}C]$Palmityl-CoA recovered in: (nmol $\times$ min^{-1} $\times$ mg protein^{-1}) | | | |
| | CO_2 | | Acid soluble products | |
Additions	$-ADP$	$+ADP$	$-ADP$	$+ADP$
None	0.01	1.06	1.89	1.37
	0.01	1.14	1.96	1.40
Malate	0.01	0.04	1.79	2.53
	0.01	0.05	1.77	2.58
Glutamate	0.01	0.25	1.70	2.19
	0.01	0.26	1.75	2.37
Malate +	0.01	0.02	1.54	2.44
glutamate	0.01	0.03	1.55	2.52

$[1-^{14}C]$Palmityl-CoA, 37 μM; (-)carnitine, 1 mM; and
mitochondria, 0.5 mg protein, were incubated with Hepes, pH 7.4,
25 mM; potassium phosphate, 5 mM; mannitol, 60 mM; and KCl,
50-60 mM; and, where noted, ADP, 2.5 mM; malate, 1 mM; 4
glutamate and 5 mM.

capacity of this enzyme in the heart is insufficient to permit
high rates of fatty acid oxidation.

Carnitine acetyltransferase represents an extra pathway for
the utilization of acetyl groups, in addition to citrate
synthase and acetyl-CoA hydrolase. This enzyme is very active
in heart mitochondria and acetylcarnitine can leave the
mitochondria via carnitine translocase (40). This possibility
is illustrated in Tables 5 and 6, which show that isolated heart
mitochondria can oxidize palmityl-CoA at a rapid rate in the
absence of malate when sufficient carnitine is present. The
isolated mitochondria contain sufficient citric acid cycle
intermediates to permit a significant rate of oxidation all the
way to CO_2 (Table 5), but more than half of the acetyl groups
formed can be transferred to carnitine (Table 6). In the
presence of malate (and ADP) acetylcarnitine formation drops
almost to nil. Evidently citrate synthase wins in the
competition when oxaloacetate is available and when citrate does
not accumulate as it does when fluorocitrate is formed from
fluoroacetylcarnitine.

TABLE 6. The effect of malate, glutamate, succinate, and ADP on
the formation of acetylcarnitine from palmityl-CoA and
carnitine in heart mitochondria.

| | [1-^{14}C]Palmityl-CoA recovered in: (nmol x min x mg protein^{-1}) | | | |
| | Acid soluble products | | Acetylcarnitine | |
Additions	−ADP	+ADP	−ADP	+ADP
None	1.01	0.72*	0.55	0.39
	0.94	0.73*	0.53	0.39
Malate	0.93	1.22	0.35	0.08
	0.90	1.23	0.33	0.06
Glutamate	0.92	1.01*	0.51	0.15
	0.91	0.98*	0.51	0.14
Malate + glutamate	0.75	1.05	0.32	0.09
	0.77	1.01	0.33	0.08
Succinate (0.5 mM)	0.32	1.07	0.06	0.06
	0.31	1.04	0.06	0.05

*In the absence of malate and in the presence of ADP significant
amounts of radioactive CO_2 is formed beside the acid soluble
products (see Table 5).
    Incubation conditions as in Table 5. The radioactivity in
acetylcarnitine was measured by addition of carrier
acetylcarnitine to the perchloric acid extract and precipitation
with ammonium reineckate. The reineckate was decomposed with 1
N HCl and acetone-ethyl ether 1:1.

    However, carnitine cannot function long as a sink for acetyl
groups in the intact tissue. The total carnitine in the heart
represents only a small fraction of the total flux of acetyl
groups in the working heart, and there is no important known
extramitochondrial metabolism of acetylcarnitine. Small amounts
of extramitochondrial acetyl-CoA may be formed by outer
carnitine acetyltransferase, but the heart has no significant
fatty acid synthesis or other metabolic uses of acetyl-CoA.
However, the formation of acetylcarnitine and extramitochondrial

acetyl-CoA will trap these cofactors in the extramitochondrial space and, as suggested by Oram et al. (4), this may have a regulatory function, decreasing the formation of long chain acyl-CoA and acylcarnitines when the rate of acetyl-CoA oxidation in the mitochondria is slowed. In this regard, it may be important that the carnitine acetyltransferase is not inhibited by malonyl-CoA in the heart (36). Therefore, acetylcarnitine formation and malonyl-CoA may act together to slow fatty acid oxidation.

A high concentration of free carnitine can be used _in vitro_ to make the β-oxidation of fatty acids in heart mitochondria independent of the citric acid cycle. Table 6 shows that the oxidation of palmityl-CoA in the presence of substrate amounts of carnitine is only moderately slower in state 4 (no ADP added) than in state 3 (ADP added). In state 3, endogenous citric acid cycle intermediates present in the isolated mitochondria evidently permit significant CO_2 production. However, in state 4 this production of CO_2 is completely suppressed. Evidently the respiratory control can suppress the citric acid cycle completely. while β-oxidation and acetylcarnitine formation continue almost unabated.

In state 3 addition of malate prevents formation of radioactive CO_2 because the added malate acts as a trapping pool. This was confirmed by column chromatography. which showed that most of the acid-soluble radioactivity was recovered in succinate and malate. However, the rate of fatty acid β-oxidation per se is unaffected by malate both in state 3 and state 4.

These results agree with previous studies on liver mitochondria showing that it is difficult to suppress β-oxidation with a high NADH/NAD ratio (41). It is much easier to suppress pyruvate oxidation (42) or the citric acid cycle (16). However, β-oxidation is not completely insensitive to competing substrates. Tables 5 and 6 show that malate plus glutamate, which is equivalent to an active malate-aspartate shuttle transporting reducing equivalents into the mitochondria, or succinate inhibit β-oxidation in the heart as they do in liver mitochondria (16), but only in a high energy state (state 4). This inhibition by glutamate plus malate can be partially overcome by a higher concentration of acyl- carnitine (not shown).

These studies show that the oxidation of fatty acids, unlike the citric acid cycle. is almost independent of the respiratory state, i.e. it is not under direct respiratory control. When

the citric acid cycle is slowed down by an increased NADH/NAD
ratio in the mitochondria, the oxidation of fatty acids is
therefore most likely slowed by secondary mechanisms such as an
increased acetyl-CoA/CoA ratio, which ties up CoA and carnitine
in the cytosol via the carnitine acetyltransferase. It has also
been suggested that accumulated acetyl-CoA may inhibit thiolase
and that the resulting accumulation of β-oxidation intermediates
gives a feedback inhibition of the acyl-CoA dehydrogenases (43).

Levels of Citric Acid Cycle Intermediates and CoA

In fasting and diabetic animals, the levels of citric acid
cycle intermediates increase in the heart and in skeletal muscle
(44). Since both have significant activities of pyruvate
carboxylase, which is stimulated by acetyl-CoA (45, 46), it is
likely that this increase is explained by an increased
acetyl-CoA/CoA ratio in the mitochondria under conditions where
the rates of fatty acid oxidation are increased. It is not
known whether this increased level of citric acid cycle
intermediates is of direct significance for the rate of fatty
acid oxidation, but since citrate is an inhibitor of glycolysis,
its increase probably facilitates the switch from glucose to
fatty acid oxidation in the fasting state.

The total level of CoA in the heart also increases in
diabetic and fasting animals (9). This seems paradoxical since
acetyl-CoA is a strong inhibitor of pantothenate kinase, the
first enzyme in the biosynthesis of CoA (47). In agreement with
this effect of acetyl-CoA, fatty acids and other acetyl-CoA
precursors inhibit the synthesis of CoA from pantothenate in the
perfused heart (48). It is not known whether this increase in
CoA is of significance for the rate of fatty acid oxidation, or
other CoA- dependent reactions in the mitochondria.

Conclusions

Fatty acids represent the predominant substrate in the heart
as in other tissues. The oxidation of long-chain acylcarnitines
is inhibited only under strongly reduced conditions in the
mitochondria. i.e. when the NADH/NAD ratio is very high. The
oxidation of other substrates, like pyruvate (glucose) and
citric acid cycle intermediates, is much more easily
suppressed. The oxidation of fatty acids in the heart (and in
other tissues) is therefore only indirectly under respiratory
control, probably via a high acetyl-CoA/CoA ratio, which may
increase the level of mitochondrial β-oxidation intermediates
(β-ketoacyl-CoA?) that inhibit the acyl-CoA dehydrogenases. A
high acetyl-CoA/CoA ratio will also make less carnitine (and
CoA?) available for acylcarnitine formation in the cytosol. The

formation of acylcarnitine may also be inhibited by malonyl-CoA which is present in the heart. The uptake of fatty acids in the heart is probably ultimately determined on the one hand by the concentration of available free fatty acids, and on the other by the availability of free CoA and a feedback inhibition of the acyl-CoA synthase by acyl-CoA.

REFERENCES

1. Evans, J.R., Opie, L.H., & Shipp, J.C. (1963): Am. J. Physiol. 205: 766.
2. Randle, P.J., Garland, P.B., Hales, C.N., Newsholm, E.A., Denton, R.M., & Pogson, C.I. (1966): Rec. Progr. Hormone Res. 22: 1.
3. Vahouny, G.V., Lilljenquist, J., Wilson, R., Liao, A., & Rodis, S.L. (1968): Arch. Biochem. Biophys. 125: 809.
4. Oram, J.F., Bennetch, S.L., & Neely. J.R. (1973): J. Biol. Chem. 248: 5299.
5. Menahan, L.A., & Hron, W.T. (1981): Eur. J. Biochem. 119: 295.
6. Bethencourt, A.V., Matos, O.E., & Shipp, J.C. (1966): Metabolism 15: 847.
7. Bohmer, T., Norum, K.R., & Bremer, J. (1966): Biochim. Biophys. Acta 125: 244.
8. Pearson, D.J., & Tubbs, P.K. (1967): Biochim. J. 105: 953.
9. Feuvrey, D., Idell-Wenger, J.A., & Neely. J.R. (1979): Circ. Res. 44: 322.
10. Oram. J.F., Wenger, J.I., & Neely. J.R. (1975): J. Biol. Chem. 250: 73.
11. Daae, L.N.W. (1973): Biochim. Biophys. Acta 306: 186.
12. Borrebaek, B., Christiansen, R., Christophersen, B.O., & Bremer, J. (1976): Circ. Res. 38: 1.
13. Borrebaek, B. (1975): Acta Physiol. Scand. 95: 44.
14. Lund, H., Borrebaek, B., & Bremer, J. (1980): Biochim. Biophys. Acta 620: 364.
15. Declercq, P.E., Debeer, L.J., & Mannaerts, G.P. (1982): Biochem. J. 202: 803.
16. Lumeng, L., Bremer, J., & Davis, E.J. (1976): J. Biol. Chem. 251: 277.
17. Norseth, J. (1980): Biochim. Biophys. Acta 617: 183.
18. Bressler, R., & Wittels, B. (1965): Biochim. Biophys. Acta 104: 39.
19. Cornelio, F., Di Donato, S., Peluchetti, D., Bizzi, A., Bertagnolio, B., D'Angelo, A., & Wiesman, U. (1977): J. Neurol. Neurosurg. Psych. 40: 170.
20. Bremer, J., & Norum. K.R. (1982): J. Lipid Res. 23: 243.
21. Scheuer, J., & Brachfeld, N. (1966): Metabolism 15: 945.
22. Augenfeldt, J., & Fritz, I.B. (1969): Can. J. Biochem. 48: 288.

23. Bieber, L.L., Markwell, M.R.K., Blair, M., & Helmrath, T.A.
    (1973): Biochim. Biophys. Acta 326: 145.
24. Brosnan, J.T., Kopec, B., & Fritz, I.B. (1971): Can. J.
    Biochem. 49: 1296.
25. Tomec, R.J., & Hoppel, C.L. (1975): Arch. Biochem.
    Biophys. 170: 716.
26. Wood, J.M. (1975): J. Biol. Chem. 250: 3062.
27. Wood, J.M., Sordahl. L.A., Lewis, R.M., & Schwartz, A.
    (1973): Circ. Res. 32: 340.
28. Snoswell. A.M., & Koundakjian, P.P. (1972): Biochem. J.
    127: 133.
29. Bremer, J. (1981): Biochim. Biophys. Acta 665: 628.
30. Stakkestad, J.A., & Bremer, J. (1983): Biochim. Biophys.
    Acta 750: 244.
31. McGarry, J.D., & Foster, D.W. (1980): Ann. Rev. Biochem.
    49: 395.
32. Saggerson, E.D., & Carpenter, C.A. (1981): FEBS Lett. 129:
    229.
33. Stephens, T.W., Cook, G.A., & Harris, R.A. (1983): Biochem.
    J. 212: 521.
34. Cook, G.A., Otto, D.A., & Cornell, N.W. (1980): Biochem.
    J. 192: 955.
35. Ontko, J.A., & Johns, M.L. (1980): Biochem. J. 192: 959.
36. Lund, H., & Bremer, J. (1983): Biochim. Biophys. Acta 750:
    164.
37. Bremer, J., & Davis, E.J. (1973): Biochim. Biophys. Acta
    326: 262.
38. Bremer, J., & Davis, E.J. (1974): Biochim. Biophys. Acta
    370: 564.
39. Singh, B., Bremer, J., & Borrebaek, B. (1982):
    Hoppe-Seyler's Z. Physiol. Chem. 363: 920.
40. Ramsay, R.R., & Tubbs, P.K. (1975): FEBS Lett. 54: 21.
41. Bremer, J., & Wojtczak, A.B. (1972): Biochim. Biophys.
    Acta 280: 515.
42. Bremer, J. (1969): Eur. J. Biochem. 8: 535.
43. Olowe, Y., & Schulz, H. (1980): Eur. J. Biochem. 109: 425.
44. Garland, P.B., & Randle, P.J. (1964): Biochem. J. 93: 678.
45. Davis, E.J., Spydevold, O., & Bremer, J. (1980): Eur. J.
    Biochem. 110: 255.
46. Peuhkurinen, K.J., Nuutinen, E.M., Pietilainen, E.P.,
    Hiltunen, J.K., & Hassinen, I.E. (1982): Biochem. J. 208:
    577.
47. Halvorsen, O., & Skrede, S. (1982): Eur. J. Biochem. 124:
    211.
48. Kreibel. D.K., Wyse, B.W., Berkich, D.A., & Neely, J.R.
    (1981): Am. J. Physiol. 240: H606.

LOCALIZATION AND FUNCTION OF LIPASES AND THEIR REACTION PRODUCTS IN RAT HEART

W. C. Hülsmann, H. Stam, and J. M. J. Lamers

Department of Biochemistry I
Erasmus University
P.O. Box 1738, 3000 DR Rotterdam, The Netherlands

Lipoprotein lipase is involved in catabolism of circulating triglycerides. Its function is exerted at the vascular endothelial surface, where the enzyme is bound and from which the enzyme is released by heparin perfusion (1-3). Natural substrates that may be used include chylomicrons and very low density lipoproteins, while artificial substrates include triglyceride-filled liposomes with phospholipid and apolipoprotein C-II on the surface. The enzyme is an -lipase that also hydrolyzes 1-acylglycerol esters of partial glycerides and phospholipids. In perfused hearts of fed rats, only about 25% of the tissue lipoprotein lipase is removed by heparin perfusion while the ability of the heart to catabolize chylomicrons is largely lost (2, 4). The study of Schotz et al. (5), who perfused rat hearts with an antibody against heart lipoprotein lipase, led to the observation that subsequent perfusion with ^{14}C-labelled chylomicron triglyceride no longer resulted in $^{14}CO_2$ formation, suggesting also that endothelial surface lipoprotein lipase, accessible to the antibody, is the functionally active fraction of the enzyme. However, small chylomicrons, very low density lipoprotein, low density lipoprotein (as well as high density lipoprotein) can enter the myocardial interstitium (6-10) so that lipoprotein lipase, shown to be present in interstitium (11, 12), could also act upon these lipoproteins. Therefore it cannot be excluded that interstitial lipoprotein lipase also contributes to lipoprotein catabolism.

27

Whereas lipoprotein lipase promotes the uptake of lipolytic
products in the cell, the lysosomal system is involved in the
mobilization of lipids stored in the cells (13). The rate of
mobilization of stored fat is larger when the lipid depot is
increased (13). The lipoprotein lipase activity during fat
feeding is also increased (14, 15), so that the fatty acid
turnover in heart is increased. In contrast to the feeding of
monoenoic very long-chain fatty acids like erucic acid, foods
rich in palmitic, oleic or linoleic acid does not cause
myocardial lipidosis. In the latter cases practically all fatty
acid taken up is oxidized. However, during limited O_2
availability or during erucic acid feeding, when the
carnitinepalmitoyltransferase reaction is inhibited (16), the
activated fatty acids cannot be oxidized by the mitochondria,
and triglyceride may be formed in the extramitochondrial space
as long as glycerol-3-phosphate is formed. When the flow is
limited, however, glycogen will soon be depleted and glucose
supply interrupted so that then free fatty acids and their
coenzyme A and carnitine derivatives accumulate (17, 18). Fatty
acid acceptor shortage does not occur during erucic acid feeding
when flow is not limited. Therefore fatty acids (and coenzyme A
and carnitine esters) only accumulate under restricted flow. In
fact, in the absence of ischemia fatty acid levels are very low
(19) and long-chain acylcarnitine absent (see below). We find
the presence of long-chain acylcarnitine a better marker for
ischemia than lowering of the phosphate potential.

RESULTS AND DISCUSSION

Release of fatty acids from cellular triglyceride stores into
the interstitium

Whereas fatty acids do not accumulate intracellularly under
aerobic conditions (19), they might attain significant levels
extracellularly under certain feeding conditions (20). The
question where interstitial fatty acids come from is important
as interstitial fluid has a lower albumin concentration than the
blood, so that detergent fatty acids (and long-chain
acylcarnitine - see below) might interfere with the cell
membranes which limit this compartment. Free fatty acids (FFA)
certainly can enter the interstitium from the blood while
complexed to albumin. This is probably harmless, as the blood
compartment generally contains sufficient albumin to bind FFA
tightly. However, FFA may also enter the interstitium from the
cells, particularly when they contain excessive stores of
long-chain fatty acid esters. This has been shown by us to
occur after erucic acid feeding to rats, particularly after
stimulation of endogenous lipolysis by glucagon or
catecholamines (20). If the interstitial fluid, which during

Langendorff perfusion can be separated from the coronary effluent (21), is produced slowly, FFA levels in the millimolar range have been measured (20). The chronic irritation of fatty acids may be the basis of myocardial fibrosis observed by many authors to occur on prolonged erucic acid feeding. Stimulation of endogenous lipolysis by catabolic hormones is accompanied by stimulation of interstitial fluid production (Table I, ref. 11). It is possible that there is a close correlation between these phenomena. A higher rate of removal of lipolysis-inhibiting fatty acid (22-24) may be expected to stimulate endogenous lipolysis. FFA removal from the cells is accomplished by secretion into the lymph (minor component - Table I), by oxidation in the mitochondria and by reesterification in the endoplasmic reticulum. In the Langendorff heart the latter amounts to 62% (25), as estimated by the effect of inhibition of glycogenolysis during glucose-free perfusion (thereby interfering with glycerol-3-phosphate synthesis) upon lipolysis (26). Hormone-stimulated fatty acid removal might be the basis of hormone-sensitivity lipolysis in heart (27, 28). Such a mechanism will normally prevent FFA overload of cells and interstitium.

TABLE I. Effects of albumin, glucagon and norepinephrine (NE) on lymph flow and lipolysis in Langendorff hearts of rats fed erucic acid.

Additions to perfusion medium	Q_i (% of total flow)	(n)	FFA	Glycerol
			(nmol/min x g wet weight)	
None	2.5+0.3*	(19)		33.8+2.3 (4)
0.2 μM glucagon	4.0+0.6	(9)		63.3+2.7 (4)
0.2 μM NE	4.2+0.3	(4)		64.3+1.9 (4)
1% albumin	1.6+0.2	(4)	17.6+2.2 (8)	–
1% albumin + 0.2 μM glucagon	2.5+0.2	(4)	22.7+2.1 (8)	–
5% albumin	0.6+0.1	(8)	–	–
5% albumin + 0.2 μM glucagon	0.9+0.1	(8)	–	–

(n) = number of experiments; *standard error of mean. Male Wistar rats were fed for 3 days with a trierucate-rich diet before sacrifice, the Langendorff perfusion technique was modified (21) to separate interstitial (Q_i) from coronary effluent. For the persuion technique followed see ref. 20. FFA and glycerol were determined in the interstitial fluid which contains more than 80% of these products (20).

Release of fatty acids within the interstitium; compartmentation
of lipoprotein lipase

Heparin addition to the perfusion medium of Langendorff
hearts in the fasted or fed states causes the immediate release
of lipoprotein lipase into the coronary effluent (Q_{rv}) and
practically not into the interstitial fluid (Q_i) (Figure 1).
Only when Ca^{2+} is omitted from the perfusion medium is a
considerable portion of lipoprotein lipase released into the
Q_i, whether heparin is present or not (compare ref. 12).   Then
an extra amount of lipoprotein lipase is also released in the
coronary effluent.   This is thought to result from a breakdown
of the glycocalyx of myocytes and opening of endothelial
plasmalemmal invaginations of capillaries (29), so that
lipoprotein lipase is released from the outside of cells, to
which lipoprotein lipase may be attached (12, 30, 31).   The
presence of lipoprotein lipase in the interstitial compartment
(Figure 1) together with triglyceride containing lipoproteins
(6-10) allow lipoprotein lipase activity to occur, leading to
the interstitial formation of FFA.

Accumulation of long-chain acylcarnitine in the sarcolemma
during ischemia

We (32) have recently reported that after a two hour
recirculating Langendorff perfusion of rat heart with
Intralipid and 5 mM carnitine, the hearts (freeze-clamped
during perfusion) contained 381 ± 35 nmoles (n=4) acid-insoluble
acylcarnitine.   Assuming a predominant cytosolic localization of
long-chain acylcarnitine (17) and a cytosolic space of 2 ml/g
dry tissue (33), we calculated a long-chain acylcarnitine
concentration of 0.8 mM in the cell.   It has been shown,
however, that long-chain acylcarnitine binds strongly to
sarcolemma (34), a finding that we have been able to confirm
(unpublished).   This phenomenon will cause high local
concentrations of these detergent molecules and probably result
in the inhibition of a number of sarcolemmal proteins and
alteration of permeability.   The latter is described by Lamers
et al. in the present volume.   We have observed that concomitant
with the accumulation of long-chain acylcarnitine,
non-heparin-releasable lipase from heart was lost (32).   This
enzyme is identical with non-releasable lipoprotein lipase (12),
the bulk of which is bound to the outside of cells and released
by Ca^{2+}-free perfusion (12, 25) (Figure 1).   Loss of
lipoprotein lipase appears to be a good marker for ischemia in
pig heart as well, as will be shown below.

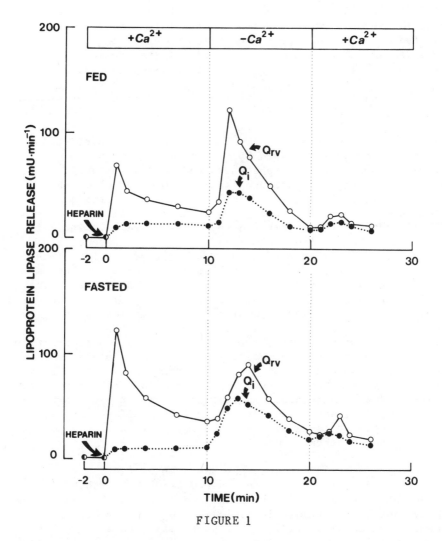

FIGURE 1

Lipoprotein lipase release from normal chow fed or fasted male
Wistar rats. For the perfusion technique see Table I.
Immediately after collection, the effluents were tested for
lipoprotein lipase activity, using an Intralipid substrate in
the presence of apolipoprotein C-II, as described in ref. 12.
Where indicated 5 U/ml heparin was added to the perfusion
medium. Calcium was present or omitted as shown.

Markers of ischemia

In the normal rat, myocardial long-chain acylcarnitine accumulation is virtually absent (Table II). The rats used had been fed olive oil 2 h prior to heart removal. In order to limit ischemia, which causes elevation of long-chain acylcarnitine levels (17, 18), we anesthetized the animals with fluothane/N_2O/O_2 (0.5:64.5:35) and attached a tracheal cannula to an artificial respirator to avoid anoxia during thoracotomy. After mobilizing the heart, the large vessels were cut and the heart rapidly frozen in isopentane at liquid N_2 temperature. The heart was crushed in a mortar cooled with liquid N_2, and deproteinized by mixing with 5% (w/v) perchloric acid. Creatinephosphate and adenine nucleotides were determined by high performance liquid chromatography. The virtual absence of long-chain acylcarnitine in heart is accompanied by a normal energy charge as is usually found when normoxic organs are rapidly frozen. Also, during Langendorff perfusion of hearts from normal rats with glucose-containing medium and during glucose-free perfusion of hearts from erucic acid fed rats, which utilize fatty acids as fuel, we find very little long-chain acylcarnitine (Table II). Therefore during the 2 h perfusions with Intralipid and carnitine (32), in which long-chain acylcarnitine accumulated, ischemia must have occurred. When the experiment was repeated with a similar medium, but fortified with 2% BSA, the long-chain acylcarnitine concentration in the heart was less [32 ± 8 nmol instead of 381 ± 35 (n=4) in the absence of BSA (details not shown)]. It is likely, therefore, that in the presence of Intralipid and lipoprotein lipase so much FFA is produced initially that in the absence of BSA ichemia develops gradually. High levels of FFA have been shown to increase capillary permeability, ultimately resulting in edema and hampered microcirculation.

The accumulation of fatty acyl detergents (long-chain acylcarnitine from the cellular contents and FFA probably predominantly from the interstitium) in plasma membranes during tissue anoxia will result in a decline in a number of plasmalemmal enzymes, including lipoprotein lipase. This is illustrated in Figure 2 for pig heart. During anesthesia and after thoracotomy, branches of the left descending coronary artery were ligated at one h intervals and samples taken from the cyanotic ischemic zones. Immediately thereafter the tissue was homogenized and sarcolemma partially purified by differential centrifugation according to Reeves and Sutko (38). This work on ischemic samples of pig heart has been carried out in cooperation with Dr. P.D. Verdouw (Thoraxcenter, Erasmus University) and will be published in detail elsewhere.

Table II. Energy-rich phosphate and carnitine derivatives in rapidly frozen rat hearts

In the first line data are shown from hearts of Wistar rats of 300 g, 27 h fasted and 15 h refed with normal chow, homogenized with olive oil (3:1 w/w), after the addition of 25 vol% water. Rats were narcotized and the hearts frozen as described in the text. In the second and third lines Langendorff hearts from rats fed normal or 3 days trierucate (TE; 40 en%) fed rats were freeze-clamped, while on the canula, with Wollenberg tongs, at liquid N_2 temperature. After crushing the hearts and mixing with 5% $HClO_4$, the perchloric acid extracts were neutralized with KOH and assayed for adenine nucleotides and creatinephosphate[35] and for acetylcarnitine spectrophotometrically[36]. Long-chain acylcarnitine was assayed after 4x washing the $HClO_4$ insoluble material (sonification and centrifugation at each step) after saponification as free carnitine. Free carnitine was assayed by a radioisotope procedure.[37] Figures are nmoles/g wet weight ± S.E.M.

	ATP	ADP	CroP	Acetyl carn.	Free carn.	Long-chain acylcarn.
Hearts of oil fed rats (n=3)	5175±79	2525±79	12283±2168	39±8	1596±98	1±1
Langendorff hearts of normal rats (n=4)	6126±58	1571±59	12745±268	16±3	1254±35	18±3
Langendorff hearts of TE fed rats (n=3)	5552±283	1572±283	8252±167	47±8	1295±78	33±6

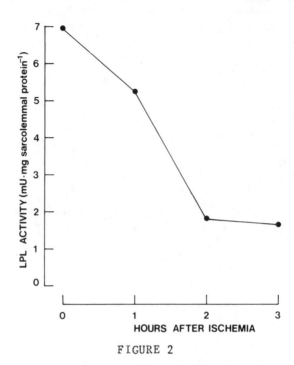

FIGURE 2

Effect of ischemia on lipoprotein lipase of pig heart. The
samples were obtained as described in the text. The lipoprotein
lipase assay was carried out with ^{3}H-trioleoylglycerol
labelled Intralipid in the presence of apolipoprotein C-II as
described (12). SL stands for sarcolemma. The specific
activity of the sarcolemmal preparation of the control sample (0
h ischemia) was 9 times higher than the specific activity of the
total homogenate from which the SL was purified (not shown).

CONCLUSIONS

     Myocardial ischemia results in the accumulation of
amphiphilic compounds: FFA, long-chain acylcarnitine,
long-chain acyl-CoA (17-19) and lysophospholipids. The latter
accumulate not only due to stimulated formation by phospholipase
action, but also by inhibited removal (39). All compounds arise
mainly intracellularly with the exception of FFA, which enters
the cell primarily by dissociation from its blood plasma vehicle
albumin, and also after its release from glycerol esters in
extracellular lipoproteins in the lipoprotein lipase reaction.
This enzyme appears to have many locations: on the vascular

endothelial cells facing the bloodstream, on the surface
membranes of cells that limit the interstitium, and within the
myocardial cells where the enzyme is synthesized. In the latter
compartment there is probably relatively little enzyme (12, 25)
(Figure 1), while its activator apolipoprotein C-II is absent at
this locus. The amphiphilic compounds accumulate in membranes,
amongst which the sarcolemma. In vitro studies reveal that FFA
(40) and the other compounds (34, 41) can inhibit
(Na^+,K^+)ATPase which, if this occurred in situ, might also
promote calcium overload by Ca^{2+}/Na^+ exchange (38). Our
recent studies (see Lamers et al., this volume) suggest that at
least FFA and long-chain acylcarnitine increase sarcolemmal
Ca^{2+} permeability in a more direct fashion as well. That FFA
increases Ca^{2+} availability to myocardial cells has been
demonstrated by us before, using contractility as an index of
intracellular Ca^{2+} (42, 43). The Ca^{2+} ionophoric properties
were thought to reside in the ability of FFA to bind Ca^{2+}, and
does not necessarily imply that FFA only functions as a Ca^{2+}
shuttle through the membrane. FFA and also their esters with
detergent properties might modulate hydrophobic domains in such
a manner that passage of Na^+ and Ca^{2+} is enhanced (compare
44). Occasionally this may lead to Ca^{2+} overload and result
in irreversible damage to the cells (45-47).

ACKNOWLEDGEMENTS

    Sigma-Tau (Rome, Italy) is thanked for support and Dr. F.
Maccari for helpful discussions. Mr. P.Ph. de Tombe (Thorax
Centre) is thanked for the HPLC determinations. Mr. W.A.P.
Breeman is thanked for expert technical assistance and Miss
Cecile Hanson for preparing the manuscript.

REFERENCES

1. Robinson, D.S. (1970): Comprehensive Biochem. 18: 51.
2. Fielding, C.J., & Havel, R.J. (1977): Arch. Pathol. Lab.
   Med. 101: 225.
3. Nilsson-Ehle, P., Garfinkel, A.S., & Schotz, M.C. (1980):
   Ann. Rev. Biochem. 49: 667.
4. Fielding, C.J., & Higgins, J.M. (1974): Biochemistry 13:
   4324.
5. Schotz, M.C., Twu, J.-S., Pedersen, M.E., Chen, C.-H.,
   Garfinkel, A.S., & Borensztajn, J. (1977): Biochim.
   Biophys. Acta 489: 214.
6. Stoke, K.T., Fjeld, N.B., Kluge, T.H., & Skrede, S. (1974):
   Scand. J. Clin. Lab. Invest. 33: 199.
7. Roy, P.-E. (1975): IN Recent Advances in Studies on
   Cardiac Structure and Metabolism, Vol. 10. (eds) P.-E. Roy,
   & G. Rona, University Park Press, Baltimore, p. 17.

8. Stam, H., Jansen, H., & Hülsmann, W.C. (1980): Biochem. Biophys. Res. Commun. 96: 899.

9. Julien, P., Downar, E., & Angel, A. (1981): Circ. Res. 49: 248.

10. Julien, P., & Angel, A. (1981): Can. J. Biochem. 59: 709.

11. Jansen, H., Stam, H., Kalkman, C., & Hülsmann, W.C. (1980): Biochem. Biophys. Res. Commun. 92: 411.

12. Hülsmann, W.C., Stam, H., & Breeman, W.A.P. (1982): Biochem. Biophys. Res. Commun. 108: 371.

13. Hülsmann, W.C., & Stam, H. (1978): Biochem. Biophys. Res. Commun. 82: 53.

14. Jansen, H., Hülsmann, W.C., van Zuylen-van Wiggen, A., Struijk, C.B., & Houtsmuller, U.M.T. (1975): Biochem. Biophys. Res. Commun. 64: 747.

15. Hülsmann, W.C., Geelhoed-Mieras, M.M., Jansen, H., & Houtsmuller, U.M.T. (1979): Biochim. Biophys. Acta 572: 183.

16. Christopherson, B.O., & Bremer, J. (1972): Biochim. Biophys. Acta 280: 506.

17. Idell-Wenger, J.A., Grotyohann, L.W., & Neely, J.R. (1978): J. Biol. Chem. 253: 4310.

18. Shug, A.L., Tomsen, J.H., Folts, J.D., Bittar, N., Klein, M.I., Koker, J.R., & Huth, P.J. (1978): Arch. Biochem. Biophys. 187: 25.

19. van der Vusse, G.J., Roemen, T.M., Prinzen, F.W., & Reneman, R.S. (1981): Basic Res. Cardiol. 76: 389.

20. Stam, H., & Hülsmann, W.C. (1981): Biochem. Int. 2: 477.

21. De Deckere, E.A.M., & Ten Hoor, F. (1975): Pflugers Archiv. 370: 103.

22. Crass, M.F. III, Shipp, J.C., & Pieper, G.M. (1975): Am. J. Physiol. 228: 618.

23. Hron, W.T., Jesmok, G.J., Lombardo, Y.B., Menahan, L.A., & Lech, J.J. (1977): J. Mol. Cell. Cardiol. 9: 733.

24. Stam, H., Geelhoed-Mieras, M.M., & Hülsmann, W.C. (1980): Lipids 15: 242.

25. Hülsmann, W.C., & Stam, H. (1983): Basic Res. Cardiol. In press.

26. Hülsmann, W.C., & Stam, H. (1980): Biochem. Biophys. Res. Commun. 88: 867.

27. Hülsmann, W.C., Stam, H., & Geelhoed-Mieras, M.M. (1979): IN Obesitas, Cellular and Molecular Aspects, Vol. 87 (ed) G. Ailhaud, INSERM, Paris, p. 179.

28. Stam, H., & Hülsmann, W.C. (1982): IN Advances in Myocardiology, Vol. 3 (eds) E. Chazov, V. Smirnov, & N.S. Dhalla, Plenum Publishing Corp., New York, p. 499.

29. Bundgaard, M., Hagman, P., & Crone, C. (1983): Microvascular Res. 25: 358.

30. Henson, L.C., Schotz, M.C., & Harary, I. (1977): Biochim. Biophys. Acta 487: 212.

31. Chajek-Shaul, T., Friedman, G., Stein, O., Olivecrona, T., & Stein, Y. (1982): Biochim. Biophys. Acta 712: 200.
32. Hülsmann, W.C., Stam, H., & Maccari, F. (1982): Biochim. Biophys. Acta 713: 39.
33. Morgan, H.E., Regen, D.M., & Park, C.R. (1964): J. Biol. Chem. 239: 369.
34. Owens, K., Kennett, F.F., & Weglicki, W.B. (1982): Am. J. Physiol. 242: H456.
35. Harmsen, E., De Tombe, P.Ph., & De Jong, J.W. (1982): J. Chromatography 230: 131.
36. Pearson, D.J., Chase, J.F.A., & Tubbs, P.K. (1969): IN Methods in Enzymology, Vol. 14 (eds) S.P. Colowick, N.O. Kaplan, & J.M. Lowenstein, Academic Press, New York, p. 612.
37. Christiansen, R.Z., & Bremer, J. (1978): FEBS Lett. 86: 99.
38. Reeves, J.P., & Sutko, J.L. (1979): Proc. Natl. Acad. Sci. USA 76: 590.
39. Cross, R.W., & Sobel, B.E. (1983): J. Biol. Chem. 258: 5221.
40. Lamers, J.M.J., & Hülsmann, W.C. (1977): J. Mol. Cell. Cardiol. 9: 343.
41. McMillin-Wood, J., Bush, B., Pitts, B.J.R., & Schwartz, A. (1977): Biochem. Biophys. Res. Commun. 74: 677.
42. Hülsmann, W.C. (1976): Basic Res. Cardiol. 71: 179.
43. Stam, H., & Hülsmann, W.C. (1978): Biochem. Biophys. Res. Commun. 82: 609.
44. Rhoads, D.E., Ockner, R.K., Peterson, N.A., & Raghupathy, E. (1983): Biochemistry 22: 1965.
45. Dhalla, N.S. (1976): J. Mol. Cell. Cardiol. 9: 661.
46. Farber, J.L. (1982): Lab. Invest. 47: 114.
47. Clusin, W.T., Buchbinder, M., & Harrison, D.C. (1983): Lancet i: 272.

ULTRASTRUCTURAL LOCALIZATION OF LIPIDS IN MYOCARDIAL MEMBRANES

N.J. Severs

Department of Cardiac Medicine
Cardiothoracic Institute
London, W1N 2DX, England

MOLECULAR STRUCTURE OF MEMBRANES

All biological membranes are constructed according to a
common plan. The central features of this plan are summarized
in the 'fluid mosaic' model proposed by Singer and Nicolson
(1). A bilayer of lipid molecules makes up the basic structure
of the membrane; proteins are embedded in and attached onto this
'backbone' (Figure 1). The properties unique to each membrane
system are determined by the exact types and amounts of its
constituent lipids and proteins. Precise chemical
identification and localization of these constituents is thus
central to our understanding of membrane function.

MEMBRANE ULTRASTRUCTURE IN THIN SECTION

When a membrane is transversely sectioned, two
electron-dense layers sandwiching a central electron-lucent
layer can often be resolved (Figure 2). This 'unit membrane'
structure arises from the interaction of the stains with the
surface groups of the membrane lipids and proteins, the
hydrophobic interior, represented by the electron-lucent core,
remaining unstained. Unit membrane structure is visible under
favorable conditions; in many instances, however, membranes are
seen as single dense lines (each corresponding to the overall
width of a single 'unit membrane') or as broader fuzzy
boundaries (in tangential view).

Details of membrane structural differentiation are
detectable by thin sectioning, especially with the aid of

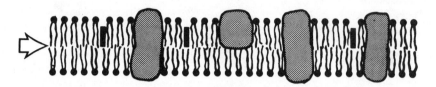

FIGURE 1

Molecular details of membrane structure. Phospholipids each have a
hydrophilic head group attached to two non-polar fatty acid tails. Black
rectangles represent the neutral lipid, cholesterol. Integral membrane
proteins (shown as large stippled globular structures) are embedded in th
lipid bilayer, sometimes spanning its entire width. Peripheral proteins,
which are only loosely attached to the membrane surface are not shown in
this diagram. The arrow indicates the path of the fracture plane in the
freeze-fracture technique.

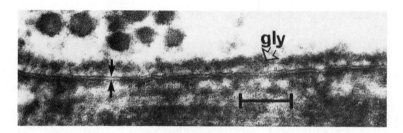

FIGURE 2

Unit membrane structure of the sarcolemma (arrows). gly, glycocalyx.
From a tannic acid-treated rabbit cardiac muscle cell. Scale bar, 100 nm

FIGURE 3. Freeze-fracture views of the sarcolemma. (a) shows a view of
the hydrophobic face of the half-membrane sheet left attached to the
protoplasm (P-face). (b) is a view of the hydrophobic face of the
half-membrane sheet left attached to the extracellular space (E-face).
Note that intramembrane particles are more abundant in the former than in
the latter. For fracture face terminology see Branton et al. (2). Rabbi
cardiac muscle cell from glutaraldehyde-fixed and glycerinated left
ventricle. Scale bar, 100 nm.

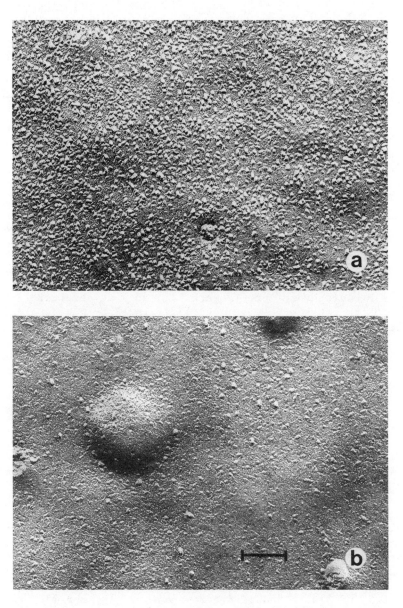

Figures 3a and 3b

special staining techniques. In many instances, such
differentiation is only hinted at (e.g. by variations in width
or staining intensity of one of the dense lines of the unit
membrane), though where extensive peripheral protein components
are involved it becomes strikingly conspicuous. In either case,
however, the precise chemical identification of the membrane
components involved can be achieved only if cytochemical methods
are combined with thin sectioning. Such methods include the use
of ligands conjugated to electron-dense markers, selective
stains, precipitation of electron-dense enzymatic products,
enzyme digestion and electron microscope autoradiography.
Through these approaches, major advances have been made in
correlating cell, organelle and membrane structure with
function, particularly with regard to the role of protein
components. However, none of these methods permits the
high-resolution localization of specific types of lipids in
membranes.

MEMBRANE ULTRASTRUCTURE IN FREEZE-FRACTURE

    The freeze-fracture technique allows membranes to be split
apart and veiwed en face. The fracture plane travels along the
membrane's hydrophobic core (Figure 1), exposing structural
detail in its interior. This detail is viewed by making a
replica. The replica is cast by shadowing a fine layer of
platinum at an angle to the specimen surface, and then
evaporating carbon from directly above to form a strengthening
coat. After removal of the cells, the replica is examined in
the transmission electron microscope.

    Freeze-fracture replicas provide compelling visual evidence
for the fluid mosaic model - they reveal the membrane as a
smooth matrix containing a rich assortment of irregularly-shaped
particles (Figure 3). Reconstitution experiments have
demonstrated that particles of this type are visible only when
proteins are incorporated into the membrane (3); pure lipid
appears completely smooth (Figure 4). The intramembrane
particles therefore represent proteins (or lipoprotein
complexes) in the hydrophobic core of the membrane (for review,
see ref. 4), as depicted in the model (Figure 1). Most natural
membranes contain a large variety of proteins but in a few
systems one protein predominates, and it is then possible to
establish the identity of individual intramembrane particles
(Figures 5 and 6). Standard freeze-fracture electron microscopy
has proved to be a highly effective tool for investigating the
structural components of membrane specializations, for example,
those of intercellular junctions (Figures 6 and 7).
Disappointingly, however, the lipid portion of the membrane is
generally visualized only as an undifferentiated background
matrix.

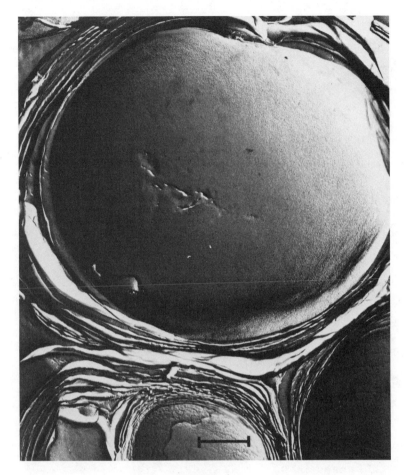

FIGURE 4

Freeze-fractured multilamellar liposome composed of
phosphatidylcholine. The fracture plane has travelled along the
hydrophobic interior of the lipid bilayer, as in natural
membranes. Note that the fracture faces are completely smooth
with no particles because of the absence of proteins. In some
artificial membrane systems, however, lipid micells (7) or
inter-membrane attachment sites (8) may give rise to structures
which superficially resemble the usual form of proteinaceous
intramembrane particles. Unpretreated specimen frozen directly
by plunging into propane (9). Scale bar, 0.5 μm.

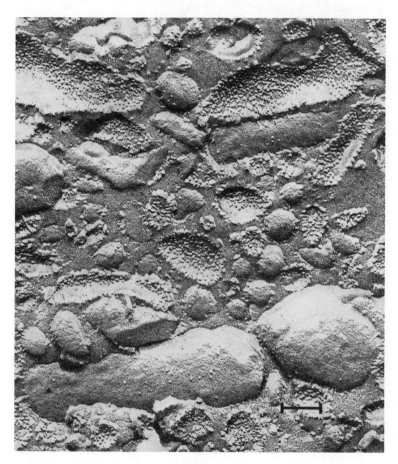

FIGURE 5

Freeze-fracture replica of isolated sarcoplasmic reticulum
vesicles. Both P-face (highly particulate) and E-face
(relatively smooth) views are visible. Because the
Ca^{2+}-ATPase is the principal integral membrane protein
present, the intramembrane particles are generally considered to
represent this protein (10, 11). Preparation isolated from
rabbit skeletal muscle (12) and directly frozen by propane
plunging (9). Scale bar. 100 nm.

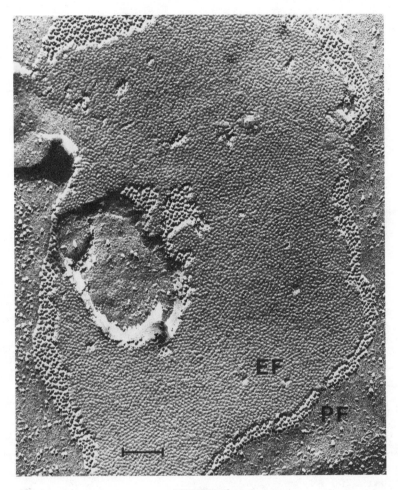

FIGURE 6

Freeze-fractured gap junction from a rabbit cardiac muscle
intercalated disc. The intramembrane particles from which this
membrane specialization is comprised are termed connexons.
Cardiac connexon proteins have recently been characterized
(13-16). In freeze-fracture, the connexons are viewed on the
P-face (PF) and their imprints on the E-face (EF) of the
adjacent membrane. From glutaraldehyde-fixed and glycerinated
left ventricle. Scale bar, 100 nm.

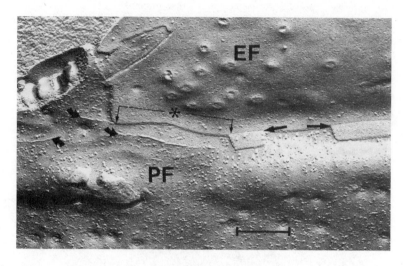

FIGURE 7

Freeze-fractured tight junction from the intercellular boundary
between two endothelial cells of a cardiac venule. This
membrane specialization appears as discontinous strands'(curved
arrows) on the P-face (PF), and as grooves (straight arrows) on
the E-face (EF). It has recently been proposed that the tight
junction strands represent lipids in micellar configuration
(17), although the more widely accepted view is that they
consist of protein. Careful inspection of P-face/E-face
boundaries (e.g. between arrows marked with asterisk) reveals an
arrangement of strands and grooves consistent with the presence
of two intramembrane fibrils rather than one (18). From
glutaraldehyde-fixed and glycerinated rabbit left ventricle.
Scale bar, 200 nm.

    As in thin-sectioning, a range of cytochemical techniques
can be combined with freeze-fracturing to gain information on
the chemical nature of the structural components viewed. It is
from advances in these techniques that attempts can now be made
to localize specific classes of lipids in biological membranes
(5, 6).

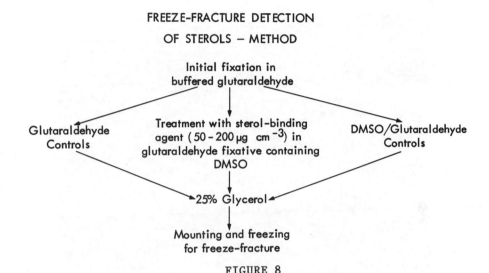

FIGURE 8

Experimental protocol for freeze-fracture detection of sterols, as used for the results illustrated in this article. An alternative approach to that summarized here is to extend the initial glutaraldehyde fixation, and then incubate the samples in buffer containing the sterol probe. Exposure of unfixed samples to the probe is not recommended because membrane and cellular damage is extensive in the absence of glutaraldehyde (5, 20).

FIGURE 9. Action of filipin (a) and tomatin (b) on a cholesterol-rich membrane, the cardiac fibroblast plasma membrane. In (a), asterisks mark zones that remain unperturbed by the agent. These zones are of two distinct types; 1) long thin bands, and 2) circular indentations. Scale bar, 200 nm.

(Following Page)

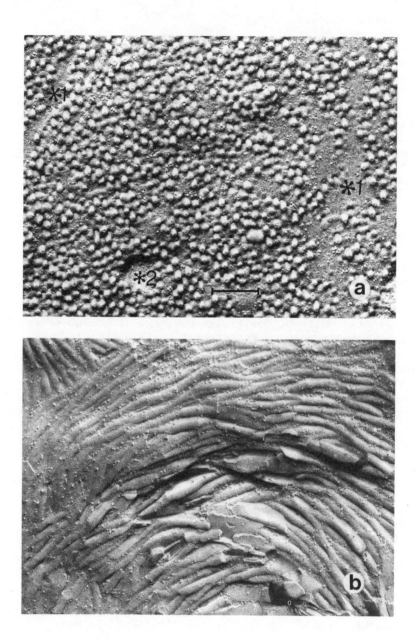

FREEZE-FRACTURE CYTOCHEMISTRY OF LIPIDS - THE PRINCIPLE

Freeze-fracture cytochemical detection of lipids relies on the induction of structural alterations in membranes by the interaction of a cytochemical probe with the target lipid molecules. These sites of altered structure appear as distinct deformations in freeze-fractured membranes and can therefore be used as labels for localizing the lipids in the membrane plane. Two classes of lipids are at present accessible to study with this approach - 3-β-hydroxysterols and anionic phospholipids. For a comprehensive discussion of this topic, the reader is referred to the review by Severs and Robenek (19).

LOCALIZATION OF STEROLS

The cytochemical probes used to detect sterols in freeze-fractured membranes are filipin (a polyene antibiotic), and tomatin and digitonin (saponins). Of these agents, filipin has been the most widely used to date because it is the least disruptive to membranes, the most sensitive to low sterol concentrations, and it provides high resolution quantifiable labelling patterns. From the practical point of view, the experimental use of these agents presents little difficulty (Figure 8). Samples are first fixed in glutaraldehyde as in the routine pretreatment procedure for freeze-fracture, and then incubated in fresh fixative containing the sterol probe. After completion of this experimental treatment, glycerination and freezing are carried out according to standard procedures. Because a small quantity of dimethylsulphoxide (DMSO) is often used to aid dissolution of the agent in the fixative, it is standard practice to process two controls in parallel; one in fixative alone and one in fixative containing DMSO.

The characteristic appearance of the deformations induced by filipin and the saponins in cholesterol-rich membranes is illustrated in Figure 9. Filipin deformations appear as circular bumps which measure ~25 nm in diameter and may protrude from either side of the membrane (Figure 9a). Saponins, on the other hand, induce hemicylindrical deformations of 40-60 nm width and variable length (Figure 9b).

Precisely how the agents induce deformations in membranes is incompletely understood. A possible mechanism of filipin action is summarized in Figure 10.

DISTRIBUTION OF CHOLESTEROL IN MYOCARDIAL MEMBRANES

Cholesterol is the principal 3-β-hydroxysterol in mammalian cellular membranes (21). In the myocardium, therefore, the effects of the agents may be attributed specifically to cholesterol rather than sterols in general.

Inspection of the filipin-treated cardiac fibroblast plasma membrane in Figure 9a reveals patches of membrane that have remained unaffected by the cholesterol probe. Two types of unlabelled domain are visible: i) long thin bands and ii) circular indentations. The former are identified as membrane areas which overlie bundles of microfilaments, and the latter as coated pits - specialized sites of the membrane engaged in receptor-mediated endocytosis. The clathrin coats of coated pits - which are so readily visualized by standard thin section electron microscopy - are not visible in freeze-fracture because of their location at the cytoplasmic surface of the membrane.

Local heterogeneities in the distribution of filipin deformations are also evident in the plasma membrane of cardiac muscle cells. As can be seen in Figure 11, gap junctions and desmosomes in the intercalated disc sarcolemma are completely resistant to filipin, despite heavy labelling in the surrounding membrane regions. Typically, the general (i.e. non-intercalated disc) sarcolemma shows a less marked response to filipin than that observed in the plasma membranes of neighbouring capillary endothelial cells and fibroblasts (Figure 12; 23). Endothelial vesicles, which are responsible for transporting materials across the endothelial wall, are usually affected in a similar manner to that characteristic of the endothelial plasma membrane. Some vesicle membranes within the endothelial cell remain unaffected, however (Figure 12).

Apart from the Golgi apparatus (24), intracellular membranes of the cardiac muscle cell show little response to filipin or tomatin. Occasional foci of affected membrane appear in the free sarcoplasmic reticulum but mitochondrial membranes are completely resistent to the treatment (Figure 13). This pattern of response is not altered following ischemia (Figure 14) despite reports of markedly increased cholesterol levels in mitochondria isolated from ischemic myocardium (25). The nuclear membranes of cardiac muscle cells are seldom affected by filipin whereas those of the capillary endothelium show a moderate to marked response (26).

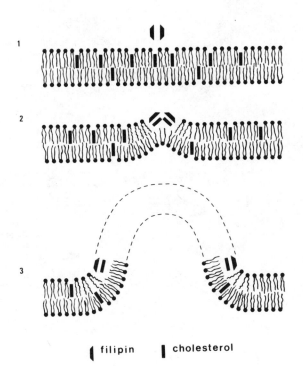

| filipin | | cholesterol |

FIGURE 10

Model of filipin action adapted from that originally discussed
by Severs et al. (22). 1) shows filipin molecules, possibly in
micellar form. in the solution external to the membrane. 2)
Binding of filipin to cholesterol in the upper monolayer of the
membrane, with an alteration in the orientation of the molecules
from a vertical to a horizontal position. This initiates
deformation of the membrane because of the increase in surface
pressure in the upper monolayer. Note the increase in fluidity
of the phospholipid molecules immediately adjacent to the
filipin-cholesterol complex. 3) Aggregation of primary filipin-
cholesterol complexes to produce an ultrastructurally-detectable
membrane deformation. The precise molecular arrangement within
the region indicated by dashes is uncertain.

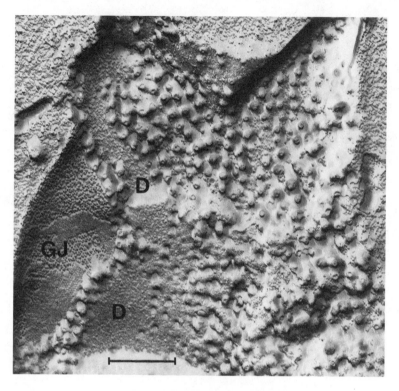

FIGURE 11

Freeze-fractured filipin-treated intercalated disc sarcolemma. Gap junctions (GJ) and desmosomes (D) are unaffected by the cholesterol probe. From rabbit left ventricle. Scale bar, 200 nm.

FIGURE 12. Freeze-fracture replica illustrating response of the plasma membranes of a cardiac muscle cell (CMC) and an endothelial cell (E) to filipin treatment. The cardiac muscle sarcolemma is only minimally affected by the probe, whereas the endothelial plasma membrane is extensively affected, both at the tissue front (ET) and at the luminal front (EL). In the endothelial cytoplasm (Cyt), most vesicles are sensitive to filipin (open arrows) though some are spared (filled arrows). ES, extracellular space; L, lumen. From rabbit left ventricle. Scale bar, 200 nm.

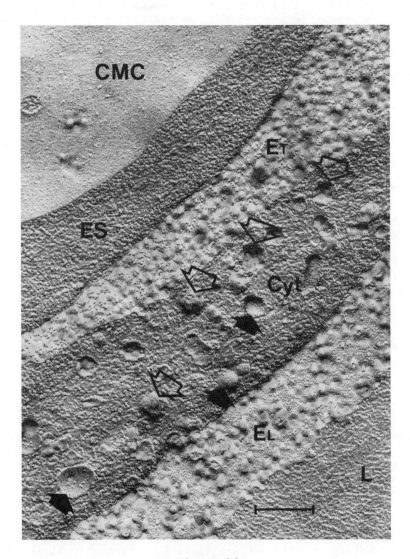

Figure 12

These observations suggest that marked heterogeneities in
cholesterol distribution exist both between and within different
membrane types. It has recently become apparent, however, that
the interpretation of filipin labelling patterns is complicated
by the possibility of false-negative responses in membrane
domains containing densely-packed integral and peripheral
proteins (19). In at least some instances, saponins can be used
to verify negative responses to filipin (22, 27). Applying this
approach to the membrane types so far investigated in the
myocardium, tomatin gives comparable results to those obtained
with filipin (28). Furthermore, in any given myocardial
membrane type for which biochemical data are available for
comparison (25, 29-31), no suspicious discrepancies in the
overall cytochemical responses are evident.

Some filipin-negative membrane domains, notably coated pits
and gap junctions, are also saponin-negative (19, 28). Since
isolated coated vesicles reportedly contain lower cholesterol
levels than those of the plasma membrane (32), the cytochemical
responses shown by their precursors might seem to be
vindicated. Enzymatic removal of the clathrin coat does not
alter the filipin insensitivity of coated pits (33) yet natural
removal of the coat from the vesicle apparently does (34). The
data on gap junctions are also puzzling; despite the agreement
in the filipin and saponin effects, isolated gap junctions
reportedly have a high cholesterol content (35, 36). However,
gap junction formation zones - in which interference with probe
action would seem unlikely because of the dearth of protein
particles present - give a negative cytochemical response just
like their mature counterparts.

Until further information on these and other membrane
domains is available, it is clear that valid interpretation of
the cytochemical results requires the exercise of extreme
caution. It should nevertheless be stated that because
interaction of the probes with 3-β-hydroxysterols is highly
specific (5), a positive cytochemical response may be taken as a
convincing demonstration of the presence of these sterols.

LOCALIZATION OF ANIONIC PHOSPHOLIPIDS

Using the peptide antibiotic polymyxin-B, attempts have been
made to localize anionic phospholipids in membranes following a
similar approach to that described for sterols. As with filipin
and the saponins, specimens are exposed to polymyxin-B before
the freezing step. There are, however, two differences in the
practical procedure that make polymyxin a less satisfactory
cytochemical probe than filipin and the saponins. First,
polymyxin treatment has to be carried out on single cell
suspensions or monolayer cultures; it has not, as yet, proved
suitable for whole tissue samples. Secondly, the experimental
treatment is given before fixation.

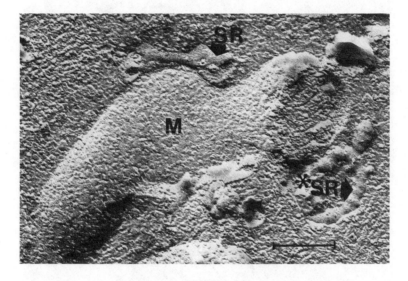

FIGURE 13

Freeze-fractured cardiac muscle mitochondrial (M) and
sarcoplasmic reticulum (SR) membranes after filipin treatment.
The former are spared though the latter are sometimes affected
(asterisk). For detailed discussion on the response of SR to
filipin, see Severs (28, 37) and Sommer et al. (38). From
rabbit left ventricle. Scale bar, 200 nm.

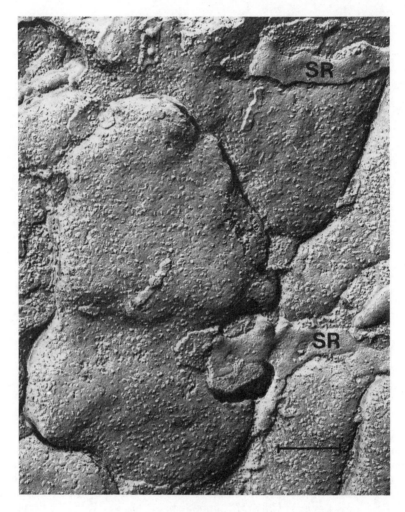

FIGURE 14

Freeze-fracture replica of filipin-treated ischemic myocardium.
The mitochondrial membranes and elements of cisternal
sarcoplasmic reticulum (SR) remain unperturbed by the agent.
From a Langendorff-perfused rabbit heart; initial
 stabilization´ perfusion with oxygenated Krebs-Henseleit
buffer. 25 min at 36º C, followed by 60 min global ischemia.
Scale bar, 200 nm.

DISTRIBUTION OF ANIONIC LIPIDS IN CARDIAC MUSCLE SARCOLEMMA

To study negatively charged phospholipids in cardiac muscle cell membranes, I, and my colleagues Trevor Powell and Victor Twist, have recently applied polymyxin treatment to suspensions of isolated myocytes. The myocytes were dissociated by in vitro perfusion of adult rat hearts with collagenase, as described by Powell et al. (39). We have previously shown that the ultrastructure of myocytes isolated by this method closely resembles that of myocytes in the intact myocardium (40).

Figure 15 illustrates the effects of polymyxin and of filipin on the sarcolemma of isolated rat myocytes. An untreated control is shown in (a); this has the usual smoothly contoured appearance of the sarcolemma studded with intramembrane particles and occasionally interrupted by caveolae. After polymyxin treatment (b), the membrane becomes somewhat ruffled, and broad (60-200 nm diameter) indentations cover the surface. These indentations are membrane deformations induced by the selective interaction of polymyxin with negatively charged phospholipids in the membrane. For comparison, the effect of filipin on the isolated myocyte sarcolemma is illustrated in (c). Small circular deformations can be seen which have a similar appearance and density to those observed in the general sarcolemma of filipin-treated myocytes in intact tissue (23).

These results indicate that anionic phospholipids – which potentially form an important source of calcium-binding sites – are widespread within the sarcolemma. The effect of polymyxin on intracellular membranes cannot be ascertained from studies on isolated myocytes, however, since the agent does not readily penetrate across the sarcolemma. No such difficulty occurs with filipin, though in tissue samples the depth of penetration of this probe is limited to several cell layers. The similar extent of filipin labelling in isolated myocytes and myocytes of the intact heart confirms that contrary to a suggestion by Sommer et al. (38), penetration problems are unlikely to account for the relatively low density of filipin deformations reported in the sarcolemma of myocytes in tissue samples (23).

CONCLUDING COMMENT

Because the freeze-fracture cytochemical approach for detecting membrane cholesterol has been adopted with great speed and enthusiasm, interpretation of the results has not always been tempered with appropriate caution. An understanding of the theoretical and practical limitations of the technique is essential if the conclusions drawn from its use are to be of value. These aspects are explored in greater detail elsewhere (19, 28). Despite some difficulties, however, freeze-fracture

cytochemistry provides fascinating insights into the
distribution of different types of lipid between and within
membranes.

ACKNOWLEDGEMENTS

    This work was supported by British Heart Foundation grant
no. 81/44. I am indebted to my colleagues, Helen Simons, Colin
Green, Trevor Powell, and Victor Twist, for collaboration in and
discussion of various aspects of these studies. The fast and
efficient photographic skills of Graham Storey enabled the
deadline for completion of the manuscript to be met.

$\longrightarrow$

FIGURE 15. Freeze-fractured sarcolemmata of isolated rat
myocytes; (a) untreated control, (b) after treatment with
polymyxin-B (200 μg cm^{-3}/20 min) and (c) after treatment with
filipin (100 μg cm^{-3}/70 min). Note that the deformations
induced by polymyxin (asterisks and arrows) are much larger than
those induced by filipin. The arrows indicate shallow
indentations; the asterisks, deeper onces in which the fracture
plane has left the membrane. Scale bar, 200 nm.

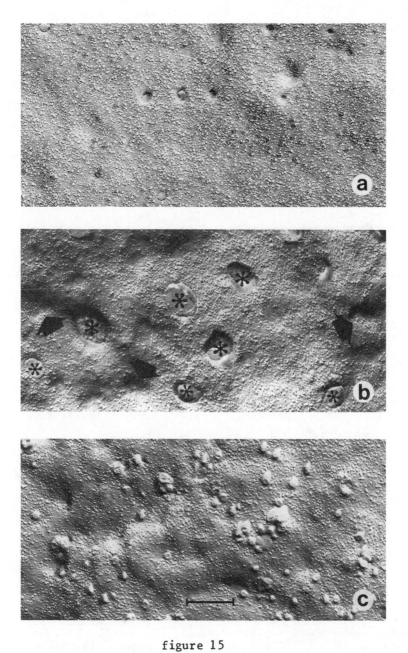

figure 15

REFERENCES

1. Singer, S.J., & Nicolson, G.L. (1972): Science 175: 720.
2. Branton, D., Bullivant, S., Gilula, N.B., Karnovsky, M.J.,
   Moor, H.. Muhlethaler, K., Northcote, D.H., Packer, B.,
   Satir, B., Satir, P., Speth, V., Staehelin, L.A., Steere,
   R.L., & Weinstein, R.S. (1975): Science 190: 54.
3. Yu, J., & Branton, D. (1976): Proc. Natl. Acad. Sci. USA
   73: 3891.
4. Bullivant, S. (1977): J. Microsc. 111: 101.
5. Elias, P.M., Friend, D.S., & Goerke, J. (1979): J.
   Histochem. Cytochem. 27: 1247.
6. Bearer, E.L., & Friend, D.S. (1980): Proc. Natl. Acad. Sci.
   USA 77: 6601.
7. Verkleij, A.J., Mombers, C., Leunissen-Bijvelt, J., &
   Ververgaert, P.H.J.Th. (1979): Nature 279: 162.
8. Miller, R.G. (1980): Nature 287: 166.
9. Severs, N.J., & Green, C.R. (1983): Biol. Cell. 47: 193.
10. Deamer, D.W., & Baskin, R.J. (1969): J. Cell Biol. 42:
    296.
11. Bray, D.F., Rayns, D.G., & Wagenaar, E.B. (1978): Can. J.
    Zool. 56: 140.
12. Madden, T.D., Chapman, D., & Quinn, P.J. (1979): Nature
    279: 538.
13. Kensler, R.W., & Goodenough, D.A. (1980): J. Cell Biol.
    86: 755.
14. Manjunath, C.K., Goings, G.E., & Page, E. (1982): Biochem.
    J. 205: 189.
15. Manjunath, C.K., Goings, G.E., & Page, E. (1982): J. Cell
    Biol. 95: 88a.
16. Nicholson, B.J., Gros, D., & Revel, J.-P. (1982): J. Cell
    Biol. 95: 104a.
17. Kachar, B., & Reese, T.S. (1982): Nature 296: 464.
18. Bullivant, S. (1976): J. Cell Biol. 70: 35a.
19. Severs, N.J., & Robenek, H. (1983): Biochim. Biophys. Acta
    (Rev. Biomembranes), 737: 373.
20. Robinson, J.M., & Karnovsky, M.J. (1980): J. Histochem.
    Cytochem. 28: 161.
21. Demel, R.A., & De Kruijff, B. (1976): Biochim. Biophys.
    Acta 457: 109.
22. Severs, N.J., Warren, R.C., & Barnes, S.H. (1981): J.
    Ultrastruct. Res. 77: 160.
23. Severs, N.J. (1981): Eur. J. Cell Biol. 25: 289.
24. Severs, N.J. (1981): Experientia 37: 1195.
25. Rouslin, W., Macgee, J., Gupte, S., Wesselman, A., & Epps,
    D.E. (1982): Am. J. Physiol. 11: H254.
26. Severs, N.J. (1982): J. Submicrosc. Cytol. 14: 441.
27. Severs, N.J., & Simons, H. (1983): Nature 303: 637.

28. Severs, N.J. (1984): IN Methods in Studying Cardiac Membranes, Vol. 2 (ed) N.S. Dhalla, CRC Press Inc., Boca Raton, in press.
29. Owens, K., Weglicki, W.G., Ruth. R.C., Stam. A.C., & Sonnenblick, E.H. (1973): Biochim. Biophys. Acta 296: 71.
30. Slack, B.E., Boegman, R.J., Downie, J.W., & Jasmin, G. (1980): J. Mol. Cell. Cardiol. 12: 179.
31. Tibbits, G.F., Sasaki, M., Ikeda. M., Shimada. K., Tsuruhara, T., & Nagatomo, T. (1981): J. Mol. Cell. Cardiol. 13: 1051.
32. Pearse, B.M.F. (1976): Proc. Natl. Acad. Sci. USA 73: 1255.
33. Feltkamp, C.A., & Van der Waerden, A.W.M. (1982): Exptl. Cell Res. 140: 289.
34. McGookey, D.J., Fagerberg, K., & Anderson, R.G.W. (1983): J. Cell Biol. 96: 1273.
35. Henderson, D., Eibl, H., & Weber, K. (1979): J. Mol. Biol. 132: 193.
36. Hertzberg, E.L., & Gilula, N.B. (1979): J. Biol. Chem. 254: 2138.
37. Severs, N.J. (1982): Cell Tiss. Res. 224: 613.
38. Sommer, J.R., Dolber. P.C., & Taylor, I. (1982): J. Ultrastruct. Res. 80: 98.
39. Powell, T., Terrar. D.A., & Twist, V.W. (1980): J. Physiol. 302: 131.
40. Severs, N.J., Slade. A.M., Powell, T., Twist, V.W., & Warren, R.L. (1982): J. Ultrastruct. Res. 81: 222.

PHOSPHOLIPASE-INDUCED ABNORMALITIES IN THE SARCOLEMMA

N. A. Shaikh, I. Parson, and E. Downar

Department of Medicine and Clinical Biochemistry
Medical Sciences Building, Room 7359
University of Toronto
Toronto, Ontario, Canada, M5S 1A8

Phospholipids are the major form of lipid in all cell
membranes and their fixed composition and disposition within
membranes are genetically predetermined. In combination with
other lipids and proteins, phospholipids are responsible for
both structural characteristics and functional properties of the
biological membranes such as fluidity (1, 2), ionic permeability
(3, 4), transport of material across cell membranes (5),
activities of a large number of membrane-bound enzymes (6) and
receptor-mediated cell responses (7, 8). Phospholipases are the
enzymatic systems responsible for the catabolism of membrane
phospholipids, and the interplay between these catabolic enzymes
and those of anabolic systems determines the turnover rate and
maintains the biological properties and fixed composition of
these lipids in membranes. Various physiological stimuli (e.g.
certain hormone-receptor interactions, increase in intracellular
Ca^{2+}, fat absorption, etc.) enhance phospholipid turnover in
membranes (8-11). In some disease conditions, membrane
phospholipid composition and metabolism are progressively
altered resulting in the functional abnormalities of the cell
(12-15).

Ischemia-induced specific electrophysiological alterations
leading to ventricular fibrillation (16) appear to be associated
with abnormal cardiac lipid metabolism (17-20). It has been
suggested that lipid abnormalities of the ischemic heart could
alter cardiac functions by changing the properties of cardiac
cell membranes and that these functional changes may contribute
to the decline in myocardial contractility, to arrhythmia and
eventual cell death (18). Some of these abnormalities have been

63

ascribed to be the consequences of ischemia-induced activation
of phospholipases, even though direct proof for such activation
is still obscure. Phospholipase activity is found in a number
of cardiac membranes (21, 22) as well as cardiac lysosomes (23)
and lysosomal enzyme activity increases in the ischemic heart
(24). Depletion in myocardial phospholipid content or
accumulation of lysophosphoglycerides and other amphiphiles have
been observed in experimental animals after coronary artery
occlusion, presumably due to phospholipase activation (12, 14,
15). Depletion of membrane phospholipid has been related to an
increased Ca^{2+} permeability of sarcoplasmic reticulum vesicles
in vitro and to the extent of irreversible damage in reperfused
myocardium. These defects could be prevented by pretreatment of
the animal with chlorpromazine, a phospholipase inhibitor (14,
25).

Reports of accumulation of lysophosphoglycerides (lyso-PL)
in ischemic myocardium (12, 15) and their increased
concentrations in effluents from ischemic isolated perfused
rabbit hearts (26) and arrhythmogenic properties of these
amphiphiles in tissue bath experiments has led Sobel and
co-workers to postulate that lysophosphoglycerides are potential
mediators of dysrhythmia (27). However, lyso-PL at their
maximum levels in ischemic heart accounts for only 160 nmoles/g
wet wt. or 0.6% of total phospholipid-phosphorus (15). A much
higher concentration of lyso-PL (approx. 10-fold) bound with
albumin is required to induce electrophysiological alterations
in normoxic Purkinje fibers in a tissue bath that are analogous
to changes in ischemic tissue in vivo (28). Unbound lyso-PL in
quantities similar to those found in ischemic myocardium or
lower amounts have recently been shown to produce electrophysiological derangements (28-30) and to induce arrhythmia in
isolated perfused hearts analogous to other detergents (31).
However, free concentrations of lyso-PL equivalent to those
employed in the forementioned experiments would not be expected
in the plasma compartment bathing cardiac tissue where these
amphiphiles would be bound with plasma albumin.

We investigated the possiblity that the accumulation of
lyso-PL or depletion of phospholipid molecules in the sarcolemma
is responsible for the electrophysiological abnormalities of
ischemic hearts by producing in vitro phospholipase-induced
abnormalities in muscle and Purkinje fibers of the sheep heart.
Under control conditions, exogenous phospholipase A_2 was
employed to produce lyso-PL in the membrane matrix, and
phospholipase C was used to achieve depletion of membrane
phospholipids (< 1.0%) without lyso-PL production. For
comparative purposes, electrophysiological effects of exogenous
free lyso-PL were also described for sheep cardiac fibers.

MATERIALS AND METHODS

Phospholipase A_2 (Naja Naja) and phospholipase C (C. welchii or B. cereus) were purchased from Sigma Chemical Co. (St. Louis, MO). Chromatographically pure lysophosphatidyl-choline (LPC) prepared from pig-liver and synthetic LPC of different fatty acid moieties were purchased from Sigma Chemical Co. and Serdery Research Laboratories Inc. (London, Ont., Canada). When necessary these lipids were further purified by thin-layer chromatography using chloroform-methanol-acetic acid-water (100:45:20:6.8, by vol.) as a developing solvent (32). Isolation of LPC from the silica gel and quantification were done essentially as described earlier (15). Gas-liquid chromatography of pig-liver LPC demonstrated the following per cent fatty acid composition (C 16:0, 32%; C 18:0, 62%; C 18:1, 2%). Mixtures of LPC resembling in fatty acid composition those of porcine heart as reported earlier (15) or of sheep moderator band (C 14:0, 3%; C 16:0, 43%; C 18:0, 42%; C 18:1, 4%; C 18:2, 3%; C 20:0 + 20:4, 4%) were prepared by proportionately mixing LPC of different fatty acid moieties in chloroform-methanol solutions. For tissue bath experiments, LPC solutions in chloroform-methanol were dried under N_2 at 37° C, dissolved in Tyrode's buffer and vortexed for 5 minutes to obtain emulsions. In some experiments, these emulsions were sonicated for 1 min. at the 50% level (high setting) of the Biosonic IV Sonicator (Bronwill Scientific). LPC solutions were prepared in larger volumes and proportionately pipetted to achieve particular molarity in 1.8 ml of tissue bath perfusate. Final LPC amounts to achieve different molarities in 1.8 ml perfusate were: 0.27 μmoles = 0.15 mM; 0.9 μmoles = 0.5 mM; 1.35 μmoles = 0.75 mM; and, 1.8 μmoles = 1.0 mM.

Sheep hearts were obtained from the abattoir at the time of sacrifice and immediately placed in ice-cold oxygenated Tyrode's buffer. The right ventricle was excised to allow dissection of both muscle and Purkinje fibers. The left ventricle was excised to obtain subendocardial muscle strips containing Purkinje fibers. The tissues were secured to the bottom of a 2 ml tissue bath and superfused with modified Tyrode's buffer oxygenated with 95% O_2, 5% CO_2 at 37° C. Buffer composition was (in mM): sodium 144, potassium 4, magnesium 1.4, calcium 1.4, chloride 125, phosphate 1.0, bicarbonate 25, and dextrose 11.

The cardiac tissue was electrically paced at one end with a surface contact bipolar probe. The stimulus was maintained at 2x threshold with a biphasic pulse width of 1 msec duration. Transmembrane action potentials were recorded using glass microelectrodes (10 to 30 Megohm tip impedance) filled with 3 M KCl and connected via driven-shield cables to high input

impedance buffer amplifiers. The action potential parameters
(resting membrane potential, RMP; amplitude, AMP; action
potential duration, APD (50 & 90%); maximum rate of rise of
phase zero, dV/dt) were analyzed, and all data recorded on an
instrumentation tape recorder. In order to minimize artifact in
the dV/dt recordings, repetitive checks were made of the
microelectrode capacitive compensation.

After continuous superfusion to stabilize the transmembrane
potentials the flow of buffer was stopped for 10-12 minutes and
action potential parameters were recorded. All subsequent test
incubations with LPC or phospholipases were done similarly in
stagnant buffer conditions. To test the effects of exogenous
LPC, the buffer flow was stopped and 0.2 ml out of 1.8 ml
perfusate (tissue bath volume) was pipetted out and this volume
was replaced with 0.2 ml of pre-warmed (37° C) LPC solutions
(9-fold concentrations of the desired molarity). The mixture
was briefly mixed by repetitive pipetting and was left
undisturbed for 10-12 minutes. This procedure ensured a
constant stagnant perfusate volume thereby avoiding impalement
adjustments and erroneous electrophysiological parameters due to
changing microelectrode compensation. In some experiments total
replacement of tissue bath fluid by LPC solutions at 37° C was
used but in these cases cell impalement required either
adjustment or re-impalement of new cells. The surface of the
tissue bath was sealed with paraffin oil when anoxic effects
were being studied. In these cases lyso-PL determinations could
not be achieved on the same fibers and parallel tissue bath
experiments without paraffin oil were used to perform these
analyses. To ensure that measured parameters were not an
isolated cell event, other cells were monitored at the end of
single cell protocols.

To test the effects of endogenously produced lyso-PL or the
depletion of membrane phospholipids, cardiac tissues were
incubated in tissue bath with phospholipase A_2 and
phospholipase C, respectively. The enzymes were dissolved in
Tyrode's buffer (37° C) and 0.2 ml aliquots were used
similarly as described above for LPC incubations. Phospholipase
activities varied from batch to batch and were monitored
before-hand under similar conditions of tissue bath
experiments. Sufficient amounts of these enzymes were then used
to achieve desired amounts of hydrolysis of the membrane
phospholipids.

At the end of each protocol, cardiac tissues were
immediately rinsed with ice-cold Tyrode's buffer to remove
entrapped perfusate containing exogenous LPC or phospholipases,
blotted dry and weighed. Depending upon the expected value for
LPC, measurement was made either by GLC or by phosphate analysis

of the isolated lipid fraction essentially as described earlier
(15).

RESULTS

Effects of Exogenous Lysophosphatidylcholine

Figure 1 shows the electrophysiological effects of different
concentrations of pig-liver LPC emulsions (unsonicated) on both
muscle and Purkinje fibers of the sheep heart. In these
experiments, moderator band (120-200 mg wet wt.) containing both
muscle and Purkinje fibers was incubated for 10 min in 1.8 ml of
pig-liver LPC prepared in Tyrode's buffer and action potential
profiles were recorded. No significant effect on
electrophysiological profiles of either muscle or Purkinje fiber
(left- hand panel) was observed when incubated for 10 min with 0
mM (control), 0.15 mM, 0.5 mM, 1.0 mM LPC emulsions in
oxygenated buffer of pH 7.35 at 37° C. In nitrogenated
acidotic conditions (right-hand panel) significant shortening of
APD (22%, p<.005) was observed but when compared to their
respective controls (0 mM LPC) LPC was ineffective in altering
any electrophysiological parameters. Similar results were
obtained when LPC emulsions of different fatty acid composition
(similar to those found in sheep or porcine hearts) were
tested. In both oxygenated and nitrogenated acidotic conditions
high concentrations of pig-liver LPC (greater than 1.5 mM)
showed significant decrease (30-50%, p<.001) in amplitude, APD,

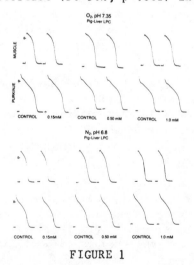

FIGURE 1

Effects of pig-liver LPC on action potential configuration of
both muscle and Purkinje fibers of the sheep heart in oxygenated
and nitrogenated acidotic buffers.

and upstroke velocity. In these instances the transmembrane
potentials continued to deteriorate even after prolonged washing
with normal oxygenated buffer, suggesting detergent-like effects
of lyso-PL.

In order to assess the possibility that unsonicated LPC
emulsions form larger particle sizes thereby reducing the
effective concentrations of LPC over the fibers, a series of
experiments were performed where sonicated synthetic
palmitoyl-LPC solutions were used. Figure 2 shows electrophysiological profiles and parameters of sheep Purkinje fibers
under such conditions. The left-hand panels show
electrophysiological profiles in oxygenated, continuous flowing
Tyrode's buffer. The middle panels show the same fibers when
incubated for 10 min with different concentrations of LPC and
the right panels show when reflow with normal oxygenated buffer
was restored. No significant changes in electrophysiological
profiles or parameters (AMP, RMP, dV/dt and APD) of Purkinje
fibers were noticed when LPC concentrations analogous to those
found in porcine ischemic myocardium (0.15 mM) or 2- to 3-fold
those amounts were used. However, at 0.75 mM LPC
concentrations, action potential parameters were altered and
continued to deteriorate even after prolonged washing with
normal buffer. After 10 min of washing, AMP, RMP, dV/dt
parameters were reduced by 40-70% of their control values.
Furthermore, sequential incubations with different amounts of
LPC (0.15-0.5 mM) increased the sensitivity of the fibers to a
lower LPC level (e.g. 0.3 mM) and enhanced the washing effect.
These observations suggest detergent-like structural damage to
the sarcolemmal membrane (removal of glycocalyx and/or
lipoproteins of sarcolemma) and that the sonicated LPC is more
potent in producing such effects than LPC emulsions. In all
these experiments LPC concentrations of the cardiac tissue did
not increase significantly (+5%) from their control levels. The
next series of experiments describes the electrophysiological
effects of raising the endogenous lyso-PL levels or depletion of
membrane phospholipid by using exogenous phospholipases.

Effects of phospholipases

Figure 3 shows typical electrophysiological profiles of both
muscle and Purkinje fibers when moderator bands were incubated
with phospholipase A_2 for 10 min in Tyrode's buffer of pH 7.35
at 37⁰ C. Only the first few layers of cardiac cells were
impaled and lyso-PL were analyzed immediately after the
completion of the incubation period. Action potential
configuration of both fibers did not alter when endogenously
produced lyso-PL levels reached 2- to 3-fold the amounts
reported for ischemic myocardium. Much higher concentrations

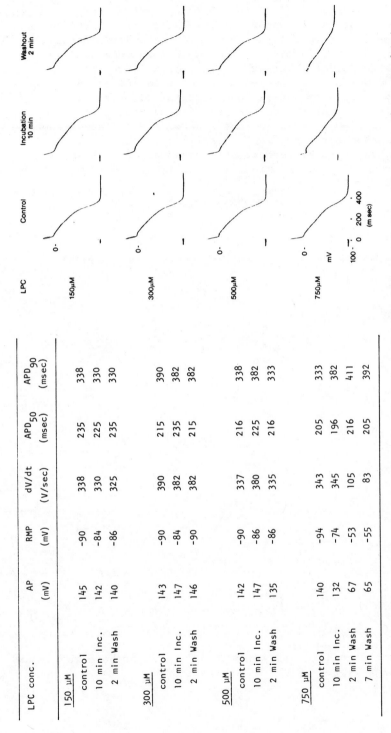

LPC conc.	AP (mV)	RMP (mV)	dV/dt (V/sec)	APD$_{50}$ (msec)	APD$_{90}$ (msec)
150 µM					
control	145	-90	338	235	338
10 min Inc.	142	-84	330	225	330
2 min Wash	140	-86	325	235	330
300 µM					
control	143	-90	390	215	390
10 min Inc.	147	-84	382	235	382
2 min Wash	146	-90	382	215	382
500 µM					
control	142	-90	337	216	338
10 min Inc.	147	-86	380	225	382
2 min Wash	135	-86	335	216	333
750 µM					
control	140	-94	343	205	333
10 min Inc.	132	-74	345	196	382
2 min Wash	67	-53	105	216	411
7 min Wash	65	-55	83	205	392

Figure 2. Effects of Exogenous Palmitoyl-LPC on Action Potential Parameters in Sheep Purkinje Fibers.

exhibited the ischemic effects. When concentrations of
endogenously produced lyso-PL equivalent to or slightly more
than ischemic concentrations were produced under controlled
conditions and the Purkinje fibers were then incubated in
nitrogenated acidotic buffer and subsequently washed with
oxygenated buffer, no changes were observed (Figure 4). Since
lyso-PL concentrations were to be determined, paraffin oil could
not be used to seal the tissue bath for maintenance of proper
anoxic conditions. This in fact reduced the effect of anoxia
which was seen for experiments described in Figure 1.
Nevertheless, lyso-PL concentration even after washing with
oxygenated buffer for 10 min remained high (0.19 mM versus
control 0.09 mM).

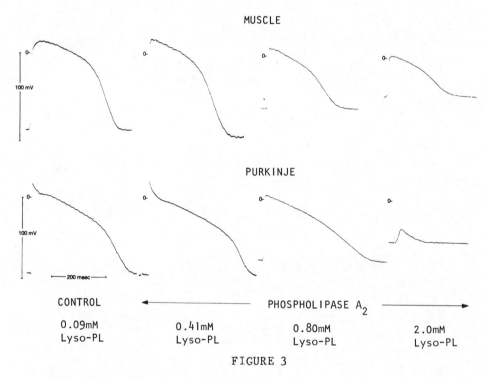

FIGURE 3

Effects of endogenously produced lyso-PL on both muscle and
Purkinje fibers of the sheep heart.

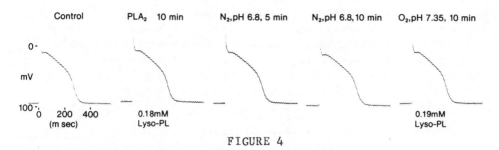

FIGURE 4

Effects of exogenous lyso-PL on action potential parameters in sheep Purkinje fibers incubated in nitrogenated acidotic buffers.

In the next series of experiments, endogenous production of much higher concentrations of lyso-PL (0.8 mM) resulted in a significant alteration of action potential parameters (Figure 5). When these preparations were subsequently washed with

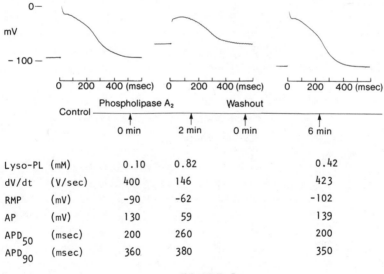

		Control	0 min	2 min	0 min	6 min
Lyso-PL	(mM)		0.10	0.82		0.42
dV/dt	(V/sec)		400	146		423
RMP	(mV)		-90	-62		-102
AP	(mV)		130	59		139
APD$_{50}$	(msec)		200	260		200
APD$_{90}$	(msec)		360	380		350

FIGURE 5

Effects of endogenously produced lyso-PL on action potential parameters in sheep Purkinje fibers.

oxygenated normal buffer, the same impaled cells showed complete
recovery in about 6 min. However the lyso-PL levels remained
abnormally high (0.42 mM). The recovery time varied for
different experiments (6-20 min) and with the extent of damage
in terms of the levels of lyso-PL produced. In our experimental
conditions, the recovery was always achieved when the endogenous
lyso-PL concentrations were not allowed to exceed more than 0.5
mM. Washing the phospholipase A_2-treated fibers with buffer
containing albumin diminished cell recovery suggesting that the
removal of hydrolysis products from the membrane plays an
important role in cell dysfunction. To test this hypothesis,
Purkinje fibers were incubated with phospholipase C under
control conditions so as to achieve very little hydrolysis of
sarcolemmal phospholipids (Figure 6). In these fibers, action
potentials were completely abolished after washing with normal
buffer and the cell became unresponsive to stimulus even after
prolonged washing (approx. 2 hrs.) with normal oxygenated
buffer. Significant differences in the phospholipid content of
whole tissue could not be demonstrated by the chemical analyses
of the phosphate content. Phospholipase C cleaves the diester
phosphate bond of phospholipid molecule to produce diglyceride
and phosphorylated base. The increase in the diglyceride
content of the incubated tissue was taken as a measure of
phospholipid hydrolysis. Diglyceride content of the fiber was

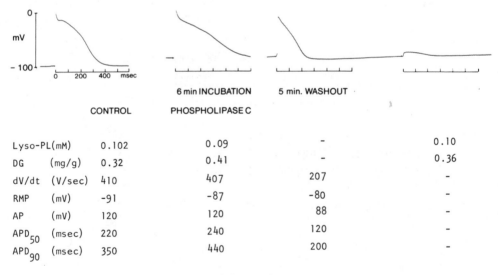

	CONTROL	6 min INCUBATION PHOSPHOLIPASE C	5 min. WASHOUT	
Lyso-PL (mM)	0.102	0.09	-	0.10
DG (mg/g)	0.32	0.41	-	0.36
dV/dt (V/sec)	410	407	207	-
RMP (mV)	-91	-87	-80	-
AP (mV)	120	120	88	-
APD_{50} (msec)	220	240	120	-
APD_{90} (msec)	350	440	200	-

FIGURE 6

Effects of membrane phospholipid depletion on action potential
parameters in sheep Purkinje fibers.

increased by 0.09 mg/g wet wt. (28%) suggesting about 0.8%
hydrolysis of membrane phospholipids. Subsequent decrease in
diglyceride content upon restoration of the flow amounts to
about 0.46% depletion in membrane phospholipid content. In
these experiments sphingomyelin was also partially hydrolyzed
but lyso-PL levels remained similar to controls.

DISCUSSION

    Lipid-induced abnormalities that may contribute to the
pathogenesis of ischemic damage in the myocardium have recently
been elegantly reviewed (18-20). Hydrolysis of membrane
phospholipids by the ischemia-induced activation of endogenous
phospholipases (33) could result in the accumulation of lyso-PL
and fatty acids and subsequent depletion of phospholipids from
membranes (34). Recently, both phospholipid depletion and
lyso-PL accumulation in and around membranes have been
implicated as important factors contributing to the functional
abnormalities of the ischemic heart (14, 25, 35). Since
phospholipids are required for a number of vital membrane
functions, their depletion could have severe consequences on
ionic transport, enzymatic activities, permeability, fluidity,
and hormone receptor-mediated cell responses. On the other
hand, lyso-PL are amphiphiles and their accumulation in and
around the sarcolemma could alter membrane-bound enzymatic
activities (36) and/or disrupt the membrane integrity by a
detergent-like effect (37). Recently lyso-PL have been reported
to induce marked electrophysiological alterations analogous to
those observed in ischemic tissue in vivo, implicating these
lipids as potential mediators of malignant dysrhythmia (27, 35,
38). We have shown earlier that lyso-PL levels increased by 60%
in an ischemic zone as compared to their pre-occlusion control
levels, this increase being similar to that reported by others
(12). Despite significant elevation in lyso-PL levels in
ischemic myocardium, their absolute quantities remained very
small (0.6% of total phospholipid-phosphorus). This led us to
suggest that these lipids alone could not be responsible for the
electrophysiological manifestation of ischemia (15). However,
the possibility that the accumulation of these amphiphilic
lipids occurs at selective membrane sites (e.g. in the vicinity
of enzymatic apparatus, at receptor sites, etc.), proposes
severe consequences for cell functions. Within the limitations
of current membrane technology, such a possibility is difficult
to ascertain.

    The arrhythmogenic nature of lyso-PL has been proposed in
tissue bath experiments where normoxic cardiac tissue has been
superfused with various concentrations of exogenously added LPC
and cell functions evaluated by determining the action potential

parameters. In some of these experiments, normoxic cardiac
tissue was continuously superfused with albumin-bound LPC in
quantities up to 10-fold higher than those present in ischemic
myocardium (12, 39) while in other experiments, the tissue was
continously superfused (29, 30, 38) or incubated with free LPC
solutions (26, 28, 35, 40) in amounts similar to or less than
those observed in ischemic tissue in situ (160 nmoles/g wet wt.
of porcine ischemic myocardium). LPC decreased maximum
diastolic potentials, peak dV/dt, amplitude, overshoot of phase
0 and action potential duration in a dose-dependent fashion
(28). Much higher amounts of LPC (2 mM) if bound with albumin
were required to induce these effects (27, 28, 39).

It is very difficult to say how much free LPC bathing the
cardiac cells would be available under in situ conditions.
Since albumin has a very high affinity for amphiphiles like
fatty acids and lyso-PL and the amounts of plasma proteins
relative to LPC is very high (8 g% protein or 4.8 g% albumin for
human plasma; 6.5 mg% LPC for porcine plasma), it is not
unreasonable to expect that all the LPC in fluids bathing the
ischemic compartment would be completely bound to plasma,
cytosolic or lymph proteins. Exposing the cardiac tissue to
free LPC solutions is therefore unphysiological and at best the
observed effects could be attributed to the detergent-like
properties of these molecules. This conclusion could also be
drawn from most of these experiments since often one particular
type of LPC (C-16) was used even though this molecular moiety
constitutes a fraction of the total lyso-PL found in ischemic
myocardium in situ. The monomeric effects of other moieties of
lyso-PL could be inferred to be different if the extent of
uptake in membranes and their effects other than detergent-like
are taken into consideration.

Bearing in mind the serious limitations of the tissue bath
studies, we performed experiments using different moieties of
lyso-PL and keeping the volume of the tissue bath to the minimum
possible (1.8 ml for 120-220 mg cardiac tissue) to simulate the
ischemic compartment. Pig-liver LPC, synthetic palmitoyl-LPC or
LPC of similar fatty acid composition to that present in sheep
or porcine heart were used. When the emulsions (vortexed
solutions) of these lyso-PL (up to 1.0 mM) were superfused in
stagnant nonflowing conditions for 10-12 min, no significant
alteration in action potential parameters were observed even in
conditions of anoxia and acidosis (Figure 1). Higher
concentrations of these amphiphilic lipids (greater than 1.5 mM)
altered transmembrane potential characteristics in a manner
similar to other detergents (unpublished results). This is
further substantiated by the fact that washing of the
pre-incubated tissue produces more deleterious effects than

incubation alone with LPC (Figure 2), suggesting removal of
lipids and/or lipoproteins from the membrane upon washing. The
concentrations of the lyso-PL required to produce significant
alteration in membrane potential were reduced to half if the
emulsions of these lipids were sonicated. This reduces the
micellar size and thereby increases the effective concentrations
of these detergent-like molecules to come in contact with
cardiac tissue. However, such micellar solutions in amounts
similar to or 2- to 3-fold the levels found in ischemic
myocardium remain ineffective in producing significant electrophysiological aterations. In all these experiments the total
amounts of lyso-PL in superfused cardiac tissue did not change
significantly. The differences in our results and those
obtained by some of the other workers (29, 30) could be
explained on the basis that in our studies a noflow incubation
rather than a continous superfusion of the cardiac tissue with
these detergent-like compounds was employed. In other studies
where a similar technique was employed (28), it is difficult to
compare the results since cardiac tissue from different
experimental animals were used and the weight of the perfused
tissue was not reported. As stated earlier (see Results), the
sequential incubation of the tissue with different amounts of
LPC and repetitive washing increases the sensitivity of the
fibers to lower LPC levels. This suggests that the ratio of
total LPC to tissue weight is important.

Assuming that the accumulation of lyso-PL in myocardial
ischemia is limited to sarcolemmal membrane, we performed
experiments to assess whether producing lyso-PL in the
sarcolemma by incubating cardiac tissue with exogenous
phospholipase A_2 mimics electrophysiological manifestation of
in situ ischemia, bearing in mind that such experimentally
produced endogenous lyso-PL may not reflect in situ conditions,
where concentrations of lyso-PL may be produced only in certain
membrane domains. These in vitro experiments nevertheless
clearly showed (Figures 3 to 5) that many fold concentration of
these amphiphiles did not alter action potential parameters.
Concentrations between 0.5 to 0.8 mM progressively altered
membrane potentials but control action potential could be
restored upon reflow with normal oxygenated buffer. Even at
this stage of complete recovery, lyso-PL concentrations
nevertheless remained abnormally high (0.3-0.42 mM). This may
reflect increased fluidity of the membrane as a consequence of
higher lyso-PL levels which were partially reacylated to diacyl
forms upon the restoration of the flow. Much higher
concentrations of endogenously produced lyso-PL (greater than
0.8 mM) drastically altered electrophysiological characteristics
and in such cases recovery upon prolonged reflow could not be
achieved indicating depletion of membrane lipids. This is in

agreement with the observations that in experiments where
complete recovery upon reflow was possible (Figure 5), washing
the cardiac tissue with normal oxygenated buffer containing
albumin deteriorated action potentials. However, the
concentrations reported above could be misleading since whole
tissue was analyzed for lyso-PL levels and the actual
concentrations in the first few layers of the cells would be
many fold higher. These results, nevertheless, strongly suggest
that the concentrations of lyso-PL reasonably expected to be
present in the sarcolemmal membranes of the ischemic myocardium
did not alter any electrophysiological characteristics. Earlier
studies employing ^{31}P NMR spectroscopy showed that when intact
erythrocytes or ghosts were treated with phospholipase A_2, the
residual phospholipids and lyso-PL remained organized in a
bilayer arrangement (41). Cholesterol, which is abundant in
membranes, can stabilize a bilayer orientation of LPC (42, 43).
Furthermore, in aqueous phases, lyso-PL and free fatty acids in
equimolar concentrations form a bilayer type of organization
(44). These studies and others (45) concluded that the
permeability barrier of the lipid core is not significantly
altered when more than half of the phospholipids are degraded to
lyso-PL in the outer membrane layer. However, lyso-PL can
modulate various enzymatic activities (36, 46, 47), although the
concentrations employed in these in vitro studies are rather
high. It is possible though difficult to document
experimentally that lyso-PL if concentrated in the
micro-environment of certain membrane bound enzymes could alter
membrane functions.

On the other hand, treatment of the cardiac tissue with
phospholipase C produced diglycerides rather than
lysophosphatides, completely abolishing action potentials
(Figure 6). Even though the depletion of membrane phospholipids
was minor (<1.0% of total phospholipid content) recovery could
not be achieved after prolonged washing with normal oxygenated
buffer. As stated earlier for phospholipase A_2 experiments,
this measured phospholipid depletion could in fact be many fold
higher at surface cell layers. The effects of phospholipases
could not be attributed to the presence of proteases in the
enzyme preparations since the levels of such activities in the
quantities of enzyme preparations used were negligible. Similar
preparations of phospholipase C were also employed by others
(48).

Thus the detrimental effects of phospholipase treatment
appear to be due primarily to loss of membrane lipids rather
than the formation of lyso-PL. Depletion of membrane
phospholipid had been shown to be associated with a marked
decrease in the activities of several membrane marker enzymes,

with an increase in tissue Ca^{2+} content in vivo, with the
development of a 6- to 50-fold increase in Ca^{2+} permeability
in sarcoplasmic reticulum and microsomal membranes (13, 14) and
with marked increase in both Ca^{2+} and K^+ permeabilities in
myoblast cell cultures (48). With the exception of two
phospholipids (phosphatidylinositol and sphingomyelin),
phospholipase C type activities toward other major phospholipid
(phosphatidylcholine and phosphatidylethanolamine) has not been
well documented, even though a report for such activity has
appeared (49). However, depletion of major membrane
phospholipids could occur progressively by the actions of
phospholipase A_2, lysophospholipases and diesterases (see
Figure 7).

The results of this study suggest that the functional
abnormalities of the ischemic myocardium could in part be
attributed to the phospholipase-induced abnormalities in the
sarcolemma. Evidence for ischemia-induced activation of
phospholipase A_2 in the intact heart has been recently
described by us elsewhere (33). Within the limitations imposed

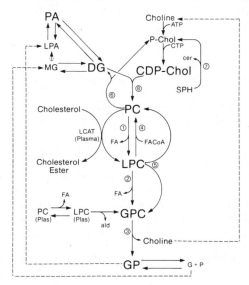

1. Phospholipase A_1 & A_2
2. Lysophospholipase
3. Glycerophosphorylcholine diesterase
4. Lysophospholipid acyltransferase
5. Lysophospholipase-transacylase
6. Phospholipase C
7. Sphingomyelinase
8. Choline phosphotransferase

Abbreviations:
PC, phosphatidylcholine; LPC, lysophosphatidylcholine; GPC, glycerophosphorylcholine; GP, glycerophosphate; SPH, sphingomyeline; FA, fatty
acid; FACoA, fatty acyl coenzyme A;
cer, ceremide; Plas, plasmalogen;
ald, fatty aldehyde; DG, diglyceride.

FIGURE 7

Schematic diagram of the metabolism of choline
phosphoglycerides.

by tissue bath experiments, it is not unreasonable to suggest
that lyso-PL alone are not responsible for the
electrophysiological abnormalities of the ischemic heart. On
the other hand, depletion of membrane phospholipids does appear
to pose potential deleterious effects on cell functions.

ACKNOWLEDGEMENTS

The authors are indebted to Mr. John Asta for obtaining the
hearts as well as his expertise in preparing samples. Also, Dr.
Thomas Chen is acknowledged for his laboratory work, and Rita
Loftsgard is appreciated for her careful typing of the
manuscript.

This work was supported by the Ontario Heart Foundation.

REFERENCES

1. Melchoir, D.L., & Steim, J.M. (1976): Annu. Rev. Biophys.
   Bioeng. $\underline{5}$: 205.
2. Boggs, J.M. (1980): Can. J. Biochem. $\underline{58}$: 755.
3. Thompson, T.E., & Henn, F.A. (1969): IN Membranes of
   Mitochondria and Chloroplasts (ed) E. Racker, Van
   Nostrand/Reinhold, New York, p. 1.
4. Papahadjopoulos, D. (1973): IN Forms and Function of
   Phospholipids (eds) G.B. Ansell, J.N. Hawthorne, & R.M.C.
   Dawson, Elsevier Scientific Publishing Co., New York, p.
   143.
5. Hawthorne, J.N. (1973): IN Forms and Function of
   Phospholipids (eds) G.B. Ansell, J.N. Hawthorne, & R.M.C.
   Dawson, Elsevier Scientific Publishing Co., New York, p.
   423.
6. Finean, J.B. (1973): IN Forms and Function of
   Phospholipids (eds) G. B. Ansell, J.N. Hawthorne, & R.M.C.
   Dawson, Elsevier Scientific Publishing Co., New York, p.
   171.
7. Michell, R.H. (1975): Biochim. Biophys. Acta $\underline{415}$: 81.
8. Hawthorne, J.N., & Pickard, M.R. (1979): J. Neurochem. $\underline{32}$:
   5.
9. Katz, A.M., & Reuter, H. (1979): Am. J. Cardiol. $\underline{44}$: 188.
10. Shaikh, N.A., & Kuksis, A. (1982): Can. J. Biochem. $\underline{60}$:
    444.
11. Shaikh, N.A., & Kuksis, A. (1983): Can. J. Biochem. Cell
    Biol. $\underline{61}$: 370.
12. Sobel, B.E., Corr, P.B., Robinson, A.K., Goldstein, R.A.,
    Witkowski, F.X., & Klein, M.S. (1978): J. Clin. Invest.
    $\underline{62}$: 546.

13. Chien, K.R., Abrams, J., Serroni, A., Martin, J.T., & Farber, J.L. (1978): J. Biol. Chem. 253: 4809.
14. Chien, K.R., Pfau, R.G., & Farber, J.L. (1979): Am. J. Pathol. 97: 505.
15. Shaikh, N.A., & Downar, E. (1981): Circ. Res. 49: 316.
16. Downar, E., Janse, M.J., & Durrer, D. (1977): Circulation 56: 217.
17. Opie, L.H. (1975): Am. J. Cardiol. 36: 938.
18. Katz, A.M., & Messineo, F.C. (1981): Circ. Res. 48: 1.
19. Liedtke, A.J. (1981): Prog. Cardiovasc. Dis. 23: 321.
20. Katz, A.M. (1982): J. Mol. Cell. Cardiol. 14: 627.
21. Weglicki, W.B., Waite, B.M., Sisson, P., & Shohet, S.B. (1971): Biochim. Biophys. Acta 231: 512.
22. Weglicki, W.B., Waite, B.M., & Stam, A.C., Jr. (1972): J. Mol. Cell. Cardiol. 4: 195.
23. Franson, R., Waite, M., & Weglicki, W. (1972): Biochemistry 11: 472.
24. Kennett, F.F., & Weglicki, W.B. (1978): Circ. Res. 43: 750.
25. Chien, K.R., Reeves, J.P., Buja, L.M., Bonte, F., Parkey, R.W., & Willerson, J.T. (1981): Circ. Res. 48: 711.
26. Snyder, D.W., Crafford, W.A., Jr., Glashow, J.L., Rankin, D., Sobel, B.E., & Corr, P.B. (1981): Am. J. Physiol. 241: H700.
27. Sobel, B.E., & Corr, P.B. (1979): IN Advances in Cardiology, Vol. 26 (ed) J.H.K. Vogel, Karger, Basel, Switzerland, p. 76.
28. Corr, P.B., Snyder, D.W., Cain, M.E., Crafford, W.A., Jr., Gross, R.W., & Sobel, B.E. (1981): Circ. Res. 49: 354.
29. Arnsdorf, M.F., & Sawicki, F.J. (1981): Circ. Res. 49: 16.
30. Clarkson, C.W., & Ten Eick, R.E. (1983): Circ. Res. 52: 543.
31. Man, R.Y.K., & Choy, P.C. (1982): J. Mol. Cell. Cardiol. 14: 173.
32. Shaikh, N.A., & Palmer, F.B. (1976): J. Neurochem. 26: 597.
33. Shaikh, N.A., & Downer, E. (1983): J. Mol. Cell. Cardiol. 15 (Suppl. 1): 171 (abstract).
34. Shaikh, N.A., & Downer, E. (1983): J. Mol. Cell. Cardiol. 15 (Suppl. 1): 170 (abstract).
35. Corr, P.B., Gross, R.W., & Sobel, B.E. (1982): J. Mol. Cell. Cardiol. 14: 619.
36. Karli, J.N., Karikas, G.A., Hatzipavlou, P.K., Levis, G.M., & Moulopoulos, S.N. (1979): Life Sci. 24: 1869.
37. Weltzein, H.U. (1979): Biochim. Biophys. Acta 559: 259.
38. Corr, P.B., Snyder, D.W., Lee, B.I., Gross, R.W., Keim, C.R., & Sobel, B.E. (1982): Am. J. Physiol. 243: H187.
39. Corr, P.B., Cain, M.E., Witkowski, F.X., Price, D.A., & Sobel, B.E. (1979): Circ. Res. 44: 822.

40. Gross, R.W., Corr, P.B., Lee, B.I., Saffitz, J.E., & Sobel,
    B.E. (1982): Circ. Res. 51: 27.
41. Van Meer, G., De Cruijff, B., Op den Kamp, J.A.F., & Van
    Deenan, L.L.N. (1980): Biochim. Biophys. Acta 596: 1.
42. Kitawaga, T., Inoue, K., & Nojima, S. (1976): J. Biochem.
    79: 1123.
43. de Gier, J., Noordam, P.C., van Echteld, C.A.J.,
    Mandersloot, J.G., Bijleveld, C., Verkleij, A., Cullis,
    P.R., & de Kruiff, B. (1980): IN Membrane Transport in
    Erythrocytes (eds) U.V. Lassen, H.H. Ussing, & J.D. Wieth,
    Alfred Benzon Symposium 14, Munksgaard, Copenhagen, p. 75.
44. Jain, M.K., van Echteld, C.J.A., Ramirez, F., de Gier, J.,
    De Haas, G.H., & van Deenen, L.L.M. (1980): Nature 284:
    486.
45. Wilbers, K.H., Haest, C.W.M., Von Bentheim, M., & Denticke,
    B. (1979): Biochim. Biophys. Acta 554: 388.
46. Mookerjea, S., & Yung, J.W.M. (1974): Can. J. Biochem. 52:
    1053.
47. Shier, W.T., & Trotter, J.T. III (1976): FEBS Lett. 62:
    165.
48. Langer, G.A., Frank, J.S., & Philipson, K.D. (1981): Circ.
    Res. 49: 1289.
49. Hostetler, K.Y., & Hall, L.B. (1980): Biochem. Biophys.
    Res. Commun. 96: 388.

A SURFACE CHARGE HYPOTHESIS FOR THE ACTIONS OF PALMITYLCARNITINE

ON THE KINETICS OF EXCITATORY IONIC CURRENTS IN HEART

A. J. Pappano and D. Inoue

Department of Pharmacology
University of Connecticut Health Center
Farmington, CT   06032   USA

The relationship between increased levels of free fatty acids (FFA) and the increased incidence of severe arrhythmias reported by Kurien and Oliver (1) in the pathogenesis of ischemic heart disease has prompted a critical examination of the mechanisms by which changes in lipid metabolism disturb the regulation of ion transport in cardiac membranes. This concept has been modified to include the possibility that long chain fatty acid derivatives (acyl carnitine; 2) and lysophosphatidyl-choline, which accumulate in the ischemic heart, can alter ion transport in cardiac membranes (reviewed in 3, 4). These reviews have also addressed the molecular mechanisms by which these lipid metabolites alter membrane structure and thereby change the function of transport proteins in the sarcoplasmic reticulum and plasma membrane.

Of particular interest is the arrhythmogenic action of palmitylcarnitine and lysophosphatidylcholine. These substances have been reported to depolarize the membrane and to reduce the amplitude, rate of rise ($\dot{V}_{max}$) and duration of action potentials in Purkinje fibers and ventricular muscle (5-7). Although there is considerable information on the derangements produced by these substances in cellular transmembrane potentials, little is known about the mechanism for the changes in biophysical properties of the plasma membrane.

Accordingly, we began a study of the mechanism for the action of palmitylcarnitine in avian ventricular muscle (8).

81

Acute mobilization of lipids by glucagon increased plasma FFA
and produced cardiotoxic effects in geese that were not
prevented by pretreatment with nicotinic acid or propranolol
(9). The glucagon-induced increase of plasma FFA was also
associated with the development of fatty deposits in the liver
and hemorrhagic lesions in the heart (10). Therefore, the avian
heart seemed to be a suitable model for ascertaining the
mechanisms of action of lipid metabolites on ion transport in
cardiac plasma membranes.

METHODS

Hatched chicks (1 to 10 days) were decapitated and the
hearts were quickly removed. The right ventricle free wall was
isolated and pinned to the bottom of a tissue chamber (3 ml
volume) with the endocardial surface uppermost. Tissues were
superfused with Tyrode's solution (mM composition: K^+, 5.4;
Na^+, 149; Ca^{2+}, 1.8; Mg^{2+}, 1.0; Cl^-, 148; HCO_{3-}, 11.9;
H_2PO_{4-}, 0.4; and glucose, 5.5) at a rate of 5 ml/min. When
equilibrated with a mixture of 95% O_2 - 5% CO_2, the Tyrode's
solution had a pH of 7.3 to 7.4; bath temperature was constant
at 37 $\pm$ 0.5° C. Preparations were equilibrated in this
solution for at least 60 minutes. In those experiments in which
membrane polarization resistance (R_{pol}) was to be measured,
thin strips of ventricle (0.3 to 0.5 mm wide, 4 to 5 mm long)
were dissected with a razor blade and placed in a single sucrose
gap chamber with 0.5 mm of tissue in the potential recording
pool. After the equilibration period, the central (2 mm) pool
was superfused with isotonic sucrose plus 0.01 mM $CaCl_2$ while
the lateral pools were superfused with Tyrode's solution.
Constant current pulses were applied across the tissue by
Ag-AgCl electrodes placed in the lateral pools. A detailed
description of this method and its limitations is given in Inoue
et al. (11).

Membrane potentials were recorded with standard
microelectrode techniques. The membrane potential was led
through a differentiator (Tektronix, Type O) with a response
linear from 0 to 500 V/sec in order to obtain the maximum rate
of rise ($\dot{V}_{max}$) of phase 0 and the plateau phase of the action
potential.

Rectangular constant voltage stimuli were applied to the
preparation through a glass insulated silver electrode (tip
diameter of 250 μm). Stimulus intensity was 1.5 to 2x diastolic
threshold at a frequency of 1 Hz for eliciting action potentials
dependent on the fast Na^+ conductance (g_{Na}) and at 0.1 Hz
for eliciting action potentials dependent on the slow Ca^{2+}
conductance (g_{Ca}).

The methods used to determine the steady-state inactivation of the Na^+-dependent (phase 0) and Ca^{2+}-dependent (plateau phase) components of the action potential have been described along with the limitations of this technique (8). Measurements of the time constant for recovery from inactivation of $\dot{V}_{max}$ were done essentially as described in a previous report from this laboratory (12). The zero point for the interval between the control action potential and the test action potential was the time at which 90% repolarization of the control action potential had occurred because there was too much uncertainty in determining the time of complete repolarization. Cardiac muscle contractions were recorded from ventricular muscle strips in the manner described previously by our laboratory (13).

Measurements are given as the mean $\pm$ SEM. Student's t-test was used to evaluate the statistical significance of sample means.

RESULTS

L-Palmitylcarnitine Modifies the Kinetics of the Fast Na^+ Channel

Membrane Actions at Resting Potential of -80 mV. L-palmitylcarnitine increased action potential duration (Figure 1A) and reduced the maximum rate of rise ($\dot{V}_{max}$; Figure 1B) of the ventricular action potential (E_m) or overshoot potential (E_{ov}). Because $\dot{V}_{max}$ of such action potentials is an index of g_{Na}, it may be concluded that palmitylcarnitine inhibited g_{Na} slightly (13% reduction of $\dot{V}_{max}$ in Figure 1B). This effect was registered at stimulus conditions that kept latency of impulse initiation constant so as to preclude the possibility that an increased latency would permit a greater proportion of inactivation (h) of g_{Na} to occur (14).

We could not detect a significant effect of stimulus frequency on the reduction of $\dot{V}_{max}$ by palmitylcarnitine. An example of one such experiment is shown in Figure 2. At a stimulus frequency of 0.1 Hz, $\dot{V}_{max}$ was 282 V/sec in the absence and 203 V/sec in the presence of palmitylcarnitine (30 μM). Palmitylcarnitine reduced $\dot{V}_{max}$ by 24% in this cell, a diminution that is greater than average. Nevertheless, increasing stimulus frequency to 1 Hz for a 60 second period did not change the amount of blockade of $\dot{V}_{max}$ caused by palmitylcarnitine. Because $\dot{V}_{max}$ is a non-linear function of g_{Na} ($\dot{V}_{max} \sim g_{Na}^{-1/2}$; 15), it is probable that we would not detect a small change of g_{Na} by this method. The variation in $\dot{V}_{max}$ measurements was $\pm$ 3% so that g_{Na} would have to be

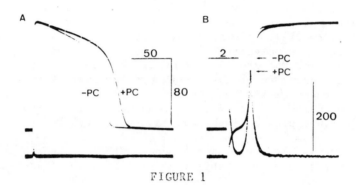

FIGURE 1

Effect of 300 μm L-palmitylcarnitine (+PC) on ventricular action
potential in 5.4 mM K$^+$-Tyrode's solution recorded at slow (A)
and fast (B) sweep speeds. Horizontal time calibrations (50
msec in A; 2 msec in B) mark zero potential; vertical voltage
calibration in A (80 mV) applies to panels A and B. Vertical
calibration for $\dot{V}_{max}$ (200 V/sec) in B applies to lowest trace
in B. (Reproduced with permission of the American Heart
Association.)

reduced by more than 2% in order to detect a frequency-
dependent action of palmitylcarnitine on fast Na$^+$ channels.
It may be concluded that stimulus frequency had no important
effect on g_{Na} in the absence or presence of palmitylcarnitine.

The depression of $\dot{V}_{max}$ by palmitylcarnitine at the normal
resting E_m (-80 mV) could be mimicked by raising the external
Ca^{2+} concentration ([Ca^{2+}]$_o$) from the usual concentration
of 1.8 mM to 5.4 mM. A comparison of the effects of elevated
[Ca^{2+}]$_o$ and of palmitylcarnitine on membrane potentials at
-80 mV is shown in Table 1. Neither palmitylcarnitine nor
elevated [Ca^{2+}]$_o$ changes the resting E_m or E_{ov} yet both
substances reduced $\dot{V}_{max}$. We do not know how $\dot{V}_{max}$ was
reduced consistently and significantly at 30 M but not at
300 μM palmitylcarnitine ($\dot{V}_{max}$ decreased in 2 out of 4 cells

Table 1. Membrane Potentials in 5.4 mM [K$^+$]$_o$

	Control	Changes Produced by Palmitylcarnitine at:		Elevated [Ca^{2+}]$_o$ at:
		30 μM (6)	300 μM (4)	5.4 mM (4)
Resting E$_m$ (mV)	-82 ± 1	0 ± 0	1 ± 1	0 ± 0
E$_{ov}$ (mV)	43 ± 1	0 ± 1	-1 ± 1	0 ± 0
V$_{max}$ (V/sec)	270 ± 13	-13 ± 5*	-8 ± 11	-54 ± 26*
APD0mV (msec)	87 ± 9	16 ± 6*	3 ± 9	-28 ± 5*
APD90% (msec)	125 ± 10	15 ± 6*	1 ± 11	-13 ± 11
V$_h$ (mV)	-60 ± 1	3 ± 1*	6 ± 3*	3 ± 1*

Measurements are given as mean ± SEM; variables are defined in the text. Number of experiments is given in parentheses.

*p < 0.05 with respect to control values.

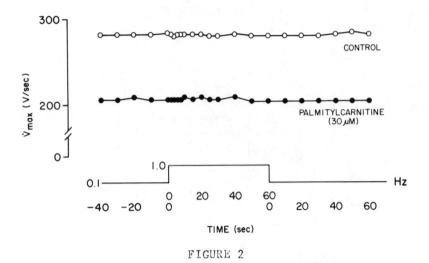

FIGURE 2

The reduction of $\dot{V}_{max}$ by palmitylcarnitine (30 μM) is
independent of frequency. In the absence of palmitylcarnitine
(0), $\dot{V}_{max}$ was 282 V/sec and did not change when stimulus
frequency was increased from 0.1 to 1 Hz for 60 seconds. In the
presence of palmitylcarnitine (●), $\dot{V}_{max}$ decreased to 208 V/sec
(a reduction of 24%) and remained at this level when stimulus
frequency was increased from 0.1 to 1 Hz for 60 seconds. In
this cell, palmitylcarnitine did not change the resting E_m
(-85 mV), reduced E_{ov} from 44 to 40 mV and increased APD_{0mV}
from 105 to 112 msec and $APD_{90\%}$ from 128 to 141 msec.

in the presence of 300 μM palmitylcarnitine). Moreover, the
increase of action potential duration at 0 mV (APD_{0mV}) and at
90% repolarization ($APD_{90\%}$) was statistically significant only
at 30 μM palmitylcarnitine. The only qualitative difference
between palmitylcarnitine and elevated $[Ca^{2+}]_o$ was
registered in the APD which was increased by the former and
decreased by the latter.

Steady-State Inactivation (h_∞) of $\dot{V}_{max}$ of Na^+-Dependent
Action Potentials. Elevated $[Ca^{2+}]_o$ shifts the inactivation
curve for i_{Na} to less negative potentials in cardiac fibers
(reviewed in 16). This effect of Ca^{2+} in cardiac fibers is
attributed to a reduction in surface negative charge first

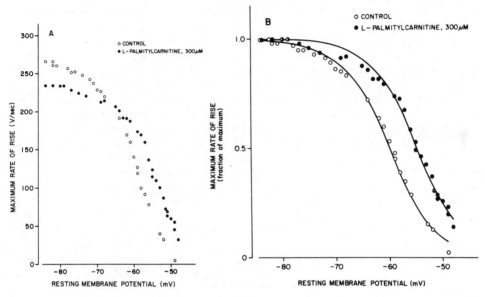

FIGURE 3

Steady-state inactivation of $\dot{V}_{max}$ in the absence (O) and presence of 300 μM palmitylcarnitine (●); same cell as in Figure 1. Absolute values of $\dot{V}_{max}$ (V/sec) vs. resting E_m (mV) are shown in A; normalized values are shown in B with $\dot{V}_{max}$ given as fraction of maximum. The lines in B are drawn according to the equation $h_\infty = 1/[1 + \exp(Z \Delta VF/RT)$ where h_∞ = steady-state inactivation of $\dot{V}_{max}$, Z = slope factor; ΔV = difference between test voltage and the voltage (V_h) at $\dot{V}_{max}$ is 0.5 of maximum, and F, R and T have their usual physical meanings (18). (Reproduced with permission of the American Heart Association.)

proposed in squid axon (17). Because palmitylcarnitine and elevated $[Ca^{2+}]_o$ acted similarly on $\dot{V}_{max}$ at −80 mV, we examined the effects of these substances on the relationship between $h_\infty\dot{V}_{max}$ and membrane voltage.

The $[K^+]_o$ was increased from 5.4 to 25 mM in order to depolarize the membrane and thereby evaluate the effect of membrane voltage on $\dot{V}_{max}$. This procedure was repeated in the same cell in the presence of palmitylcarnitine and the results of a typical experiment are shown in Figure 3 (same cell as in Figure 1). Palmitylcarnitine reduced $\dot{V}_{max}$ by 13% at the resting E_m of −84 mV (Figure 3A). As elevated $[K^+]_o$ depolarized the membrane, $\dot{V}_{max}$ diminished and the steady-state values of $\dot{V}_{max}$ in palmitylcarnitine crossed over the control values at −65 mV so that at more positive voltages, $\dot{V}_{max}$ was greater in the presence of palmitylcarnitine. When fraction values of $\dot{V}_{max}$ were plotted as a function of membrane voltage (Figure 3B), the half maximum value of $\dot{V}_{max}$ (V_h) shifted by 5 mV from −60 to 55 mV to more positive potentials in the presence of palmitylcarnitine without a change of slope. The positive shift of V_h by palmitylcarnitine was observed consistently and was concentration dependent (Table 1).

Elevation of $[Ca^{2+}]_o$ from 1.8 to 5.4 mM, as expected, shifted the steady-state inactivation of V_{max} to more positive potentials; the average shift was 3 ± 1 mV in 4 cells (Table 1). Because elevated $[Ca^{2+}]_o$ reduced $\dot{V}_{max}$ at −80 mV, the $h_\infty\dot{V}_{max}$ vs. voltage curve in 5.4 mM $[Ca^{2+}]_o$ crossed over the control curve (1.8 mM) at around −69 mV.

Time Constant for Recovery from Inactivation of $\dot{V}_{max}$ (τ_{Rec}). Gettes and Reuter (19) reported that elevated $[Ca^{2+}]_o$ not only shifted the $h_\infty\dot{V}_{max}$ vs. voltage relation to more positive potentials but also accelerated the recovery of $\dot{V}_{max}$ from inactivation (that is, τ_{Rec} decreased). Measurements in normal Tyrode's solution indicated that τ_{Rec} averaged 26 ± 5 msec (Table 2). Elevation of $[Ca^{2+}]_o$ to 5.4 mM did not change τ_{Rec} (28 ± 9 msec) significantly from that observed in 1.8 mM $[Ca^{2+}]_o$, a result that confirms that reported by Gettes and Reuter (19). For this reason and because it is unlikely that τ_{Rec} can be diminished to values significantly less than this at potentials more negative than −80 mV (reviewed in 16), the cells were depolarized in order to slow recovery from inactivation. In the presence of 10.8 mM $[K^+]_o$ at normal $[Ca^{2+}]_o$, the membrane depolarized and $\dot{V}_{max}$ was significantly reduced (Table 2). Moreover, τ_{Rec} increased significantly to 69 ± 8 msec, a result consistent with those obtained by Gettes and Reuter (19) and by this laboratory (12).

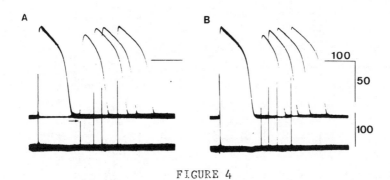

FIGURE 4

Palmitylcarnitine (300 μM) reduced τ_{Rec} in ventricular cell depolarized to -68 mV in 10.8 mM K^+-Tyrode's. Calibrations for time, voltage and $\dot{V}_{max}$ are given as in Figure 1. Panel A shows recovery of $\dot{V}_{max}$ (first interpolated $\dot{V}_{max}$ signal indicated by arrow) from inactivation at constant voltage in control. The first test action potential had $\dot{V}_{max}$ of 69 V/sec at an interval of 33 msec. Panel B shows results obtained in palmitylcarnitine. At this voltage, palmitylcarnitine had no significant effect on E_{ov} (42 mV), $\dot{V}_{max}$ increased slightly (202 to 213 V/sec), and APD_{OmV} (82 msec) and $APD_{90\%}$ (100 msec) did not change. $\dot{V}_{max}$ of the first test action potential was 119 V/sec at an interval of 24 msec. The τ_{Rec} was significantly reduced by palmitylcarnitine from 53 to 22 msec (see Figure 5).

Experimental determination of τ_{Rec} is shown in Figure 4 in the absence (A) and presence (B) of palmitylcarnitine. Peak values of $\dot{V}_{max}$ for test pulses regained the control value with two time constants. This is shown graphically in Figure 5 where 85% of the recovery occurred with τ_{Rec} of 50 msec in the absence of palmitylcarnitine. The slower phase of recovery accounted for 15% of the total and had a τ_{Rec} of 140 msec. [Recovery from inactivation could be described by two exponentials in 6 out of the 12 cells in the control group with an average time constant of 112 ± 10 msec for the slower phase. That recovery from inactivation of cardiac Na^+ channels may

Table 2. τ_{Rec} of V_{max} of Na^+ Channels

N	$[K^+]_o$	$[Ca^{2+}]_o$	E_m(mV)	E_{ov}(mV)	V_{max}(V/sec)	APD (msec) at: 0mV	90%	τ_{Rec}(msec)
8	5.4	1.8	-79±1	41±1	230±22	101± 8	130± 8	26±5
12	10.8	1.8	-65±1*	39±1	184±11*	94± 7	118± 7	69±8*
4	10.8	1.8 + Palmityl-carnitine (300µM)	-66±1	39±2	153±25	109±14	135±15	35±8*
8	10.8	5.4	-65±1	46±1*	188±17	86±10	103± 7	35±7*

N is the number of cells studied at concentrations of $[K^+]_o$ and $[Ca^{2+}]_o$ given as mM.

*P ≤ 0.05 when compared to control value given in line immediately above for 10.8 mM $[K^+]_o$, 1.8 mM $[Ca^{2+}]_o$ in the absence and presence of palmitylcarnitine. Data obtained in 10.8 mM $[K^+]_o$, 5.4 mM $[Ca^{2+}]_o$ are compared to those in 10.8 mM $[K^+]_o$, 1.8 mM $[Ca^{2+}]_o$.

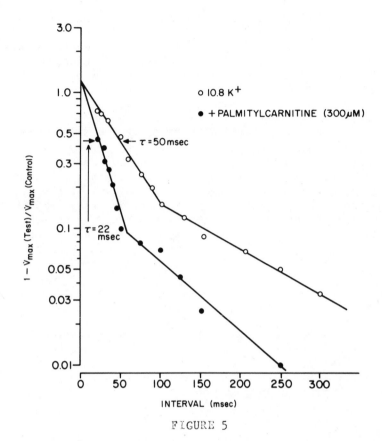

FIGURE 5

Graphical representation of results from Figure 4 illustrating reduced τ_{Rec} by palmitylcarnitine. Ordinate: $1 - (\dot{V}max_{test}/\dot{V}max_{control})$ on logarithmic scale; abscissa: time in msec after attainment of 90% repolarization (= 0 msec) on linear scale. There are two exponential phases for $\dot{V}_{max}$ recovery. The τ_{Rec} of the faster phase in the absence (0) and presence (●) of palmitylcarnitine is shown with τ_{Rec} of 50 and 22 msec, respectively.

occur according to two exponential processes has been reported by others (20-23).] In the presence of palmitylcarnitine there was no significant change of resting E_m or of APD, while $\dot{V}_{max}$ increased from 202 to 213 V/sec (Figure 4B). Recovery from inactivation in the presence of palmitylcarnitine could also be described by two exponentials with the faster phase

accounting for 90% of the total and the slower phase accounting
for 10%. The τ_{Rec} of the faster phase was 22 msec in
palmitylcarnitine, a significant reduction in recovery from
inactivation. (In the presence of palmitylcarnitine, 2 out of 4
cells displayed two exponential phases of recovery; the slower
phase had τ_{Rec} of 84 $\pm$ 14 msec.)

The effects of palmitylcarnitine on membrane potentials in
10.8 mM $[K^+]_o$ are summarized in Table 2. The amphiphile did
not change the resting E_m, E_{ov}, $\dot{V}_{max}$ or APD
significantly. Although $\dot{V}_{max}$ tended to deline in
palmitylcarnitine, the change was not significant. This may be
explained by the observation that the cross-over of the h $\dot{V}_{max}$
vs. membrane voltage relationship occurred at around −65 mV (see
Figure 3) and therefore $\dot{V}_{max}$ might be expected to increase or
decrease relative to control. The τ_{Rec} of the faster phase
was reduced by about 50% in the presence of palmitylcarnitine to
35 $\pm$ 8 msec.

A significant reduction of τ_{Rec} was also observed when
$[Ca^{2+}]_o$ was increased to 5.4 mM in the presence of 10.8 mM
$[K^+]_o$ (Table 2). As with palmitylcarnitine, elevated
$[Ca^{2+}]_o$ reduced τ_{Rec} by about 50% to 35 $\pm$ 8 msec without
changing the resting E_m, $\dot{V}_{max}$ or APD significantly. Unlike
palmitylcarnitine, E_{ov} of the action potential increased
significantly to 46 $\pm$ 1 mV in 5.4 mM $[Ca^{2+}]_o$ (Table 2).
This may be explained by a larger i_{si} produced by elevated
$[Ca^{2+}]_o$ which can carry a large inward current through i_{si}
channels.

L-Palmitylcarnitine Modifies the Kinetics of the Slow Ca^{2+} Channel

Membrane Actions at Resting Potential of −40 mV. Activation
of i_{si} channels that generate Ca^{2+}-dependent action
potentials was achieved by depolarizing the preparations with 25
mM K^+-Tyrode's solution. The fast Na^+ channels are
completely inactivated at potentials more positive than −45 mV
(12) so that the Ca^{2+}-dependent action potential can be
studied directly. Under these conditions, the cells displayed
Ca^{2+}-dependent action potentials in the absence of
catecholamines and E_{ov} of these action potentials changed by
30 mV/10-fold changes of $[Ca^{2+}]_o$ (24). The $[Ca^{2+}]_o$ was
reduced to 0.9 mM to permit detection of the effects of
palmitylcarnitine and elevated $[Ca^{2+}]_o$ (8).

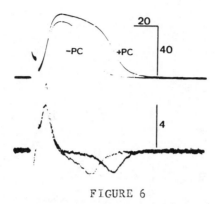

FIGURE 6

Palmitylcarnitine (30 µM) increases the magnitude of the
Ca^{2+}-dependent action potential in 25 mM K^+-Tyrode's
solution with 0.9 mM Ca^{2+}. Calibration format is the same as
in Figure 1. In the presence of palmitylcarnitine (+PC), the
amplitude, duration and $\dot{V}_{max}$ of the Ca^{2+}- dependent action
potential increased. (Reproduced with permission of the
American Heart Association.)

Palmitylcarnitine increased the amplitude, $\dot{V}_{max}$ and
duration of Ca^{2+}-dependent action potentials; a representative
experiment is shown in Figure 6. The effect of
palmitylcarnitine on the Ca^{2+}-dependent action potential was
similar to that observed with the Na^+-dependent action
potential insofar as the resting E_m was not changed and a
steady-state effect was reached in about 15 minutes. A summary
of the concentration-dependent effects of palmitylcarnitine on
the Ca^{2+}- dependent action potential is given in Table 3. It
is evident in the results shown in Table 3 that elevation of
$[Ca^{2+}]_o$ to 5.4 mM mimicked the stimulatory effects of
palmitylcarnitine on the amplitude, $\dot{V}_{max}$ and duration of the
Ca^{2+}-dependent action potential.

Table 3. L-Palmitylcarnitine and Calcium on Ca^{2+}-Dependent Action Potentials

| | Control (17) | Changes Produced by | | |
| | | Palmitylcarnitine at | | Ca^{2+} at |
		$3 \times 10^{-5}M$ (6)	$3 \times 10^{-4}M$ (6)	5.4 mM (5)
Resting Em (mV)	-41 ± 0	0 ± 0	1 ± 1	0 ± 1
Eov (mV)	10 ± 1	5 ± 1*	9 ± 3*	24 ± 2*
V_{max} (V/sec)	4.5 ± 0.6	2.4 ± 0.9*	4.9 ± 2.1*	4.3 ± 0.6*
APD-0mV (msec)	37 ± 5	8 ± 2*	28 ± 5*	25 ± 7*
V_h (mV)	-32 ± 0	3 ± 1*	3 ± 1*	6 ± 2*

Measurements are given as mean ± SEM with the number of cells shown in parentheses. Abbreviations are explained in text.

*p < 0.05 with respect to control values.

Adapted from Inoue and Pappano (1983).

Steady State Inactivation (f_∞) of $\dot{V}_{max}$ of Ca^{2+}-Dependent Action Potentials. The increased magnitude of the Ca^{2+}-dependent action potential caused by palmitylcarnitine could arise from either a change in the kinetics (d, activation variable; f, inactivation variable) or in the driving force (resting E_m-reversal potential) on i_{si}. A change of driving force seemed unlikely because the resting potential did not change. However, a change of i_{si} kinetics by palmitylcarnitine was supported by the results shown in Figure 7 (same cell as in Figure 6). The cell was depolarized by raising $[K^+]_o$ continuously from 25 mM to 60 mM and the potential-dependent reduction of $\dot{V}_{max}$ had a sigmoid shape in the absence and presence of palmitylcarnitine (Figure 7A). In the presence of palmitylcarnitine, however, $\dot{V}_{max}$ of the Ca^{2+}-dependent action potential increased at the resting E_m (-42 mV) and its inactivation was shifted to more positive potentials (Figure 7A). The positive shift by palmitylcarnitine is also evident in the normalization of the f_∞-V relationship (Figure 7B). The lines in Figure 7B were drawn according to the equation given in the figure legend and had the same slope factor (k = 2). The membrane voltage at which $\dot{V}_{max}$ was 0.5 maximum (V_h) shifted by 3 mV to more positive potentials in the presence of palmitylcarnitine and was observed consistently (Table 3). Again, the effect of palmitylcarnitine was mimicked by elevation of $[Ca^{2+}]_o$ to 5.4 mM which also shifted V_h by 6 mV to more positive potentials (Table 3). It is noteworthy that isoproterenol, which also increases the amplitude, $\dot{V}_{max}$ and duration of Ca^{2+}-dependent action potentials, did not change V_h (8), a result similar to that reviewed by Reuter (25) in voltage clamp experiments. Therefore, the positive shift of V_h by palmitylcarnitine and elevated $[Ca^{2+}]_o$ is probably not an artifact of the increased $\dot{V}_{max}$ that simply permits its detection at more positive potentials.

Force of Contraction. Because palmitylcarnitine increased the amplitude, $\dot{V}_{max}$ and duration of Ca^{2+}-dependent action potentials, it would be expected that the amphiphile increase the force of contraction. This supposition was borne out as shown in Figure 8. Palmitylcarnitine increased the force of contraction in a concentration-dependent manner. Maximal effects of palmitylcarnitine occurred in 15 minutes in right ventricular muscle strips superfused with Tyrode's solution (5.4 mM K^+) and excited at a frequency of 1 Hz. At 15 minutes in palmitylcarnitine, the force of contraction had increased to 151 $\pm$ 20% (3 x 10^{-5} M) and to 242 $\pm$ 45% (3 x 10^{-4} M). Propranolol (3 x 10^{-7} M) was present in all but one of the experiments (3 x 10^{-4} M palmitylcarnitine increased force to 228% of control values in this experiment) so that the positive inotropic effect of palmitylcarnitine was probably independent

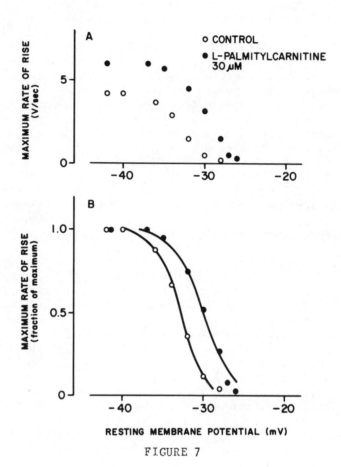

FIGURE 7

Palmitylcarnitine shifts the $f_\infty \dot{V}_{max}$-V relationship to more positive potentials. Results are taken from the same cell shown in Figure 6. Panel A: ordinate in V/sec; abscissa in mV. Palmitylcarnitine (●) increased $\dot{V}_{max}$ to 6 V/sec from a control (O) value of 4 V/sec. Panel B: "normalized" plot of results in panel A with $\dot{V}_{max}$ given as fraction of maximum. The lines are drawn according to the equation $f_\infty = 1/[1 + \exp(V_m - V_h/k)]$ where f_∞ = steady-state inactivation of $\dot{V}_{max}$, V_m = test voltage, V_h = voltage at which $\dot{V}_{max}$ is 0.5 of maximum and k = slope factor. V_h shifted from -33 mV (control) to -30 mV in the presence of palmitylcarnitine. (Reproduced with permission of the American Heart Association.)

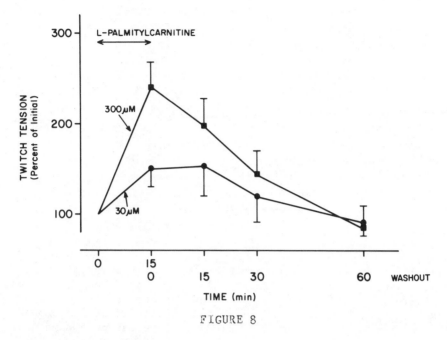

FIGURE 8

Palmitylcarnitine increased the force of contraction in a
concentration-dependent manner. Ordinate: twitch tension as
percent of initial (=100%); abscissa: time in minutes. Tissues
stimulated at 1 Hz in normal Tyrode's solution were exposed to
either 30 μM or 300 μM L-palmitylcarnitine for 15 minutes.
Washout of palmitylcarnitine continued for 60 minutes and is
marked by the lower set of numbers (0.15, 30 and 60 minutes).

of β-adrenergic receptor activation. Removal of palmitylcarnitine was associated with a slow reversal of the positive
inotropic effect; initial twitch tension was attained between 30
and 60 minutes of washout (Figure 8). It is noteworthy that the
time course for onset and dissipation of palmitylcarnitine
action on the force of contraction was the same for its
electrophysiological effects.

L-Palmitylcarnitine and Background K+ Conductance (g_{K1})

The ability of palmitylcarnitine to increase plateau
amplitude and duration has been attributed to an effect on i_{si}
kinetics. However, the amphiphile may act indirectly on the

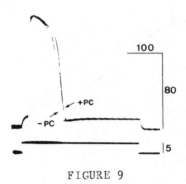

FIGURE 9

Lack of effect of palmitylcarnitine on electrotonic potentials.
A 325 msec depolarizing current pulse of 5 μA was applied across
a single sucrose gap on evoked action potentials in the absence
(-PC) and presence (+PC) of 30 μM palmitylcarnitine. Although
APD was increased L-palmitylcarnitine, there was no change in
the amplitude of the electrotonic potential at 325 msec.
Calibrations for time and voltage and zero potential are given
as in Figure 1.

Ca^{2+}-dependent action potential by reducing an outward
current. Such a mechanism has been considered to explain the
effects of lysophosphatidylcholine on Purkinje fibers (5).

To test the hypothesis that palmitylcholine affected
voltage-dependent g_{K1}, experiments were done with the single
sucrose gap technique. The results of a typical experiment are
shown in Figure 9. In the absence of palmitylcarnitine (Figure
9, -PC), a 5 μA depolarizing current pulse evoked an action
potential with an E_{ov} of 37 mV and APD_o and APD_{90} of 59
and 81 msec, respectively. At 15 minutes in palmitylcarnitine
(Figure 9, +PC), the APD_o and APD_{90} had each increased by 10

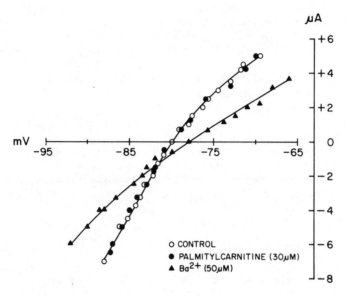

FIGURE 10

Current-voltage (I-V) relationship for cell shown in Figure 9 in
the absence (0) and presence (●) of L-palmitylcarnitine.
Ordinate: applied current in μA (depolarizing current is
positive); abscissa: membrane potential in mV. Neither the
resting E_m (-80 mV) nor the I-V relationship was changed by
palmitylcarnitine. Addition of 50 μM Ba^{2+} depolarized the
membrane to -78 mV and increased R_{pol} from a control value of
1.2 KΩ to 3.0 KΩ.

msec while E_{ov} and resting E_m were unchanged. The
steady-state electronic potential evoked a 5 μA depolarizing
current was the same (11 mV) in the absence and presence of

palmitylcarnitine. The lack of effect of palmitylcarnitine on
resting membrane conductance is shown more clearly in Figure 10
which illustrates the current-voltage (I-V) relationship for the
same cell in Figure 9. The control I-V relationship displayed
inward-going rectification; polarization resistance (R_{pol}) was
estimated from the slope of the membrane voltage changes
produced by hyperpolarizing currents. Neither inward-going
rectification nor R_{pol} (1.2 KΩ) was changed by
palmitylcarnitine (Figure 10). Addition of 50 μM Ba^{2+}, which
reduced g_{K1}, increased R_{pol} to 3.0 KΩ and depolarized the
membrane from -30 to -78 mV. The Ba^{2+}-induced depolarization
is attributable to the reduction of g_{K1}.

These results indicate that palmitylcarnitine does not
change plateau amplitude and duration by reducing g_{K1} which
is voltage-dependent. However, these experiments do not exclude
the possibility that the amphiphile increases the plateau
amplitude and duration by reducing a time-dependent outward
current (i_x).

DISCUSSION

Our results indicate that L-palmitylcarnitine and elevated
$[Ca^{2+}]_o$:

1) reduced $\dot{V}_{max}$ of the Na^+-dependent phase of the
   ventricular action potential at the resting potential of -30
   mV,

2) shifted the $h_\infty \dot{V}_{max}$-V relationship to more positive
   potentials,

3) reduced τ_{Rec} from inactivation of fast Na^+ channels,

4) increased the amplitude, $\dot{V}_{max}$ and duration of the
   Ca^{2+}-dependent phase of the ventricular action potential,

5) shifted the $f_\infty \dot{V}_{max}$-V relationship to more positive
   potentials, and

6) increased the force of cardiac contractions.

Taken altogether, these results are consistent with the
hypothesis that palmitylcarnitine affects excitatory Na^+ and
Ca^{2+} channels in the heart by reducing surface negative charge
in a manner qualitatively similar to that of elevated
$[Ca^{2+}]_o$.

The manner by which $[Ca^{2+}]_o$ can modify surface negative
charge and thereby affect the kinetics of membrane ionic
currents has been addressed by Frankenhaeuser and Hodgkin (17)
and by Hille et al. (26). Discussion will focus on how
$[Ca^{2+}]_o$ affects the kinetics of fast Na^+ channels as an
example but the argument can also be applied to the i_{si}
channel. The Na^+ channel can exist in 3 states, resting (R)
or closed, open (O) and inactivated (I). Sodium ions flow down
their electrochemical gradient to produce an inward current only
when the Na^+ channel is in the open state. The relationships
among states of the Na^+ channel are as follows:

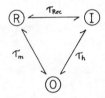

At very negative resting potentials, Na^+ channels are in the R
state. Rapid depolarization shifts a large fraction of the
channels to the O state by virtue of a voltage-dependent
increase of the opening rate constant, α_m. [The rate
constants α and β, which are functions of voltage, temperature
and Ca^{2+}, regulate the activation (m) and inactivation (h) of
the Na^+ channel with time constants defined as: $\tau_m = (\alpha_m
+ \beta_m)^{-1}$ and $\tau_h = (\alpha_h + \beta_h)^{-1}$.] Maintained
depolarization shifts the Na^+ channel to the I state because
of the eventual increase of β_h. The effects of elevated
$[Ca^{2+}]_o$ are qualitatively similar to those of membrane
hyperpolarization (17, 26) and include: 1) a reduction of α_m
thereby slowing the transition of Na^+ channels from R $\longrightarrow$ O
(τ_m is increased). The reduction of $\dot{V}_{max}$ by elevated
$[Ca^{2+}]_o$ at -80 mV is consistent with this view, 2) a
reduction of β_h thereby slowing the transition of Na^+
channels from O $\longrightarrow$ I (τ_h is increased). This mechanism is
consistent with the positive shift of the steady-state

inactivation curve for $\dot{V}_{max}$ of Na^+-dependent action
potentials. (This mechanism may also explain the positive shift
of the f_∞-V relationship for the Ca^{2+}-dependent action
potential.)

In their analysis, Frankenhaeuser and Hodgkin (17) found no
difference between τ_h and the removal of inactivation.
However, it has been reported that the time constant for
recovery from inactivation (τ_{Rec}) exceeds τ_h in cardiac
fibers at depolarized potentials (reviewed in 16). In their
experiments on mammalian cardiac fibers, Gettes and Reuter (19)
reported that the voltage-dependent increase of τ_{Rec} could be
overcome by elevated $[Ca^{2+}]_o$, a result attributed to the
effect of Ca^{2+} on surface negative charge. Our results were
essentially the same as those of Gettes and Reuter insofar as
elevated $[Ca^{2+}]_o$ reduced τ_{Rec} particularly in depolarized
fibers. Summarily, the similar effects of palmitylcarnitine and
elevated $[Ca^{2+}]_o$ on voltage- and time-dependent properties
of $\dot{V}_{max}$ of Na-dependent action potentials can be taken as
evidence that the amphiphile, like elevated $[Ca^{2+}]_o$, affects
the kinetics of Na^+ channels by reducing surface negative
charge. A similar model can be applied for the effects of
palmitylcarnitine and elevated $[Ca^{2+}]_o$ on the kinetics of
i_{si} channel operation. Although our results focus primarily
on the possible effects of the amphiphile and elevated
$[Ca^{2+}]_o$ on inactivation of Na^+ and Ca^{2+} channels, we
cannot exclude an action on activation. Our recording
techniques are not suited to such an analysis.

Two observations deserve comment because they are not
consistent with this hypothesis. First, palmitylcarnitine
tended to increase APD while elevated $[Ca^{2+}]_o$ tended to
decrease APD. This may be explained by the ability of elevated
$[Ca^{2+}]_o$, but not of palmitylcarnitine, to increase outward
time-dependent current and thereby accelerate repolarization
(27-29). Second, palmitylcarnitine had no effect on g_{K1} in
spite of its ability to affect i_{Na} and i_{si} through a
reduction of surface negative charge. Whereas elevated
$[Ca^{2+}]_o$ should screen surface negative charge at K^+ as
well as at Na^+ channels (17), it has been concluded that the
local electrical fields at K^+ channels are smaller than at
Na^+ channels in peripheral nerve (26). Perhaps a similar
condition is operative at resting K^+ channels in heart muscle;
this could explain the lack of effect of palmitylcarnitine on
g_{K1}. It should be noted that the inability of
palmitylcarnitine to change g_{K1} can be viewed as evidence in
favor of the amphiphile's action on g_{si} alone to increase the
amplitude, $\dot{V}_{max}$ and duration of Ca^{2+}-dependent action
potentials.

Several laboratories have reported concentration-dependent effects of palmitylcarnitine on the Ca^{2+}-ATPase activity and Ca^{2+}-binding capacity of cardiac and skeletal muscle sarcoplasmic reticulum (SR) membranes (30-32). The binding of Ca^{2+} to SR membranes was reported to increase in the presence of low concentrations of palmitylcarnitine (30). If palmitylcarnitine had a similar effect on Ca^{2+} binding to plasma membrane, one would have a plausible mechanism for the ability of palmitylcarnitine to reduce surface negative charge. However, we cannot exclude the possibility that incorporation of palmitylcarnitine into the lipid regions around Na^+ and Ca^{2+} channels acts directly to reduce surface negative charge by virtue of the cationic head of the molecule. In either case, the incorporation of palmitylcarnitine into the lipid bilayer of the plasma membrane would be a necessary step to account for the amphiphile's actions on ionic currents. The interaction of palmitylcarnitine and lysophosphatidylcholine with cardiac plasma membranes has been attributed to incorporation of the amphiphiles in the lipid bilayer (reviewed in 3, 4) and has been tested in experiments with cardiac membranes (33).

It is instructive to compare our results in the avian heart with those obtained in the mammalian heart regarding the biochemical and electrophysiological actions of palmitylcarnitine on ion transport. Palmitylcarnitine inhibited Na^+,K^+-ATPase of mammalian heart, an action attributed to delipidation of phospholipids essential for enzyme function, and this has been offered as a mechanism for inhibition of ion transport (30). We did not detect membrane depolarization in avian hearts and therefore cannot implicate inhibition of active Na^+ and K^+ transport by palmitylcarnitine in the avian ventricle. In this connection, accumulation of palmitylcarnitine in ischemic mammalian heart apparently was insufficient to inhibit the Na^+,K^+-ATPase because tissue K^+ content did not change (2, 34). Rather, it has been speculated that the accumulated palmitylcarnitine disturbed myocardial Ca^{2+} metabolism (34).

Our results in avian heart muscle appear to be dissimilar with those obtained in mammalian heart. In ventricular muscle and Purkinje fibers from mammals, palmitylcarnitine depolarized the membranes and blocked fast Na^+ channels by voltage-dependent inactivation (7). Whatever the mechanism for depolarization, it may be concluded that avian ventricular muscle is less sensitive to this effect of palmitylcarnitine. However, this result should not obscure the possibility that the amphiphile has similar actions in avian and mammalian hearts. For example, the reduction of $\dot{V}_{max}$ of the Na^+-dependent component of the action potential is greater than might be

expected on the basis of depolarization alone (7). This view is
supported by the observation that low concentrations of lysophosphatidylcholine (10 to 20 μM), which acts like
palmitylcarnitine, reduced V_{max} without changing the resting
potential of Purkinje fibers (5). Moreover, depolarized
Purkinje fibers and ventricular muscle could generate
Ca^{2+}-dependent action potentials in the presence of palmitylcarnitine (35). Although the effect of amphiphiles on the
properties of Ca^{2+}-dependent action potentials was not
reported (35), it is conceivable that the Ca^{2+}-dependent
action potentials persisted in mammalian cardiac fibers for the
reasons offered to explain the action of palmitylcarnitine on
these action potentials in avian heart (8).

The concept that abnormal concentrations of acyl carnitine
injures the ischemic heart by altering ion transport and
contractility has attracted much attention (reviewed in 3, 4,
36). Insofar as our results are consistent with a surface
charge hypothesis for the electrophysiological actions of
palmitylcarnitine, it may be concluded that the amphiphile
exerts a membrane stabilizing effect like that of Ca^{2+}.
Palmitylcarnitine differs from local anesthetics (membrane
stabilizers) insofar as the latter block $\dot{V}_{max}$ in a
frequency-dependent manner, shift the $h_{\infty}\dot{V}_{max}$-V relationship to
more negative potentials and increase τ_{Rec}. Because the
effects of palmitylcarnitine on kinetics of i_{Na} are opposite
those obtained with the antiarrhythmic drugs quinidine and
lidocaine (37), it may be supposed that palmitylcarnitine is
arrhythmogenic. However, it is difficult to draw such a
conclusion until we have a better understanding of the
disposition of palmitylcarnitine in the extracellular
environment of normal (non-ischemic) and ischemic heart cells.
Although V_{max} of the Na^+-dependent component of the action
potential is reduced by palmitylcarnitine at very negative
resting potentials, the non-linear relationship between
conduction velocity (θ) and $\dot{V}_{max}$ ($\theta \sim \dot{V}_{max}^{1/2}$) should permit
little change in conduction of non-ischemic cells. It also
seems unlikely that the amphiphile could reduce τ_{Rec} of
non-ischemic cells sufficiently to diminish the refractory
period so that premature impulses might be more readily
conducted. If the resting potential were about -65 mV in
ischemic tissue, palmitylcarnitine would tend to reduce the
refractory period because it decreased τ_{Rec}. Actually, τ_{Rec}
in palmitylcarnitine at 10.8 mM K^+ was as brief as that
observed in control cells in 5.4 mM K^+. Accordingly,
palmitylcarnitine might be expected to make the refractory
period of depolarized cells similar to that of cells at their
normal resting potential and thereby reduce inhomogeneity of
refractory periods between ischemic and non-ischemic tissues.

The ability of palmitylcarnitine to increase the entry of Ca^{2+} through i_{si} channels and thereby augment the force of contraction could be considered beneficial if one supposed that decreased contractility associated with ischemia is deleterious. However, the increased force of contraction would require additional O_2 consumption for its maintenance, a potentially harmful outcome for ischemic myocardium.

ACKNOWLEDGEMENTS

Supported by USPHS Grants HL-13339 and HL-22135 (A.M. Katz)

REFERENCES

1. Kurien, V.A., & Oliver, M.F. (1966): Lancet 2: 122.
2. Liedtke, A.J., Nellis, S., & Neely, J.R. (1978): Circ. Res. 43: 652.
3. Katz, A.M., & Messineo, F.C. (1981): Circ. Res. 48: 1.
4. Corr, P.B., & Sobel, B.E. (1982): IN Ventricular Tachycardia: Mechanisms and Management (ed) M.E. Josephson, Futura Publishing Co., Mount Kisco, N.Y., p. 97.
5. Arnsdorf, M.F., & Sawicki, G.J. (1981): Circ. Res. 49: 16.
6. Corr, P.B., Cain, M.E., Witkowski, F.X., Price, D.A., & Sobel, B.E. (1979): Circ. Res. 44: 822.
7. Corr, P.B., Snyder, D.W., Cain, M.E., Crafford, W.A., Gross, R.W., & Sobel, B.E. (1981): Circ. Res. 49: 354.
8. Inoue, D., & Pappano, A.J. (1983): Circ. Res. 52: 625.
9. Hoak, J.C., Connor, W.E., & Warner, E.D. (1968): J. Clin. Invest. 47: 2701.
10. Hoak, J.C., Connor, W.E., & Warner, E.D. (1967): J. Clin. Invest. 46: 1071.
11. Inoue, D., Hachisu, M., & Pappano, A.J. (1983): Circ. Res. 53: 158.
12. Iijima, T., & Pappano, A.J. (1979): Circ. Res. 44: 358.
13. Higgins, D., & Pappano, A.J. (1981): Circ. Res. 48: 245.
14. Walton, M., & Fozzard, H.A. (1979): Biophys. J. 25: 407.
15. Marcus, N.C., & Fozzard, H.A. (1981): J. Mol. Cell. Cardiol. 13: 335.
16. Carmeliet, E., & Vereecke, J. (1979): IN Handbook of Physiology, Section 2: The Cardiovascular System, Vol. I. The Heart (ed) R.M. Berne, American Physiological Society, Bethesda, Maryland, p. 269.
17. Frankenhaeuser, B., & Hodgkin, A.L. (1957): J. Physiol. (London) 137: 218.
18. Jack, J.J.B., Noble, D., & Tsien, R.W. (1975): Electric Current Flow in Excitable Cells, Clarendon Press, Oxford.
19. Gettes, L.S., & Reuter, H. (1974): J. Physiol. (London) 240: 703.

20. Weld, F.M., & Bigger, J.T. (1975): Circ. Res. 37: 630.
21. Brown, A.M., Lee, K.S., & Powell, T. (1981): J. Physiol. (London) 318: 479.
22. Cohen, C.J., Bean, B.P., Colatsky, T.J., & Tsien, R.W. (1981): J. Gen. Physiol. 78: 383.
23. Saikawa, T., & Carmeliet, E. (1982): Pflugers Arch. 394: 90.
24. Hachisu, M., & Pappano, A.J. (1983): J. Pharmacol. Exp. Ther. 225: 112.
25. Reuter, H. (1982): IN Normal and Abnormal Conduction in the Heart (eds) A.P. Paes de Carvalho, B.F. Hoffman, & M. Lieberman, Futura Press, Mount Kisco, NY, p. 277.
26. Hille, B., Woodhull, A.M., & Shapiro, B.I. (1975): Phil. Trans. R. Soc. Lond. B. 270: 301.
27. Isenberg, G. (1975): Nature 253: 273.
28. Bassingthwaighte, J.B., Fry, C.H., & McGuigan, J.A.S. (1976): J. Physiol. (London) 262: 15.
29. Kass, R.S., & Tsien, R.W. (1976): J. Gen. Physiol. 67: 599.
30. Adams, R.J., Cohen, D.W., Gupte, S., Johnson, J.D., Wallick, E.T., Wang, T., & Schwartz, A. (1979): J. Biol. Chem. 254: 12404.
31. Messineo, F.C., Pinto, P.B., & Katz, A.M. (1982): IN Advances in Myocardiology, Vol. 3 (eds) E. Chazov, V. Smirnov, & N.S. Dhalla, Plenum Publishing Corp., New York, p. 407.
32. Pitts, B.J.R., Tate, C.A., Van Winkle, W.B., Wood, J.M., & Entman, M.L. (1978): Life Sci. 23: 391.
33. Gross, R.W., Corr, P.B., Lee, B.I., Saffitz, J.E., Crawford, W.A., & Sobel, B.E. (1982): Circ. Res. 51: 27.
34. Feuvray, D., Idell-Wenger, J.A., & Neely, J.R. (1979): Circ. Res. 44: 322.
35. Corr, P.B., Snyder, D.W., Lee, B.I., Gross, R.W., Keim, C.R., & Sobel, B.E. (1982): Am. J. Physiol. 243: H187.
36. Opie, L.H. (1979): Am. Heart J. 97: 375.
37. Hondeghem, L.M., & Katzung, B.G. (1977): Biochim. Biophys. Acta 472: 373.

MODULATION OF MEMBRANE FUNCTION BY LIPID INTERMEDIATES:

A POSSIBLE ROLE IN MYOCARDIAL ISCHEMIA

J. M. J. Lamers, J. T. Stinis,
A. Montfoort and W. C. Hülsmann

Departments of Biochemistry I and Pathological
Anatomy I
Erasmus University, P.O. Box 1738
3000 DR Rotterdam, The Netherlands

The specific biochemical derangements that lead to the rapid loss of contractile function and enhancement of cardiac excitability after the interruption of myocardial bloodflow are not yet settled. However, it may involve either a cellular depletion of high energy compounds (1), an accumulation of noxious products such as H^+ ions and lipid intermediates (2-6), and/or alteration in the functional properties of subcellular membranes (7-10). Abnormalities found in membrane preparations purified from the ischemic heart are most likely irreversible defects. These destructive changes may be caused by degradation of membrane phospholipids or proteins by activated phospholipases and proteases, respectively.

Some cellular factor(s) or metabolic product(s), occuring as a consequence of reduced coronary perfusion, could also contribute to the observed degeneration of membrane function. Large accumulations of long chain fatty acids and their derivatives: fatty acyl CoA-thio esters, fatty acylcarnitine esters have been demonstrated in ischemic myocardium due to oxygen deficiency of the mitochondria (2, 3). These compounds are active detergents and bind extensively to membranes (11-13). A large body of evidence (11, 13-17) now indicates that these intermediates alter functional properties of myocardial membranes in vitro, and that these changes may contribute in the decline of myocardial contractility and the

generation of arrhythmias. By this mechanism, the lipid
intermediates may also cause intracellular Ca^{2+} overload,
which may lead to cell death (18-20).

Long chain fatty acids and acylcarnitines have been found to
inhibit $(Na^+ + K^+)$ATPase in sarcolemma isolated from cardiac
muscle (11, 14, 21). In these studies $(Na^+ + K^+)$ATPase
enriched membrane particles were prepared by using a
surface-active agent (desoxycholate) to solubilize and a high
dilution into detergent-free media to reprecipitate them. After
this treatment Ca^{2+} transport is no longer measurable because
the membrane particles are not well sealed. There are no
studies available on the influence of lipid intermediates on
sarcolemmal Ca^{2+} transporting systems such as the Ca^{2+} pump
and the electrogenic Na^+/Ca^{2+} antiporter. In the present
study the sarcolemmal membranes were not treated with
surface-active agents during isolation in order to attempt to
maintain in vitro the native environment of the sarcolemma as
much as possible. In a previous study we showed that cardiac
sarcolemmal vesicles contain large amounts of latent
$(Na^+ + K^+)$ATPase activity, which was attributable to tightly
sealed right side-out oriented vesicles (22). These vesicles
have also been shown to sequester Ca^{2+} ions intravesicularly,
when a gradient of Na^+ ions is imposed across their membranes
(23). An ATP-dependent Ca^{2+} transport system was also shown
to be present, which was ascribed exclusively to sarcolemma as
the accumulated Ca^{2+} was promptly and completely released in
exchange for Na^+ (22, 24). This Ca^{2+} pumping activity
indicates the presence of a significant amount of sealed
inside-out sarcolemmal vesicles in the preparation. In the
present study the effects of lipid intermediates on sarcolemma
enzyme activity and ion permeability are investigated.

MATERIAL AND METHODS

Sarcolemma was isolated from pig heart by the procedure
described by Reeves and Sutko (25) except that 0.5 mM phenyl
methane sulfonyl fluoride, a protease inhibitor, was added to
all media. The preparation was highly enriched in sarcolemma as
revealed by the high specific activity of ouabain-sensitive
$(Na^+ + K^+)$ATPase: 50-75 μmoles/h/mg if preincubated with 0.3
mg SDS or 0.5 mg alamethicin per mg membrane protein (compare
22, 26). Cross contamination with sarcoplasmic reticulum
membranes was minimal as controlled by Na^+- and Ca^{2+}-
dependent ^{32}P-incorporation into 120 kD proteins separated on
polyacrylamide gel electrophoresis (22).

Assay of Na$^+$/Ca^{2+} exchange and passive Ca^{2+} permeability

Na$^+$/Ca^{2+} was measured in sarcolemmal vesicles loaded
with 160 mM NaCl (20 mM MOPS pH 7.4) by preincubation in this
salt medium at 37° C for 20 min essentially according to the
method previously described (23). To estimate Ca^{2+} uptake, a
10 µl aliquot (12.5 µg protein) was added to 200 µl 160 mM KCl
or NaCl medium containing 20 mM MOPS (pH 7.4) and 50 µM
^{45}CaCl$_2$ (0.1 Ci/mmol). The ^{45}Ca uptake reaction was
terminated at 15, 30, 60 and 120 sec by Millipore filtration (50
µl) and washed twice with ice-cold 160 mM KCl, 20 mM MOPS (pH
7.4) containing 0.1 mM LaCl$_3$. ^{45}Ca uptake reactions in NaCl
were used as blank values and subtracted from corresponding time
values in dilution with KCl. The passive efflux from preloaded
vesicles was estimated by dilution of 50 µl sample of a 2 min
Na$^+$/Ca^{2+} exchange reaction into 1.2 ml 160 mM KCl, 20 mM
MOPS (pH 7.4) containing 0.1 mM EGTA at 37° C. Samples of 200
µl stopped by Millipore filtration after 15 sec, 1, 3, 5 and 10
min were used for estimation of the release rate.

ATPase assays

(Na$^+$+K$^+$)ATPase activity was determined by incubating
12.5 µg membrane protein (either preincubated in 0.25 mg/ml SDS,
20 mM imidazol, pH 7.4 or not) in 200 µl medium containing 50 mM
Tris-maleate (pH 7.4), 100 mM NaCl, KCl concentration as
indicated, 2.5 mM MgCl$_2$, 1 mM EGTA, 2 mM [γ-^{32}P]-ATP (0.25
mCi/mmol). Reactions were carried out in the absence or
presence of 1 mM ouabain. (Ca^{2+}+Mg^{2+})ATPase reactions were
done in 200 µl medium containing 12.5 µg membrane protein, 0.1
mM [γ-^{32}P]-ATP (0.01 Ci/mmol), 50 mM Tris-maleate (pH 6.8),
100 mM KCl and 5 mM MgCl$_2$ at 37° C. Free Ca^{2+} was
controlled in the subµM range by buffering with 100 µM EGTA
(27).

Assay of cyclic AMP-dependent protein kinase

Phosphorylations were carried out by adding 10 µM
[γ-^{32}P]-ATP (20 Ci/mmol) to 50 µl media containing 5 µg
membrane protein, 50 mM KCl, 10 mM MOPS (pH 7.4), 20 mM
K-phosphate, 5 mM MgCl$_2$, 0.5 mM EGTA, 5 µM cyclic AMP and 10
mM theophylline. Incubations were carried out for 2 min at
25° C and terminated by adding SDS-β-mercaptoethanol-glycerol
mixture, further incubated at 95° C for 10 min and analyzed
for SDS-PAGE (15%) as described previously (28, 29).

Assay of [22]Na release from [22]Na-preloaded vesicles

Membrane samples (500 µg protein) were preincubated for 20 h at 0-4° C in 60 µl medium containing 160 mM [22]NaCl (0.4 mCi/mmol), 20 mM MOPS (pH 7.4). [22]Na efflux was initiated by adding a 5 ul aliquot of this suspension into 200 ul medium containing 160 mM KCl, 20 mM MOPS (pH 7.4). Samples of 50 ul were withdrawn for the estimation of vesicular [22]Na content by Millipore filtration as described for the assay of Na^+/Ca^{2+} exchange.

Preparation of the oleate-albumin complexes

Oleic acid was dissolved in a hot solution of 160 mM KCl at concentrations of 0, 2.8, 14 and 19.6 mM by adding an equivalent amount of KOH. One volume of these hot oleate solutions were added dropwise to one volume of 2.8 mM albumin (made fatty acid poor by the method of Chen, 30) in 160 mM KCl and 40 mM MOPS (pH 7.4). This procedure gave oleate-albumin complexes with molar ratios of 0, 1, 5 and 7, respectively. Aliquots were added to the assay media to produce a 0.14 mM albumin concentration.

Materials

Radioactive [γ-^{32}P]-ATP, [45]Ca, [22]Na were obtained from Amersham International PLC (Amersham, U.K.). A23187 was purchased from Boehringer (Mannheim, West Germany). Alamethicin was a kind gift from Dr. J.E. Grady (The Upjohn Company, Kalamazoo, MI). L-palmitoylcarnitine was a gift from Sigma-Tau (Rome, Italy).

RESULTS

Effect of palmitoylcarnitine on Na^+/Ca^{2+} antiporter

Palmitoylcarnitine produced a concentration-dependent inhibitory effect on the sarcolemmal Na^+/Ca^{2+} antiporter as illustrated in Figure 1. Almost complete inhibition was obtained at 100 µM and half-maximal inhibition was seen at 15 µM palmitoylcarnitine. At 25 µM the ratio of acylcarnitine to sarcolemma protein was 0.45 µmol/mg. Similarly, it was shown previously (15, 31) that palmitoylcarnitine at this ratio was a potent inhibitor of ATP-dependent Ca^{2+} sequestration by the sarcoplasmic reticulum Ca^{2+} pump. From the results presented in Figure 1 it can be inferred that the initial rate of the Na^+/Ca^{2+} antiporter is extremely high. However, it is apparent from the first time point at 15 sec and the last at 2 min that the initial rate and the maximum Ca^{2+} uptake are both

affected by the lipid intermediate. To test the possibility
that palmitoylcarnitine caused the sarcolemmal vesicles to
become leaky, Ca^{2+} uptake was allowed to proceed for 1 min
before addition of palmitoylcarnitine. Palmitoylcarnitine
stimulated Ca^{2+} release to the same extent that it inhibited
the initial rate of Na^+/Ca^{2+} exchange (results not shown).
To further differentiate the effects of palmitoylcarnitine on
either the Na^+/Ca^{2+} antiporter or the Ca^{2+} and Na^+
permeability of the sarcolemma, the lipid intermediate was
tested on the passive Ca^{2+} release. Vesicles were preloaded
with Ca^{2+} by the Na^+/Ca^{2+} antiporter and, after 2 min
incubation (compare Figure 1), the sarcolemmal vesicles were
rapidly diluted in 160 mM KCl containing 0.1 mM EGTA. This
dilution step reduced the external Na^+ and Ca^{2+}
concentrations to extremely low values. Unpublished experiments
have shown that the addition of 50 mM Na^+ released the Ca^{2+}
within 1 min, indicating that the Ca^{2+} is still removable by
reversed Na^+/Ca^{2+} exchange. Without Na^+ the passive
Ca^{2+} efflux is measured and, as seen in Figure 2,
palmitoylcarnitine addition resulted in a rapid release of
accumulated $^{45}Ca^{2+}$ within the first min of the measurements.

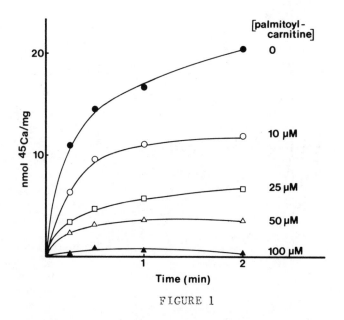

FIGURE 1

Effect of palmitoylcarnitine on Na^+/Ca^{2+} antiporter activity
in cardiac sarcolemmal vesicles.

The efficiency of stimulation of Ca^{2+} release by acylcarnitine is even higher than that of inhibition of the Na^+/Ca^{2+} exchange (compare Figures 1 and 2). However, this difference is probably due to the higher ratio of acylcarnitine to sarcolemmal protein in the Ca^{2+} release experiments if similar amphiphile concentrations are compared. These results appear to indicate that the inhibition of the Na^+/Ca^{2+} exchange by acylcarnitine is due to an effect on leakiness of the vesicles to Ca^{2+} ions.

Effect of palmitoylcarnitine on (Ca^{2+}+Mg^{2+})ATPase

The effect of palmitoylcarnitine on ATP-dependent Ca^{2+} uptake was also studied and inhibition by this amphiphile – again very likely due to Ca^{2+} permeability increase – was found at a concentration that was similar to that which inhibited the Na^+/Ca^{2+} antiporter. The Ca^{2+}- dependent ATP hydrolysis driving this Ca^{2+} accumulation exhibited a rate that was about 10-fold higher than that of the Ca^{2+} uptake. The low coupling ratio (ratio of the amount of Ca^{2+} taken up and ATP hydrolyzed), which has been found repeatedly (23, 24,

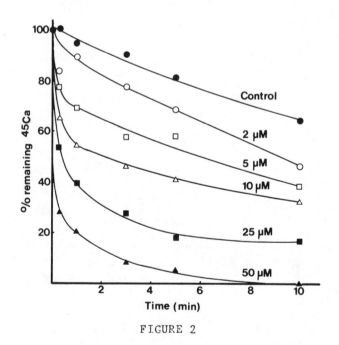

FIGURE 2

Effect of increasing concentrations of palmitoylcarnitine on the passive Ca^{2+} release in sarcolemma.

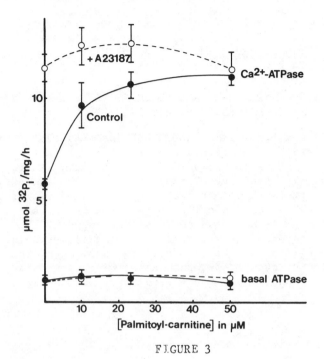

FIGURE 3

Effect of palmitoylcarnitine on the sarcolemmal
$(Ca^{2+}+Mg^{2+})$ATPase, either stimulated by the Ca^{2+}-ionophore
A23187 or not. The activity was assayed with (12 µM
Ca^{2+}_{free}) or without Ca^{2+} (basal ATPase).

28, 32), indicates that the inside-out oriented particles in the
sarcolemmal preparation contain a relatively large amount of
unsealed vesicles. In contrast to its effect on the
ATP-dependent Ca^{2+} uptake, 50 µM palmitoylcarnitine stimulated
the $(Ca^{2+}+Mg^{2+})$ATPase 1.9-fold (Figure 3). The ATPase was
estimated at saturating Ca^{2+} concentration of 12 µM after it
had been shown that the Ca^{2+}-affinity of the enzyme (K_a=0.35
µM) was not affected by the lipid intermediate (results not
shown). The concentrations of palmitoylcarnitine that reduced
Na^+/Ca^{2+} exchange activity and increased $(Ca^{2+}+Mg^{2+})$-
ATPase activity were both in the range of 10-50 µM (compare
Figures 1 and 3). As this finding suggests a possible
relationship between the stimulation of the $(Ca^{2+}+Mg^{2+})$-
ATPase and increased leakiness of the vesicles for Ca^{2+} ions,
we tested the specific Ca^{2+} ionophore A23187, which indeed
caused a similar increase of enzyme activity. Palmitoyl-

carnitine had no clear additive effect when tested in the
presence of the Ca^{2+} ionophore. These data suggest the
intravesicularly accumulated Ca^{2+} is inhibiting the
$(Ca^{2+}+Mg^{2+})$ATPase.

Influence of palmitoylcarnitine on sarcolemmal $(Na^{+}+K^{+})$ ATPase and cyclic AMP-dependent protein kinase

The membrane preparation used contains vesicular particles
as demonstrated by the operation of the Na^{+}/Ca^{2+} antiporter
and Ca^{2+} pump. Because the vesicles are tightly sealed, they
exhibit several latent enzyme activities. In earlier work (22,
26), we and others showed that the activities of latent enzymes
such as $(Na^{+}+K^{+})$ATPase, adenylate cyclase and cyclic
AMP-dependent protein kinase could be increased if the vesicles
were pretreated with the peptidic ionophore alamethicin.
Alamethicin eliminates the permeability barriers of the vesicles
for $[\gamma-^{32}P]$-ATP, cyclic AMP, and, as we will show later, for
monovalent cations. From these results it was concluded that

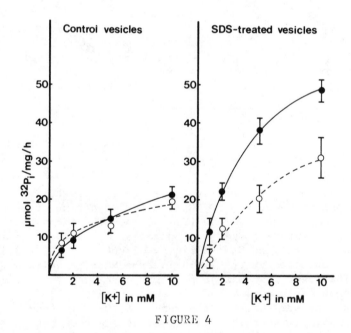

FIGURE 4

Cardiac sarcolemmal $(Na^{+}+K^{+})$ATPase measured in control and
SDS-treated vesicles either in the presence (O) or absence (●)
of 25 μM palmitoylcarnitine.

the method now used to isolate sarcolemmal vesicles yields
predominantly right side-out oriented vesicles (22, 26).
Palmitoylcarnitine at 0.4 μmol/mg membrane protein (25 μM), a
concentration that markedly increased the Ca^{2+} permeability as
shown in Figure 2, did not significantly affect the sarcolemmal
(Na^++K^+)ATPase (Figure 4). The potency of free fatty acids
to inhibit sarcolemmal (Na^++K^+)ATPase increased if
suboptimal K^+ concentrations were used for estimation of the
enzyme activity (14). Therefore, in the present work, we
attempted to study the possible effect of low K^+ concentration
on the palmitoylcarnitine interaction with the
(Na^++K^+)ATPase. Even if K^+ concentrations lower than 10
mM were used for estimating the ouabain-sensitive ATPase, no
clear effect of palmitoylcarnitine on the enzyme was observed
(Figure 4). SDS pretreatment of the vesicles (0.3 mg/mg
membrane protein) typically increased (Na^++K^+)ATPase
activity 2.4-fold, a degree of stimulation that is similar to
that found with alamethicin (results not shown). Under these
experimental conditions, which measured overt plus latent
activity, 37% inhibition was caused by the addition of 25 μM
acylcarnitine (Figure 4). This finding suggests that the
activity of (Na^++K^+)ATPase, when present in the
microenvironment provided by the sarcolemma, is resistent to
perturbation by palmitoylcarnitine. Apparently the detergent
effect of SDS may be sufficient for the lipid intermediate to
enter the lipid bilayer and to readily affect the
(Na^++K^+)ATPase.

Another enzyme that was markedly stimulated by alamethicin
in cardiac sarcolemmal vesicles is the intrinsic cyclic
AMP-dependent protein kinase of type II (Figure 5). Unpublished
observations revealed that SDS could not be used to unmask the
protein kinase because of the concomitant inactivation of the
enzyme by the detergent. From the results shown in Figure 5 it
can be seen that there are several substrate proteins for cyclic
AMP-dependent protein kinase in the sarcolemma: phospholamban-
like protein or otherwise named calciductin (9 kD molecular
weight) and some minor proteins of 55, 26 and 15 kD molecular
weight. As demonstrated in Figure 5, there is no complete
parallelism between alamethicin-activation of the
^{32}P-incorporation into the 9 and 15 kD proteins. Analogous
results have been reported earlier and it was suggested that
this non-parallelism is due to the presence of subpopulations of
sarcolemmal vesicles (22, 29, 33). At any rate,
palmitoylcarnitine, up to concentrations of 50 and 100 μM (0.4
and 0.8 μmole/mg membrane protein), could not unmask the protein
kinase. In some unpublished experiments it was shown that no
concomitant detergent inactivation of the cyclic AMP-dependent
protein kinase occurred. This was tested by adding palmitoyl-

carnitine to alamethicin-treated sarcolemmal vesicles. Thus,
palmitoylcarnitine at relatively high concentrations (50-100 µM)
did not increase the permeability of the sarcolemmal vesicles
for $[\gamma-^{32}P]$-ATP and cyclic AMP. These results are in
agreement with the data illustrated in Figure 4, in which no
stimulation of $(Na^+ + K^+)$ATPase by acylcarnitine could be
observed.

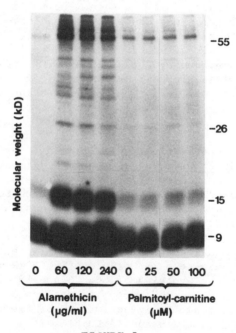

FIGURE 5

Effect of alamethicin and palmitoylcarnitine on the intrinsic
cyclic AMP-dependent protein kinase of cardiac sarcolemma.
Autoradiographs of ^{32}P-protein patterns obtained after running
on 15% SDS-PAGE are shown.

Effect of oleate-albumin complexes with different ratios on
sarcolemmal Ca^{2+} permeability

To study the effect of high concentrations of free fatty
acids on some of the Ca^{2+} transport properties of cardiac
sarcolemma, fatty acid was added to the membranes in the form of
fatty acid-albumin complexes similar to those delivered from the
plasma to the cardiac cell in vivo (34, 35). Albumin has two
very strong binding sites and a number of weak binding sites for
free fatty acid so that the amount of unbound fatty acid
increases exponentially as fatty acid-albumin ratios are
increased. Once transported through the sarcolemma, free fatty
acid is also believed to be bound to "Z-proteins" or
incorporated into cellular membranes. Fatty acid-albumin ratios
of 4 or more are very unusual in plasma, even in disease.
However, due to low albumin concentration in interstitium
compared to that of plasma, interstitial and intracellular
accumulation of free fatty acid, during hampered β-oxidation,
very likely lead to high concentrations of unbound fatty acid.
We found previously (14) that fatty acid-albumin ratios higher
than 5 were inhibitory to sarcolemmal (Na^++K^+)ATPase
purified from myocardium using deoxycholate. Similar results
comparing molar ratios of 0, 1, 5 and 7 were obtained with the
present sarcolemmal preparation. Only the complex of ratio 7
effectively produced almost complete inhibition of
(Na^++K^+)ATPase at 10 mM K^+ (0.14 mM albumin, results not
shown) in either control or SDS-treated vesicles. It was
therefore of interest to examine whether fatty acid under the
same conditions is able to affect the Ca^{2+} permeability and
Na^+/Ca^{2+} exchange activity of the vesicles. Although
albumin (0.14 mM) itself increased slightly, but reproducibly,
the Ca^{2+} permeability, as illustrated in Figure 6, only the
oleate-albumin ratio of 7 dramatically increased the Ca^{2+}
efflux rate from sarcolemmal vesicles. It is interesting to
note that the oleate-albumin complex of ratio 5 somewhat
decreased the Ca^{2+} permeability of the vesicles compared to
that seen when albumin alone was present. This effect of a low
concentration of unbound fatty acid on Ca^{2+} permeability may
be related to the inhibition by low concentrations of oleic acid
of Ca^{2+} release from sarcoplasmic reticulum vesicles, as
observed previously by Katz et al. (36). Our results with
increased sarcolemmal Ca^{2+} permeability caused by free fatty
acid are consistent with the results of Cheah (37) in
sarcoplasmic reticulum vesicles. There is no clear explanation
for the effect of bovine serum albumin itself on the sarcolemmal
Ca^{2+} permeability; it may be due to contamination of the
albumin preparation with cations (Ca^{2+} or Na^+) which were
not removed after extensive dialysis. These cations could have
initiated Ca^{2+} release by operation of Ca^{2+}/Ca^{2+} or

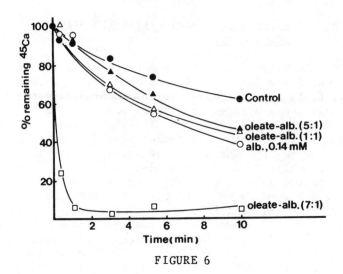

FIGURE 6

Effect of oleate-albumin complexes with different molar ratios on the passive Ca^{2+} release in sarcolemmal vesicles.

Ca^{2+}/Na^+ exchange (38). As was expected from the results obtained in studying fatty acid effects on the Ca^{2+} permeability, only the oleate-albumin complex of ratio 7 was inhibitory to the Na^+-dependent Ca^{2+} influx in sarcolemmal vesicles (data not shown).

Effect of lipid intermediates on Na^+ permeability of sarcolemma

Electrophysiological studies have indicated that the sarcolemma is impermeable to Na^+ and Ca^{2+} except during the action potential. The net direction and rate of the in vivo operating Na^+/Ca^{2+} antiporter is dependent on both the Na^+ gradient and the membrane potential, which are regulated by the activity of the Na^+/K^+-ATPase (23). Therefore the possibility that palmitoylcarnitine or free fatty acid could alter the Na^+ gradient by a direct ionophoretic action was investigated by $^{22}Na^+$ flux studies. Due to the extremely low amounts of Na^+ crossing the sarcolemmal membrane in exchange for Ca^{2+}, relative to the absolute Na^+ concentration intra- and extravesicularly, it was not possible to load the vesicles with $^{22}Na^+$ by Ca^{2+}/Na^+ exchange for the study of passive $^{22}Na^+$ release. For this reason sarcolemmal vesicles were loaded with $^{22}Na^+$ by preincubation in 160 mM $^{22}NaCl$ for 20 h at 0-4° C. To increase the sensitivity of the $^{22}Na^+$ measurement it was necessary to use a very concentrated vesicle suspension (about 8 mg/ml) in the preincubation phase, after which $^{22}Na^+$ efflux was initiated by rapid 40-fold dilution in 160 mM KCl medium. A disadvantage of this method is that, due to the passive loading with $^{22}Na^+$, a large part of the $^{22}Na^+$ may be present at sarcolemmal binding sites for this cation and not free in the intravesicular medium. If the fraction of bound Na^+ is assumed to be negligible, the isotope space of the sarcolemmal vesicles is calculated to be about 2 μl/mg protein, which is well in the usual range found for the sarcolemmal vesicles (39). First the ability of the sarcolemmal fraction to exchange $^{22}Na^+$ for external Ca^{2+} was tested. As can be seen from the results in Table 1, 1 mM $CaCl_2$ caused 20% more Na^+ release than in the control situation after 1 min. As was the case for the passive Ca^{2+} leakage (compare Figures 2 and 6), the Na^+ release rate was in the order of minutes, which we believe is characteristic for non-mediated (not by carrier or voltage-dependent channel) permeation. The peptidic ionophore alamethicin released almost all Na^+ within 10 sec, the first time point in Millipore filtration. Both palmitoylcarnitine at 50 μM (0.25 μmol/mg membrane protein) and oleate-albumin complex

TABLE 1. $^{22}Na^+$ release from cardiac sarcolemmal vesicles.

| | N^b | $^{22}Na^+$ content in nmoles/mg | | | |
		10 sec	1 min	2 min	45 min
Control	7	320±25	278±18	225±17	36±13
25 μM palm.carnitine	7	340±25	283±29	244±25	27±10
50 μM palm.carnitine	5	263±21[a]	211±23[a]	181±11[a]	–
1 mM oleate-albumin (7:1)	3	259±42	209±33[a]	168±29[a]	17±5[a]
1 mM $CaCl_2$	7	285±28	217±32[a]	172±29[a]	6±1[a]
0.1 mg/ml alamethicin	4	10± 2[a]	6± 1[a]	6±1[a]	–

[a] Values differ significantly from the corresponding control values.
[b] N means the number of experiments.

of ratio 7 were able to increase the Na^+ permeability of the vesicles. At least for palmitoylcarnitine Na^+ and Ca^{2+} permeability of the vesicles are seen to increase in parallel, when results obtained at similar palmitoylcarnitine/membrane protein ratios are compared.

GENERAL DISCUSSION

Although the Ca^{2+} uptake under the experimental conditions described in this paper is referred to as sarcolemmal uptake, the possibility that a vesicle preparation with mainly inside-out sarcolemmal vesicles would be affected by the lipid intermediates in a manner different from that of right side-out vesicles cannot be overlooked. The cardiac sarcolemmal vesicles were isolated in vesicular form; because they were tightly sealed and predominantly of right side-out orientation, intrinsic (Na^++K^+)-ATPase and cyclic AMP-dependent protein kinase exhibited considerable latency. In an idealized situation, where no leaky vesicles are present, the carriers and enzymes are allowed to operate depending on the orientation of the sarcolemmal vesicle (Figure 7). It is important to note that the Na^+/Ca^{2+} antiporter has been shown to operate symmetrically in both directions (38, 40). Thus in the present report, passive Ca^{2+} and Na^+ efflux is measured from both inside- and right side-out vesicles. The effects of palmitoylcarnitine and oleate-albumin complexes on (Na^++K^+)ATPase and $(Ca^{2+}+Mg^{2+})$ATPase in native sarcolemmal vesicles probably were exerted at the cytosolic side of the sarcolemmal membrane. Again, for this analysis, it must be assumed that no leaky vesicles were present. The finding that palmitoylcarnitine at 0.4 $\mu mol/mg$ protein did not significantly inhibit (Na^++K^+)ATPase could be related to this problem of sidedness of the vesicles. Accumulation of palmitoylcarnitine in vivo will most likely exert its membrane perturbing effect at the cytosolic side of the sarcolemmal membrane. On the other hand, high amounts of fatty acids are supposed to occur in either the cytosolic or interstitial compartment during an ischemic episode in the heart because fatty acids accumulate not only by the hampered β-oxidation in the mitochondria, but also by increased intracellular lipolysis and apolipoprotein C II-dependent lipoprotein lipase action in the interstitium (35, 41). Moreover the low protein (albumin) concentration in the interstitial space further contributes in the accumulation of high concentrations of unbound fatty acid in this compartment.

We have demonstrated that SDS-unmasked (Na^++K^+)ATPase is significantly inhibited by 0.4 µmol palmitoylcarnitine/mg protein which, according to the scheme presented in Figure 7, would mean that the amphiphile is effective only at the outer side of the sarcolemmal membrane. This would imply that the inhibition of the vectorial enzyme (Na^++K^+)ATPase by palmitoylcarnitine has no pathophysiological relevance, unless the detergent accumulates under pathological conditions in the interstitial fluid. An alternative explanation would be that the detergent SDS may have altered the membrane structure and lipid domains rendering (Na^++K^+)ATPase into a palmitoylcarnitine-sensitive form. Some evidence for this alternative explanation can be found in the report of Adams et al. (11) which demonstrated a difference between palmitoyl-carnitine concentration-response curves for two cardiac preparations of (Na^++K^+)ATPase (citrate and deoxycholate fraction). At any rate, our results with native sarcolemmal vesicles agree with those of Owens et al. (17), who showed no effect of palmitoylcarnitine on (Na^++K^+)ATPase using concentrations of the lipid intermediate up to 10 µmol/mg

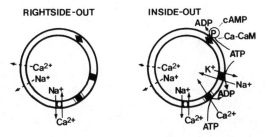

FIGURE 7

Schematic picture of operation of ion fluxes, carrier and enzyme systems depending on the orientation of the sarcolemmal vesicles.

protein. Finally, it should be questioned whether vesicle
sidedness is important for studying the effect of lipid
intermediates on vectorial membrane properties as the
amphiphiles studied are lipophilic in character and therefore
may rapidly pass the membrane having acess to both sides.

The other sarcolemmal membrane enzyme that might have been
attacked only from the cytosolic side of the membrane is the
$(Ca^{2+}+Mg^{2+})$-ATPase. As found earlier by Adams et al. (11)
for sarcoplasmic reticulum $(Ca^{2+}+Mg^{2+})$ATPase, 10-50 μM
palmitoylcarnitine (0.16-0.80 μmol/mg protein) produced a
concentration-dependent stimulation of the sarcolemmal enzyme.
Niggli et al. (42) and Gietzen et al. (43) recently reported
that amphiphilic lipids can mimic the effect of calmodulin on
purified erythrocyte $(Ca^{2+}+Mg^{2+})$ATPase and brain
phosphodiesterase. Previously it was shown by us (27) and by
Caroni and Carafoli (24) that calmodulin is also involved in the
regulation of the sarcolemmal $(Ca^{2+}+Mg^{2+})$ATPase. The
possibility of a calmodulin-like effect of palmitoylcarnitine on
the $(Ca^{2+}+Mg^{2+})$ATPase in the present preparation is very
unlikely because calmodulin is tightly bound and not easily
removed, in contrast to the loosely bound entity of erythrocyte
$(Ca^{2+}+Mg^{2+})$ATPase and brain phosphodiesterase. The findings
that the $(Ca^{2+}+Mg^{2+})$ATPase of sarcolemma was stimulated to
the same extent by the Ca^{2+} ionophore A23187 and that
palmitoylcarnitine increased the Ca^{2+} permeability of the
sarcolemma, suggest that a Ca^{2+} ionophoric mechanism of action
explains the acylcarnitine effect. It is important to note that
the effect on the $(Ca^{2+}+Mg^{2+})$ATPase cannot be attributed to
unmasking of the enzyme (alteration of the vesicle permeability
for the substrate ATP), in view of the inability of
palmitoylcarnitine, up to concentrations of 0.8 μmol/mg protein,
to unmask $(Na^{+}+K^{+})$ATPase and cyclic AMP-dependent protein
kinase.

The present study has demonstrated that the in vitro effects
of palmitoylcarnitine, an endogenously occurring long chain
fatty acid acyl-ester, are deleterious to the Ca^{2+} and Na^{+}
permeability of the sarcolemma. These findings confirm previous
reports on effects of palmitoylcarnitine on Ca^{2+} release in
isolated sarcoplasmic reticulum membranes (15, 31). It is
questionable if high concentrations of palmitoylcarnitine are
present under ischemic conditions in the heart. From the values
given by Idell-Wenger et al. (2) it can be calculated that the
"cytosol" content of acylcarnitine in normal and ischemic heart
is 0.15 and 0.73 μmol/g wet weight. Pitts et al. (15) estimated
the amount of palmitoylcarnitine relative to sarcoplasmic
reticulum from these values by assuming the presence of 3 mg
sarcoplasmic reticulum protein/g wet weight of heart. They

calculated ratios of 0.03 and 0.16 μmol palmitoylcarnitine/mg sarcoplasmic reticulum in normal and ischemic heart, respectively. If these calculations are also applicable to the sarcolemma, the present results indicate that acylcarnitine could be expected to cause considerable effects on Ca^{2+} permeability of sarcolemma in the ischemic heart. Recent experiments carried out in our laboratory (Hülsmann et al., this volume) have demonstrated that acylcarnitine in control hearts is undetectable when artificial respiration of rats is carried out prior to freezing of the heart. Thus the relative increase of myocardial content of palmitoylcarnitine during ischemia may be more extreme than previous measurements would suggest. Finally, other direct effects of palmitoylcarnitine on sarcolemma-bound enzymes, e.g. $(Na^{+}+K^{+})$ATPase, $(Ca^{2+} + Mg^{2+})$ATPase and Ca^{2+}-calmodulin-dependent protein kinase (5, 11, 17, 21, 44) are usually seen at higher concentrations of the lipid intermediate in comparison to the effect on ion permeability.

From the present work it can be concluded that high concentrations of fatty acid also increase Ca^{2+} and Na^{+} permeability of sarcolemma. As we showed previously (14) free fatty acids are also very potent inhibitors of $(Na^{+}+K^{+})$-ATPase. Both effects of free fatty acid may have causal significance for the derangements of cardiac cell function seen in ischemia (4, 5). Marked accumulation of free fatty acid has been observed in biopsies taken from ischemia areas of the left ventricular wall of dog hearts (45). Fatty acid complexes of molar ratios 6 or higher added to perfusates in Langendorff perfused hearts, even under normoxic conditions, produced depression of contractility (46). Many inhibitory effects of free fatty acids on plasma membrane transport phenomena have also been described (47, 48) in tissues other than heart. In conclusion, our data are in full accord with the hypothesis that lipid intermediates accumulating in cardiac ischemia might influence membrane and thereby muscle function.

ACKNOWLEDGEMENTS

The authors wish to thank Miss A.C. Hanson for assistance in the preparation of the manuscript.

REFERENCES

1. Kübler, W., & Katz, A.M. (1977): Am. J. Cardiol. 40: 467.
2. Idell-Wenger, J.A., Grotyohann, L.W., & Neely, J.L. (1978): J. Biol. Chem. 253: 4310.

3. Shug, A.L., Thomsen, J.H., Folts, J.D., Bittar, N., Klein,
   M.I., Koke, J.R., & Huth, P.J. (1978): Arch. Biochem.
   Biophys. 187: 25.
4. Opie, L.H. (1979): Am. Heart J. 97: 375.
5. Liedtke, A.J. (1981): Prog. Cardiovasc. Dis. 23: 321.
6. Corr, P.B., Gross, R.W., & Sobel, B.E. (1982): J. Mol.
   Cell. Cardiol. 14: 619.
7. Schwartz, A., Wood, J.M., Allen, J.C., Bornet, E.P., Entman,
   M.L., Goldstein, M.A., Sordahl, L.A., Suzuki, M., & Lewis,
   R.M. (1973): Am. J. Cardiol. 32: 46.
8. Beller, G.A., Conroy, J., & Smith, T.W. (1976): J. Clin.
   Invest. 57: 341.
9. Chien, K.R., Reeves, J.P., Buja, M., Bonte, F., Parkey,
   R.W., & Willerson, J.T. (1981): Circ. Res. 48: 711.
10. Bersohn, M.M., Philipson, K.D., & Fukushima, J.I. (1982):
    Am. J. Physiol. 242: C288.
11. Adams, R.J., Cohen, D.W., Gupte, S., Johnson, J.D., Wallick,
    E.T., Wang, T., & Schwartz, A. (1979): J. Biol. Chem. 254:
    12404.
12. Karnovsky, M.J. (1979): Am. J. Pathol. 97: 212.
13. Katz, A.M., & Messineo, F.C. (1981): Circ. Res. 48: 1.
14. Lamers, J.M.J., & Hülsmann, W.C. (1977): J. Mol. Cell.
    Cardiol. 9: 343.
15. Pitts, B.J.R., Tate, C.A., Van Winkle, B., Wood, J.M., &
    Entman, M.L. (1978): Life Sci. 23: 391.
16. Messineo, F.C., Pinto, P.B., & Katz, A.M. (1980): J. Mol.
    Cell. Cardiol. 12: 725.
17. Owens, K., Kennett, F.F., & Weglicki, W.B. (1982): Am. J.
    Physiol. 242: H456.
18. Dhalla, N.S., Das, P.K., & Sharma, G.P. (1978): J. Mol.
    Cell. Cardiol. 10: 363.
19. Farber, J.L. (1981): Life Sci. 29: 1289.
20. Clusin, W.T., Buchbinder, M., & Harrison, D.C. (1983): The
    Lancet i: 272.
21. Wood, J.M., Bush, B., Pitts, B.J.R., & Schwartz, A. (1977):
    Biochem. Biophys. Res. Commun. 74: 677.
22. Lamers, J.M.J., & Stinis, J.T. (1982): IN Advances in
    Studies on Heart Metabolism (eds) C.M. Caldarera & P.
    Harris, CLUEB, Bologna, p. 41.
23. Lamers, J.M.J., & Stinis, J.T. (1981): Biochim. Biophys.
    Acta 640: 521.
24. Caroni, P., & Carafoli, E. (1981): J. Biol. Chem. 256:
    3263.
25. Reeves, J.P., & Sutko, J.L. (1980): Science 208: 1461.
26. Jones, L.R., Maddock, S.W., & Hathaway, D.R. (1981): J.
    Biol. Chem. 255: 9971.
27. Lamers, J.M.J., Stinis, J.T., & De Jonge, H.R. (1981): FEBS
    Lett. 127: 139.
28. Lamers, J.M.J., & Stinis, J.T. (1980): Biochim. Biophys.
    Acta 624: 443.

29. Lamers, J.M.J., & Weeda, E. (1983): IN Methods in Studying Cardiac Membranes (ed) N.S.Dhalla, CRC Press, Inc., Florida, in press.
30. Chen, R.F. (1967): J. Biol. Chem. 242: 173.
31. Messineo, F.C., Pinto, P.B., & Katz, A.M. (1982): IN Advances in Myocardiology, Vol. 3 (eds) E. Chazov, V. Smirnov, & N.S. Dhalla, Plenum Publishing Corp., New York, p. 407.
32. Lamers, J.M.J., & Stinis, J.T. (1979): Life Sci. 24: 2313.
33. Manalan, A.S., & Jones, L.R. (1982): J. Biol. Chem. 257: 10052.
34. Spector, A.A., & Fletcher, J.E. (1978): IN Disturbances in Lipid and Lipoprotein Metabolism (eds) J.M. Dietschy, A.M. Gotto, & J.A. Ontko, Am. Physiol. Soc., Bethesda, p. 229.
35. Stam, H. (1983): J. Drug Res. 8: 1.
36. Katz, A.M., Messineo, F.C., Miceli, J., & Nash-Adler, P.A. (1981): Life Sci. 28: 1103.
37. Cheah, A.M. (1981): Biochim. Biophys. Acta 648: 113.
38. Slaughter, R.S., Sutko, J.L., & Reeves, J.P. (1983): J. Biol. Chem. 258: 3183.
39. Gilbert and Meissner, G. (1983): Arch. Biochem. Biophys. 223: 9.
40. Philipson, K.D., & Nishimoto, A.Y. (1982): J. Biol. Chem. 257: 5111.
41. Hülsmann, W.C., Stam, H., & Maccari, F. (1982): Biochim. Biophys. Acta 713: 39.
42. Niggli, V., Adunyah, E.S., & Carafoli, E. (1981): J. Biol. Chem. 256: 8588.
43. Gietzen, K., Xü, Y.-H., Galla, H.-J., & Bader, H. (1982): Biochem. J. 207: 637.
44. Katoh, N., Wrenn, R.W., Wise, B.C., Shoji, M., & Kuo, J.F. (1981): Proc. Natl. Acad. Sci. USA 78: 4813.
45. Van der Vusse, G.J., Roemen, Th.H.M., Prinzen, F.W., Coumans, W.A., & Reneman, R.S. (1982): Circ. Res. 50: 538.
46. Stam, H., & Hülsmann, W.C. (1978): Basic Res. Cardiol. 73: 208.
47. Lamers, J.M.J., & Hülsmann, W.C. (1975): Biochim. Biophys. Acta 394: 31.
48. Rhoads, D.E., Ockner, R.K., Peterson, N.A., & Raghupathy, E. (1983): Biochemistry 22: 1965.

FATTY ACID EFFECTS ON SARCOPLASMIC RETICULUM FUNCTION IN VITRO

F. C. Messineo, M. Rathier, J. M. Watras, H. Takenaka,
and A. M. Katz

Department of Medicine
Division of Cardiology
University of Connecticut Health Center
Farmington, CT 06032 U.S.A.

When heart muscle is rendered ischemic or hypoxic, changes
in lipid and phospholipid metabolism result in the accumulation
of amphiphilic compounds, including non-esterified fatty acids
(FA), fatty acylcarnitine esters, and lysophosphatides (1-5).
These amphiphilic substances, possibly by interacting with
membrane lipids, can alter the functional properties of a
variety of membrane systems in vitro; and this interaction has
been postulated as a possible mechanism for ischemic heart
muscle dysfunction in vivo. (See references 6-8 for reviews).
The mechanism by which amphiphiles alter membrane function in
vitro, however, remains unclear. The calcium sequestration
properties and ATPase activity of sarcoplasmic reticulum
membrane vesicles (SR) isolated from skeletal muscle are
modified by both non-esterified fatty acids and acylcarnitines
(9-11). The present report describes studies examining the
effect of oleic and palmitic acids on the properties of calcium
sequestration and ATPase activity of SR in order to elucidate
the mechanisms by which structurally dissimilar fatty acids can
alter differently SR calcium sequestration. The results suggest
that fatty acids can influence calcium permeability of SR or
change the amount and characteristics of the sequestered
calcium. These qualitative effects appear to depend upon
aliphatic change structure whereas the quantitative potency of
the effects appear to depend, in part, on the relative amounts
of added amphiphile to membrane phospholipid.

127

METHODS

Crude or "light" (enriched in longitudinal tubule derived
membranes) sarcoplasmic reticulum vesicles were prepared by
methods described previously (12, 13). Calcium sequestration by
6 to 12 μg/ml SR protein was determined in 120 mM KCl, 1 mM
MgCl, 1 mM Mg ATP, 8 to 13 μM ^{45}CaCl$_2$, and 40 mM histidine
buffer (pH 6.8) at 25° C. Reactions were initiated by the
addition of sarcoplasmic reticulum and terminated by Millipore
filtration as previously described (12, 14). ATPase activity
and phosphoprotein levels were determined by the methods of
Shigekawa (15) and Takenaka et al. (14). Reaction conditions
were as described for calcium sequestration except the reactions
were initiated with either 1 mM (γ^{32}P) MgATP for ATPase
determinations or 50 μM (γ^{32}P) ATP for EP levels.

RESULTS

When present from the onset of the reaction M concentrations of palmitic acid (C16 saturated) stimulated and oleic
acid (C18 cis Δ9) inhibited calcium sequestration by SR
membranes (Table 1). When added at similar concentrations to
calcium filled vesicles palmitic acid promoted further calcium
sequestration while oleic acid induced calcium release (data not
shown). Although the inhibitory effect of oleic acid on calcium
sequestration is concentration dependent in the presence of a
fixed amount of SR membrane (16), the finding that the effect of
16 M oleic acid could be attenuated from 78% inhibition in the
presence of 6 μg/ml SR protein to 21% inhibition in the presence
of 48 μg/ml (Table 2) suggests that these fatty acid effects are
dependent on the mole ratio of amphiphile to membrane
phospholipid.

Despite opposite effects on the amount of calcium
sequestered, both palmitic and oleic acids, at a concentration
of 18 M, stimulated SR ATPase activity from 0.74 ±
0.04 μmol/mg·min to 2.12 ± 0.23 and 1.81 ± 0.14 μmol/mg·min,
respectively (Table 1). The amount and distribution of the
phosphoprotein intermediates of the SR ATPase protein were not
affected by the presence of either fatty acid. Therefore, the
divergent effects of these fatty acids on calcium sequestration
was not reflected by their effects on either ATPase activity or
phosphoenzyme distribution (Table 1).

When added to calcium-filled sarcoplasmic reticulum vesicles
under conditions where low concentrations of ATP cannot support
calcium influx, oleic acid promotes further calcium release
whereas palmitic acid has no effect (data not shown). These

TABLE 1

EFFECT OF PALMITIC AND OLEIC ACID ON SARCOPLASMIC RETICULUM FUNCTION IN VITRO

	Control	18μM Palmitic	18μM Oleic Acid
Ca sequestration (nmol/mg)	126 ± 5	174 ± 10	73.6 ± 6
ATPase activity (μmol Pi/mg.min)	.74 ± .04	1.81 ± .14	2.12 ± .23
Total EP (nmol/mg)	3.51 ± .18	3.28 ± .22	3.20 ± .22
ADP insensitive EP nmol/mg	0.98 ± 0.11	0.94 ± 0.12	1.12 ± 0.12

Calcium sequestration and ATPase activity of 12 μg/ml SR determined as described in Methods and carried out at 25° C in 120 mM KCl, 40 mM histidine buffer (pH 6.8), 10 μM added CaCl2, 1 mM MgCl2. Reactions were initiated by addition of 1 mM (γ32P)MgATP. EP was determined under identical conditions except the labeled MgATP concentration was 50 μM. Fatty acids were present from the onset of the reaction. Values are mean ± S.E.M. of 5 determinations for calcium sequestration and ATPase activity and 17-20 determinations for EP.

Table 2. Effect of increasing SR membrane lipid on the
inhibition of Ca sequestration by 16 μM oleic acid
expressed as percent control.

6 μg/ml	12 μg/ml	24 μg/ml	48 μg/ml
(2.66)	(1.33)	(0.67)	(0.33)
22%	47%	71%	79%

Numbers in parentheses represent the mole ratio of fatty acid to
membrane phospholipid. Conditions were as described in Methods
and a crude SR preparation was utilized.

results suggest that oleic acid inhibits calcium sequestration
by increasing a passive calcium permeability whereas palmitic
acid under these conditions has no effect on calcium
permeability.

The unusual ability of palmitic acid to enhance SR calcium
sequestration was not observed in the absence of ATP or when
control calcium sequestration was inhibited completely by the
presence of the calcium ionophore A23187 (Figure 1). This
ionophore when added to control calcium-filled vesicles causes
the immediate release of all but approximately 10 nmole/mg of
the sequestered calcium; in contrast, approximately 120 nmole/mg
of the calcium sequestered in the presence of 18 M palmitic
acid is not released by A23187 (Figure 1, Table 3).

DISCUSSION

The studies presented in this report demonstrate that
micromolar concentrations of non-esterified fatty acids can
alter both calcium sequestration and ATPase activity of
sarcoplasmic reticulum vesicles in vitro (Table 1). The effect
of these compounds on calcium sequestration is not solely
dependent on fatty acid concentration but related to the ratio
of amphiphile to SR protein or lipid. Since Lee et al. (16)
have suggested that fatty acid binding to the SR ATPase protein
is saturated at approximately 10 μM, the finding that oleic acid
induced inhibition of calcium sequestration decreases with
increasing protein concentration suggests that the oleic acid
effect is not due to a direct action of the fatty acid on the
ATPase protein, but may reflect a secondary effect mediated
through an interaction with SR phospholipid.

The double bond at position 9 in the aliphatic chain of
oleic acid imparts a 30 degree angle to the molecule; and this
structure results in a compound that inhibits calcium

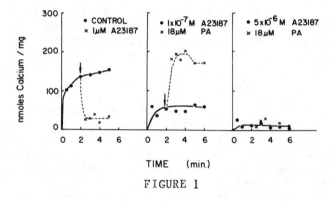

FIGURE 1

The effect of A23187 added to Ca-filled vesicles (left) or
present from the onset of the calcium sequestration reaction
(middle and right). Palmitic acid was added 2 mins. after the
onset of the reactions initiated in the presence of A23187. Ca
sequestration by 6 μg/ml SR was carried out as described in
Methods except for the presence of 5 mM MgATP.

Table 3. Calcium released by A23187 in the presence and absence
of palmitic acid.

Calcium sequestered	140 ± 5 (4)	209 ± 11 (9)
Calcium released by A23187 (nmol/mg)	129.3	91
A23187 "insensitive" calcium	10.7 ± 0.8 (4)	118 ± 12 (4)

The amount of calcium sequestered by 12 g/ml sarcoplasmic
reticulum vesicles in the presence or absence of 18 M palmitic
acid was measured 5 min. after the start of the reaction and 1
min. later in 120 mM KCl, 40 mM histidine buffer (pH 6.8), 5 μM
added $CaCl_2$, and 1 mM MgATP + 1 mM $MgCl_2$, or 5 mM MgATP.
Values are mean $\pm$ S.E. for the n listed in parentheses.

sequestration while the straight aliphatic chain palmitic acid,
of similar molecular length, enhances calcium sequestration.
These findings suggest that fatty acids may exert their
different effects by inserting into different phospholipid
domains within the SR membrane. The unchanged phosphoprotein
intermediate amounts and the similar stimulation of SR ATPase by
both compounds, however, argues that this particular effect on
the ATPase reaction may not be secondary to preferential
insertion of the fatty acids into different SR lipid domains
(17).

The abilities of oleic acid to inhibit calcium
sequestration, to promote calcium release from calcium filled
vesicles, to enhance the calcium release observed during ATP
depletion, and to stimulate SR ATPase activity all support the
view that this fatty acid increases membrane permeability to
calcium. However, whether oleic acid is altering a regulated
membrane permeability such as a channel or, by a detergent-like
action, is disrupting the structural integrity of the membrane
as an ion barrier is not clear from this study (18).

Palmitic acid, however, does not appear to enhance calcium
sequestration by inhibiting the permeability of the SR membrane
to calcium. Furthermore, the finding that palmitic acid does
not enhance calcium sequestration in the absence of ATP or when
sequestration has been inhibited by A23187 argues against
palmitic acid promoting calcium binding to the outer membrane
surface of the vesicle (Figure 1). The ability of palmitic acid

to enhance calcium sequestration, therefore, requires that calcium be transported and concentrated in the SR vesicle interior. The generation of an A23187-insensitive calcium pool within the vesicle by palmitic acid (Table 3) suggests that this compound is interacting, possibly complexing, with a portion of the intravesicular calcium to generate a second pool of sequestered calcium and thereby enhance the total calcium sequestered by the SR membrane. The recent report demonstrating that micromolar concentrations of palmitic acid, but not oleic acid, can lower the ionized calcium concentration in aqueous solution further supports this view (19).

The findings reported here demonstrate that the effects of non-esterified fatty acids on isolated intact SR membrane function are complex; and these effects are dependent on both fatty acid aliphatic chain structure and the relative amounts of fatty acid and membrane present. Therefore, any potential role for the accumulation of these compounds in the deterioration of myocardial membrane function during ischemia must consider individual amphiphile structure as well as the total membrane compartment with which these amphiphiles will interact.

ACKNOWLEDGEMENTS

Supported by research grants HL-22135 and HL-21812 from the National Institutes of Health. Dr. Messineo is a Clinical Investigator (HL-00911) of NIH-NHLBI.

REFERENCES

1. Idell-Wenger, J., & Neely, J. (1978): IN Disturbances in Lipid and Lipoprotein Metabolism (eds) J. Dietschy, A. Gott, and Centko, American Physiological Society, Bethesda, MD p. 269.
2. Shaikh, N. A., & Downar, E. (1981): Circ. Res. 49: 316.
3. Van der Vusse, G. J., Roemen, Th. H. M., Prinzen, F. W., Coumans, W. A., & Reneman, R. S. (1982): Circ. Res. 50: 538.
4. Liedtke, A. J., Nellis, S., & Neely, J. R. (1972): Circ. Res. 13: 652.
5. Sobel, B. E., Corr, P. B., Robison, A. K., Goldstein, R. A., Witkowski, F. X., & Klein, M. S. (1978): J. Clin. Invest. 62: 546.
6. Katz, A. M., & Messineo, F. C. (1980): Circ. Res. 48: 1.
7. Liedtke, A. J. (1981): Prog. Cardiovasc. Dis. 23: 321.
8. Katz, A. M. (1982): J. Mol. Cell. Cardiol. 14: 627.
9. Messineo, F. C., Pinto, P. B., & Katz, A. M. (1980): J. Mol. Cell. Cardiol. 12: 725.

10. Adams, R. J., Cohen, D. W., Gupte, S., Johnson, J. D., Wallick, S. T., Wang, T., & Schwartz, A. (1979): J. Biol. Chem. 254: 12404.
11. Messineo, F. C., Rathier, M., Favreau, C., Watras, J., & Takenaka, H. (1984): J. Biol. Chem. 259: 1336.
12. Katz, A. M., Repke, D. I., & Hasselbach, W. (1977): J. Biol. Chem. 252: 1938.
13. Caswell, A. H., Lau, Y. H., & Brunschwig, J. P. (1970): Arch. Biochem. Biophys. 176: 417.
14. Takenaka, H., Adler, P. A., & Katz, A. M. (1982): J. Biol. Chem. 257: 12649.
15. Shigekawa, M., & Dougherty, J. P. (1978): J. Biol. Chem. 253: 1458.
16. Lee, A. G., East, J. M., Jones, O. T., McWhirter, J., Rooney, E. K., & Simmonds, A. C. (1982): Biochemistry 21: 6441.
17. Klausner, R., Kleinfeld, A., Hoover, R., & Karnovsky, M. (1980): J. Biol. Chem. 255: 1286.
18. Helenius, A., & Simons, K. (1975): Biochim. Biophys. Acta 415: 29.
19. Watras, J., Messineo, F.C., & Herbette, L. (1984): J. Biol. Chem. 259: 1319.

FACTORS INFLUENCING THE METABOLIC AND FUNCTIONAL ALTERATIONS INDUCED BY ISCHEMIA AND REPERFUSION

R. Ferrari, F. Di Lisa, R. Raddino, C. Bigoli, S. Curello,
C. Ceconi, A. Albertini*, and O. Visioli

*Chair of Cardiology and Institute of Chemistry
School of Medicine
University of Brescia, Brescia, Italy

Myocardial ischemia describes a condition that exists when fractional uptake of oxygen in the heart is not sufficient to maintain the rate of cellular oxidation. This leads to an extremely complex situation which has been extensively studied in recent years. Part of this complexity is due to the fact that experimental myocardial ischemia results in a non-homogeneous tissue damage which depends on the duration of the ischemic period, degree of coronary flow reduction and substrate availability.

Many authors have pointed out that there are wide differences in flow across an infarction area of myocardium (1, 2). It has been suggested that surrounding the severely damaged area (where coronary flow can be reduced to zero) may exist a region of moderate damage (where coronary flow is moderately reduced) separating it from the normally perfused non-ischemic tissue (3). Histological analyses have shown that adjacent individual heart cells may be differently affected. An ischemic zone, therefore, is a mixture of dead, dying and normal cells, subjected to a wide range of reduction in blood flow. The degree of coronary flow reduction during ischemia may influence the extent of ischemic damage, as it can provide some oxygen supply to the ischemic cell and remove metabolic products from the interstitial space.

Another important factor that may influence the degree of ischemic damage is the substrate composition of the coronary perfusate. High levels of fatty acids (FFA) have been found to be deleterious for the ischemic myocardium (4, 5), whilst glucose has been found to be protective (6). The mechanism of the toxic effects of FFA during ischemia is not completely understood. Fatty acids increase myocardial oxygen consumption when compared to carbohydrate (7), which may be detrimental during ischemia, when the oxygen supply is severely damaged. Alternatively, the toxic effect of fatty acids may be related to the intracellular accumulation of their intermediates (8, 9).

In this study the effects of different degrees and duration of coronary flow reduction on the metabolic and mechanical function of the isolated and perfused rabbit hearts have been investigated, and the effects of glucose, palmitate and the combination of the two substrates on the metabolic and mechanical function of the isolated and perfused hearts have been compared. Hearts were perfused under moderate ischemic conditions for 30 minutes, after which the effects of post-ischemic reperfusion were followed. Because the accumulation of free fatty acid intermediates has been associated with histological evidence of mitochondrial destruction (10), mitochondria were isolated and their function assessed by measuring calcium content, oxygen consumption, and the capacity to phosphorylate adenosine diphosphate.

METHODS

Perfusion of the Hearts

Adult New-Zealand white rabbits (2.5 to 3.0 kg) were stunned by a blow on the head. The hearts were rapidly excised and perfused by the non-recirculating Langendorff technique (11). A period of 30 minutes equilibration during which hearts were perfused with Krebs-Henseleit solution (12) equilibrated with 95% O_2 - 5% CO_2 was allowed before any experimental intervention. Hearts were then electrically paced at 180 beats/min as previously described (13) and subjected to three different degrees of global ischemia. Moderate ischemia was induced by reducing the coronary flow rate to 3 ml/min (12% of control value); severe ischemia by reducing the coronary flow to 1 ml/min (4% of control value); while in a third series of experiments coronary flow was completely abolished to provide no flow ischemia (total ischemia). Left ventricular wall temperature was maintained at 35 to 36° C, irrespective of coronary flow.

In separate groups of experiments the hearts were reperfused
after each period of ischemia. Reperfusion was for 30 minutes
at the aerobic, pre-ischemic coronary flow of 25 ml/min with
Krebs-Henseleit solution. In these experiments, when moderate
or severe ischemia was induced, the perfusate consisted of
Krebs-Henseleit buffer, equilibrated with 95% O_2 - 5% CO_2
and with glucose as substrate (11 mM). When the effects of FFA
on the ischemic myocardium were tested, the hearts were
separated in three groups depending on the substrate utilized:
glucose 11 mM (group 1); palmitate 1.2 mM (group 2); glucose
11 mM + palmitate 1.2 mM (group 3). In group 2 glucose was
replaced with an equimolar concentration of mannitol.
Palmitate, as sodium salt, was bound to 3% bovine serum albumin
as described by Oram (14), and palmitate concentration
determined on the final perfusate by the procedure of Ducombe
(15). The hearts were either perfused under aerobic conditions
for 60 minutes, made ischemic for 30 minutes (by reducing
coronary flow from 25 to 3 ml/min), or made ischemic for 30
minutes and then reperfused for 30 minutes. During reperfusion,
glucose 11 mM was always the only substrate.

Left Ventricular Pressure Measurements

To obtain an isovolumetrically beating preparation, a fluid
filled balloon was inserted into the left ventricular cavity via
the atrium. The intraventricular balloon was then connected by
a fluid filled polyethylene catheter to a Statham pressure
transducer (P 23 D 6) for the determination of left ventricular
pressure.

Isolation of Mitochondria

Mitochondria were isolated at the end of each perfusion by
differential centrifugation with conventional homogenization
methods as previously described, using either a KCl, BSA and
EDTA-containing medium or a medium containing sucrose and
ruthenium red (16).

Oxygen Consumption Measurements

Rates of oxygen consumption were monitored polarographically
at 25° C using a Clark electrode. The reaction media were
idential to those previously described (16, 17).

Protein Determination

Protein determination was made as described by Bradford,
following hypotonic shock (18).

Mitochondrial ATP Production

ATP synthesis was initiated by adding ADP to provide a final concentration of 0.5 mM. Samples were taken before and at 6, 15, 30, 45, 60, 120 and 180 seconds after adding the ADP. They were then mixed with 50 1 of 10% perchloric acid on ice. Precipitated protein was separated by centrifugation and the ATP content of the supernatant determined enzymatically (19).

Mitochondrial Calcium Content

Mitochondrial calcium content was determined by atomic absorption spectrometry. Mitochondrial pellets were digested overnight in 500 1 HNO_3. $CaCO_3$ was used as the standard.

Tissue ATP and CP

The perfusion of the hearts in which ATP and CP levels were to be measured were terminated by freeze clamping with aluminum tongs (20). The frozen muscle was then pulverized, homogenized and assayed for ATP and CP as previously described (19).

Tissue Calcium

At the end of the perfusion period duplicate samples of left ventricular muscle were taken and digested in 1 ml/g wet wt. of nitric acid (HNO_3). The extracts were diluted in 25 ml of deionized water and the calcium content was assayed spectrophotometrically using a Perkin Elmer atomic absorption spectrometer (mod. 306). Lanthanum trichloride was added to provide a final concentration of 0.1 percent. Total tissue water was obtained by drying to constant weight at 95° C.

CPK Activity

During each perfusion, the coronary effluent was collected in chilled glass vials and assayed, on the same day, for CPK (creatine phosphokinase). CPK activity was determined by the method of Oliver (21).

Statistical Analysis

Results are expressed as mean $\pm$ standard error of the mean. Tests of significance were made using Student's t tests, taking P = 0.05 as the limit of significance.

RESULTS

Effects of Duration and Degree of Coronary Flow Reduction

In the isolated rabbit hearts perfused under aerobic
condition at coronary flow of 25 ± 1.72 ml/min for 120 minutes
with oxygenated Krebs-Henseleit buffer (with glucose 11 mM as
substrate), the developed pressure remained constant for the
first 60 minutes of perfusion and was only slightly decreased
after 120 minutes (Figure 1a). When coronary flow was reduced
from the unrestricted rate of 25 ml/min to 3 ml/min (Figure 1b)
or abolished (Figure 2), developed pressure rapidly fell to near
zero. Contractile activity ceased completely 10 minutes after
the coronary flow was reduced to 1 ml/min (data not shown) or
0 ml/min (Figure 2). In contrast, 70 minutes after reduction of
coronary flow to 3 ml/min, developed tension was still 6% of
control values and ventricular activity ceased completely only
80 minutes after the onset of low flow perfusion (Figure 1b).

When coronary flow was reduced to 3 ml/min, resting pressure
did not change significantly during the first 40 minutes, after
which started to increase (Figure 1b). This pattern is in
contrast to that seen with 1 ml/min ischemia (data not shown) or
zero flow ischemia in which resting pressure began to rise as
early as 20 minutes after the onset of ischemia (Figure 2).

Reperfusion after 30 minutes of ischemia resulted in a rapid
decline of resting pressure in all groups. When the ischemic
period was prolonged to 60 minutes, reperfusion resulted in a
small, further increase in resting pressure, followed by a
decline towards control (Figure 1b). However, after 30 minutes
of reperfusion following 60 minutes of no flow ischemia, resting
pressure was still increased (Figure 2), while for the 3 ml/min
group it was almost at the control values (Figure 1b).
Reperfusion after 90 minutes of ischemia resulted in a marked
increase in resting pressure in the total ischemia group (Figure
2). In the 3 ml/min group, resting pressure started to decline
after an initial increase, and at the end of 30 minutes of
reperfusion was 5 ± 0.9 mmHg (Figure 1b). Reperfusion of the
ischemic hearts resulted in some restoration of their capacity
to generate active tension (Figures 1b and 2), the percentage of
recovery being inversely proportional to the duration of the
ischemic period (Table 1). Table 1 and Figures 1 and 2 show
that the degree of developed pressure recovered during
reperfusion was also inversely proportional to the degree of
reduction of coronary flow, the highest percentage of tension
recovery occurring in the group with coronary flow rate
maintained at 3 ml/min and the lowest in the group with no
coronary flow.

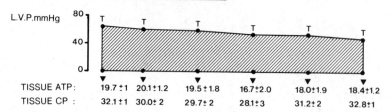

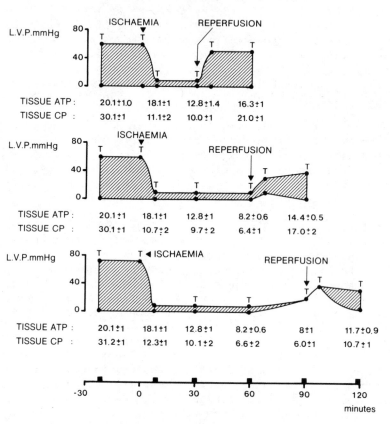

FIGURE 1

Effect of the duration of moderate ischemia and subsequent
reperfusion on mechanical function and tissue ATP and CP content
in isolated and perfused rabbit hearts. Data are mean ±
standard error of at least six separate experiments. Under
control and reperfusion conditions the hearts were perfused with
Krebs-Henseleit buffer at a mean of coronary flow of 25 ml/min.
Ischemia was induced by reducing coronary flow to 3 ml/min.
Tissue ATP and CP are expressed as µmoles/g dry wt.

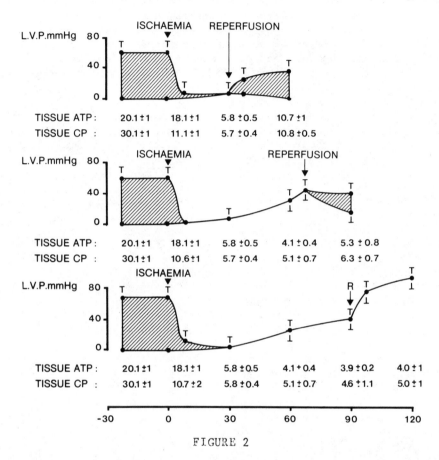

FIGURE 2

Effect of duration of the total ischemic period and subsequent reperfusion on mechanical function and tissue ATP and CP content of the isolated and perfused rabbit hearts. The data are the mean values ± standard error of at least six separate experiments. Under control and reperfusion conditions the hearts were perfused with Krebs-Henseleit buffer at a mean of coronary flow of 25 ml/min. Ischemia was induced by abolishing completely coronary flow. Tissue ATP and CP are expressed as μmoles/g dry wt.

Figure 1a shows that tissue ATP and CP levels were virtually constant during 120 minutes of aerobic perfusion. As expected, 30 minutes of ischemia reduced ATP and CP levels significantly. The fall in ATP and CP concentration after 30 minutes of ischemia was proportional to the severity of the ischemic condition, the decline in CP being greater than that for ATP. The decline in ATP and CP concentrations, however, was not proportional to the duration of ischemia as there was not a significant difference between the ATP and CP values after 60 and 90 minutes of ischemia.

The effects of reperfusion on absolute values of ATP and CP content of the hearts are shown in Figure 1 and 2, and the percentage of ATP recovered after 30 minutes of reperfusion in Table 2. Restoration of coronary flow after 30 minutes of ischemia resulted in a significant (P<0.05) increase of ATP and CP contents in both groups when compared with the ischemic values obtained before reperfusion. In none of the hearts, however, were the ATP and CP concentrations restored completely to the aerobic control value. The percentage of recovery of ATP after reperfusion was inversely proportional to the duration of the ischemic period, and the percentage of ATP recovered after reperfusion was also inversely proportional to the degree of reduction of coronary flow (Table 2). Figure 3 shows that there was an association between the tissue ATP content measured at the end of 30 minutes of reperfusion and the maximum recovery of developed pressure after 30 minutes of reperfusion.

TABLE 1. Percentage Recovery of Developed Pressure During Reperfusion

Duration of Ischemia (Min) before Reperfusion	30	60	90
Moderate low flow ischemia (3 ml/min)	100	65	53
Severe low flow ischemia (1 ml/min)	83	39	21
No flow ischemia	62	20	0

The percentage of developed tension recovered after 30 minutes of reperfusion is calculated with respect to the pressure developed before the onset of ischemia.

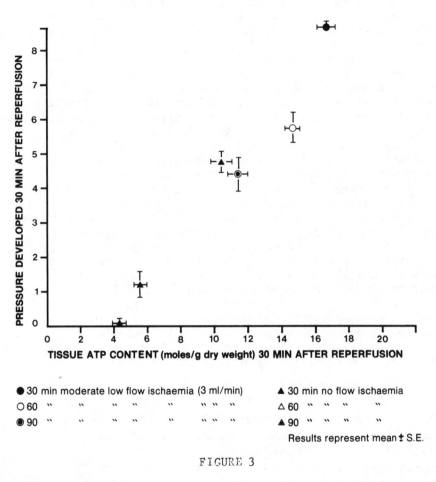

Results represent mean ± S.E.

FIGURE 3

Relation between tissue ATP content and recovery of developed pressure after reperfusion.

Effects of Fatty Acid During Ischemia

Figure 4 shows the effects of 30 minutes of moderate ischemia (3 ml/min) followed by reperfusion, using glucose as the only substrate, while Figure 5 shows the effects of the same period of ischemia when palmitate was the only substrate during ischemia. Figure 4 shows that, as expected, when coronary flow was reduced from the unrestricted rate of 25 ml/min to 3 ml/min, developed pressure fell rapidly towards zero. Resting pressure did not change significantly during ischemia or reperfusion, and CPK release during ischemia was not significantly different from that observed during aerobic perfusion. Thirty minutes of moderate ischemia significantly reduced tissue ATP and CP levels, CP declining to a greater extent than ATP. The data illustrated in Figure 4 also show that when glucose was present, reduction of coronary flow from 25 ml/min to 3 ml/min did not significantly modify tissue and mitochondrial calcium content, or isolated mitochondrial function measured in terms of rate of respiration during ATP synthesis (QO_2) and total ATP production. Reperfusion resulted in a prompt recovery of active pressure generation. During the first 10 minutes of reperfusion there was a transient increase of CPK concentrations in the coronary effluent that was followed by a decline towards control, pre-ischemic values. Re-establishment of coronary flow also resulted in a signficiant, but incomplete, recovery of tissue ATP and CP concentrations. Reperfusion did not significantly affect tissue and mitochondrial calcium concentrations or isolated mitochondrial function. Figure 5 shows that when palmitate was used as the only substrate during ischemia, reduction of coronary flow to 3 ml/min induced a rapid decline of developed pressure, contractile activity of the hearts ceased completely 5 minutes after the onset of ischemia.

TABLE 2. Percentage of Recovery of Tissue ATP during Reperfusion

Duration of Ischemia (Min) before Reperfusion	30	60	90
Moderate low flow ischemia (3 ml/min)	90	79.3	64.5
Severe low flow ischemia (1 ml/min)	74.9	38.1	37.4
No flow ischemia	59	29.2	23.7

The percentage of ATP recovery after 30 minutes of reperfusion is calculated with respect to the values obtained before the onset of ischemia.

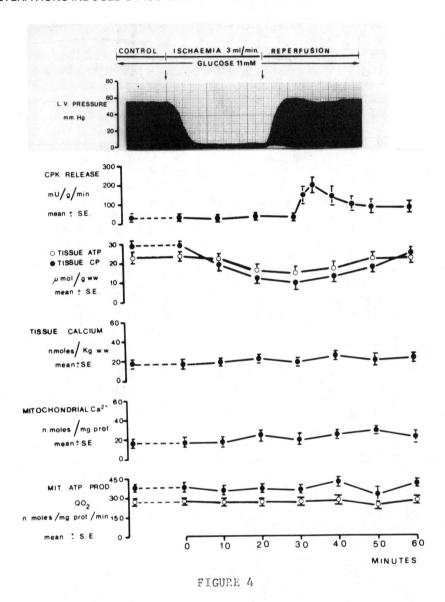

FIGURE 4

Effect of moderate ischemia and reperfusion on mechanical and
metabolic function of isolated, perfused rabbit hearts.
Substrate during ischemia was 11 mM glucose. Under control and
reperfusion conditions hearts were perfused with Krebs-Henseleit
buffer containing 11 mM glucose as substrate. Data are mean ±
standard error of at least six experiments. P is the
significance of the difference between values obtained during
aerobic perfusion and those obtained during ischemia and
reperfusion.

At this time resting pressure was unchanged. However, 10
minutes after the onset of ischemia resting pressure began to
rise progressively and, by the end of 30 minutes, had increased
to 79 $\pm$ 11 mmHg. During ischemia there was significantly more
release of CPK than when glucose was used as substrate (compare
with Figure 4). Tissue ATP and CP were severely reduced after
30 minutes of ischemia. Tissue calcium was unchanged after
ischemia, while mitochondrial calcium content was increased
after 30 minutes of ischemia. Mitochondrial QO_2 and ATP
production were also reduced after 30 min. of ischemia.
Reperfusion of these hearts with a perfusate containing 11 mM
glucose as substrate resulted in a small, insignificant decline
of resting pressure and a minor recovery of developed pressure
(compare with Figure 4). Reperfusion also resulted in a marked
release of CPK into the coronary effluent. (The scales of CPK
release are different in Figures 4 and 5.) Readmission of
coronary flow did not result in a recovery of tissue ATP and CP
concentrations, but were followed by a large, significant
increase of tissue and mitochondrial calcium content.
Mitochondria isolated after 30 minutes of post-ischemic
reperfusion were virtually incapable of phosphorylating ADP to
ATP.

Addition of 11 mM glucose to palmitate as substrate during
the ischemic period provided some protection from the effects
shown in Figure 5. Resting pressure did not increase during
ischemia and reperfusion, and on readmission of coronary flow
there was a greater recovery of active pressure generation
(Figure 6). The decline of tissue ATP and CP during ischemia
was significantly reduced, and there was some recovery of both
these nucleotides during reperfusion (Figure 5). Mitochondrial
calcium did not increase during ischemia and tissue and
mitochondrial calcium overloading during post-ischemic
reperfusion were almost abolished. Isolated mitochondrial
function was maintained either after ischemia or after
reperfusion.

DISCUSSION

Effect of Duration and Degree of Coronary Flow Reduction

These results indicate that the extent of ischemic damage,
and whether or not reperfusion is beneficial or detrimental to
ischemic myocardium, depends upon the severity and the duration
of ischemia. Increasing the severity and the duration of the
ischemic period reduces the recovery of normal myocardial
function on reperfusion.

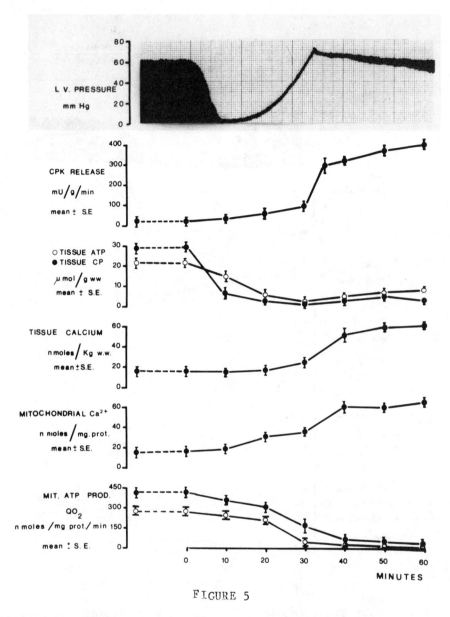

FIGURE 5

Effect of moderate ischemia and reperfusion on mechanical and
metabolic function of isolated, perfused rabbit hearts.
Substrate during ischemia was 1.2 mM palmitate. Under control
and reperfusion conditions hearts were perfused with
Krebs-Henseleit buffer containing 11 mM glucose as substrate.
Data are mean ± standard error of at least six experiments.
P is the significance of the difference between values obtained
during aerobic perfusion and those obtained during ischemia and
reperfusion.

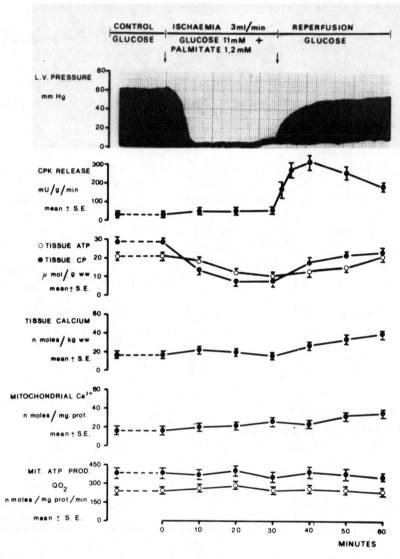

FIGURE 6

Effect of moderate ischemia and reperfusion on mechanical and
metabolic function of isolated, perfused rabbit hearts.
Substrates during ischemia were 11 mM glucose and 1.2 mM
palmitate. Under control and reperfusion conditions hearts were
perfused with Krebs-Henseleit buffer containing 11 mM glucose as
substrate. Data are mean ± standard error of at least six
experiments. P is the significance of the difference between
values obtained during aerobic perfusion and those obtained
during ischemia and reperfusion.

The reduction or the abolition of coronary flow induced a
very rapid cessation of contraction, followed by a progressive
rise in resting tension. Increasing the degree of coronary flow
reduction had no effect on the decine of developed pressure, but
increased the rise of resting tension. The decline of active
pressure generation induced by ischemia has important metabolic
consequences because it removes an enormous energy drain on the
cell, as the maintenance of contraction utilizes almost 75% of
total cellular ATP production. It is possible that the residual
ATP content during the first 30 minutes of ischemia was
sufficient to maintain basic cellular functions, such as control
of cell volume, maintenance of ionic homeostasis and
preservation of ultrastructure (22, 23), thereby allowing
recovery of metabolic and mechanical function on reperfusion.
It is clear from our results, that residual coronary flow plays
an important role even in this early stage of ischemia as the
recovery on reperfusion was greater for the hearts exposed to
moderate ischemia than for those made total ischemic (Figures 1
and 2). The finding of an incomplete restoration of ATP and CP
content even after reperfusion of the hearts made ischemic for
30 minutes at 3 ml/min (Figure 1), is probably due to a
reduction of adenine nucleotide pool in the ischemic cell (24),
rather than to a defect of mitochondrial ATP producing capacity,
which was, in fact, unchanged (Figure 4).

Extending the ischemic period to 60 and 90 minutes resulted
in progression of the ischemic damage, as resting pressure
increased further, and ATP and CP levels decreased further
(Figures 1 and 2). The progression of ischemic damage seems to
be delayed by the presence of residual coronary flow. When
coronary flow was reduced by 78% from control levels for 90
minutes, ATP and CP levels were better maintained than when
coronary flow was completely abolished for the same period of
time (Figures 1 and 2). It is possible that during low flow
ischemia (3 ml/min) the hearts reached a new state where the
rate of cellular ATP hydrolysis is reduced by the depressed
mechanical activity to almost match the lower ATP production.
Under ischemic conditions, however, several metabolic pathways
continue to utilize the free energy provided by ATP. They
include reactions involved in the maintenance of ion disribution
and cell volume (25), enzyme reactions such as adenylate cyclase
(26), myokinase (27), fatty acid synthetase (28), and protein
kinase (29). In addition, ATP is essential for maintenance of
normal cell structure, biosynthesis of proteins, nucleic acids,
complex carbohydrates and lipids. It is also necessary,
indirectly, for mitochondrial oxidative phosphorylation as ATP
provides for the entry of glucose into the glycolytic pathway
and the activation of fatty acids. In the 3 ml/min group,
however, the residual ATP was not sufficient to prevent the

increase in resting pressure, an abnormality which depends on
both ATP and tissue calcium (30, 31).

Residual ATP may just suffice to support basic cellular
functions, such as maintenance of ionic homeostasis and
preservation of ultrastructure. Readmission of flow at the
stage of ischemic damage where cellular membranes are presumably
still intact, some cellular supplies of ATP are available, and
pathways of electron transport and oxidative phosphorylation are
simply blocked and not damaged, should result in a re-
energization of the electron transport pathway. This, in turn,
should lead to at least a partial restoration of oxidative
phosphorylation and ATP production, with a resumption of
contractile activity. There is, in fact, an association between
these two parameters, as shown in Figure 3.

Extending the period of total ischemia to 60 and 90 minutes
resulted in a further depletion of the high energy phosphate
stores. This suggests that in this group of experiments ATP
consumption during ischemia exceeded ATP production. Under
severe ischemic conditions, there is almost no possibility of
ATP production. Oxygen uptake is abolished, and anaerobic
glycolysis is severely inhibited by the intracellular
accumulation of H^+, NADH and lactate (32). Theoretically some
ATP synthesis could be coupled to the reverse flux of ions
through an ATP-dependent ion pump such as the Ca-ATPase of the
sarcoplasmic reticulum or the Na-K ATPase of the sarcolemma. It
is still uncertain if an ischemic episode brings about the
conditions necessary for reversing the ATPase-dependent calcium
flux across the sarcoplasmic reticulum, but, in any case, it is
unlikely that the amount of ATP produced by this process is of
great importance. Reperfusion after 90 minutes of severe
ischemia did not lead to a re- establishment of the cell
function; but instead produced further an increase of resting
pressure and no recovery of developed pressure or high energy
phosphate groups. A number of mechanisms have been suggested to
explain these findings. From our previous studies (13, 17, 33,
34) it appears that mitochondrial function plays an important
role in the molecular mechanism of reperfusion damage after
prolonged periods of ischemia. In particular, it has been
proposed (35), and confirmed by us (13, 33), that with the
readmission of coronary flow after a prolonged period of severe
ischemia there is an abundant supply of external calcium that
enters the myocardium. At this stage, the cell membrane no
longer acts as a permeability barrier to ions such as calcium.
The mechanism of this alteration is unclear; it may be related,
as it will be discussed in more detail later, to the detergent
action of FFA metabolites, to lesions caused by the action of
free radicals generated by the re-introduction of oxygen (37),

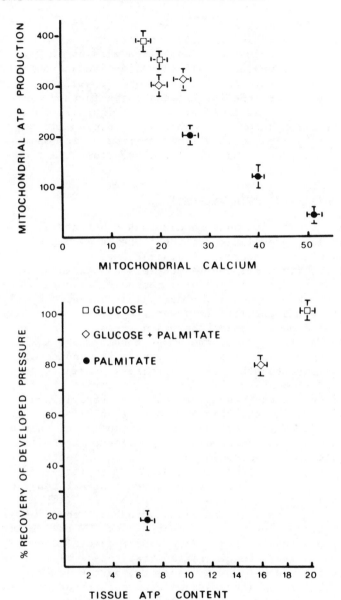

FIGURE 7

Relationship between mitochondrial calcium content and
mitochondrial ATP production after different conditions of
perfusion. Mitochondria were isolated in medium containing
ruthenium red and in the absence of a chelating agent, so that
they would retain their endogenous calcium. Results are
expressed as the mean ± standard error.

or the severe ATP reduction. Whichever mechanism is involved,
this leads to an increased calcium concentration at the time
when mitochondria are re-energized by readmission of O_2. When
given the choice of producing ATP via oxidative phosphorylation
or accumulating calcium, cardiac mitochondria will
preferentially perform the latter, causing a further decrease in
ATP synthesis (36). The data reported in Figure 7, showing an
inverse correlation between mitochondrial calcium content and
ATP production by mitochondria isolated from hearts made
ischemic with different substrates and reperfused, are an
indirect confirmation of this hypothesis.

Effects of Substrate During Ischemia

From our results it would appear that substrate availability
is important in the evolution of the ischemic damage of the
isolated and perfused hearts. Glucose alone, or in association
with palmitate, minimized the deleterious consequences of
inadequate oxygenation and restored mechanical function on
reperfusion (Figures 4 and 6). When palmitate was the only
substrate, ischemia resulted in severe impairment of metabolic
and mechanical function and there was no recovery on
reperfusion. In this group, there was a remarkable and
progressive increase of diastolic pressure 10 minutes after the
onset of ischemia, together with a progressive reduction in
tissue ATP and CP content. Tissue calcium during the first 20
minutes of ischemia was unchanged, but mitochondrial calcium was
increased, indicating that the presence of palmitate during
ischemia induced an intracellular redistribution of calcium.
Cytosolic calcium concentration increased, the extramitochondrial calcium concentration being the major factor
determining calcium accumulation (38, 39). An increase of
cytosolic calcium, together with a decrease of ATP can explain
the increase in resting pressure (Figure 5) (23). This
alteration of intracellular calcium homeostasis could be
dependent on: (a) severe reduction of tissue ATP as ATP is
necessary to prevent the redistribution of calcium down
previously established concentration gradients; (b) an increased
sarcolemmal membrane cation permeability, particularly for
calcium, leading to an increased calcium uptake during ischemia;
or, (c) an increased release of calcium from the sarcoplasmic
reticulum to the cytosol.

When palmitate is the only substrate, the accelerated
development of ischemic abnormalities indicates the existence of
some alteration not occurring when glucose, or glucose +
palmitate, are substrates. The following discussion examines
the question: Why should palmitate, during ischemia, induce an
earlier and more severe ATP and CP depletion than glucose?

In our experiments this effect does not depend on mechanical factors, as the hearts developed exactly the same pressure before the onset of ischemia and the decline of contractility in the early stage of ischemia was the same, independently of the substrate utilized. It does not depend on changes in osmolarity, as the hearts perfused with palmitate received an equimolar concentration of mannitol. The most likely explanation, therefore, is related to the ability of exogenous glucose to enhance glycolytic ATP production and to the deleterious effect of palmitate on mitochondrial function. Under conditions of moderate ischemia, as chosen in this study, the rate of anaerobic glycolysis has been shown to be accelerated (40).

Our earlier results indicate that during 3 ml/min ischemia some of the ATP is derived from oxidative metabolism, as the substitution of N_2 for O_2 in the perfusate resulted in a reduction of the ATP and CP levels. When palmitate was used as the only ischemic substrate, anaerobic glycolysis could not occur and the isolated mitochondrial function, including ATP production after 20 and 30 minutes of ischemia, was significantly reduced while with glucose it was unchanged. Although function of isolated mitochondria is not necessarily representative of their function in the cell, these data suggest that the residual oxidative ATP production was reduced when palmitate was used as substrate.

The reason why mitochondrial function should be altered when palmitate is substrate is not completely understood. An association between accumulation of FFA intermediates and histological mitochondrial destruction has been reported which could be the result of a detergent effect on mitochondrial membrane (10, 41). Alternatively, function could be altered as the consequence of increased mitochondrial calcium concentration. Figure 7 shows an inverse relationship between mitochondrial calcium content and ATP-producing capacity, and it is known that Ca^{2+} ions play an important role in the regulation of mitochondrial metabolism (42-44). The capacity to oxidize oxoglutarate and other substrates diminishes when mitochondria are overloaded with calcium (45). An increased calcium concentration, together with high levels of long-chain acyl CoA has also been shown to inhibit the adenine nucleotide translocator (46-48) which reduces the capacity for ATP transport from the mitochondria to the cytosol that further decreases the cytosolic ATP pool.

The maintenance of the normal calcium homeostasis implies the movement of Ca^{2+} against gradients, and therefore is an energy-dependent process. It is quite likely that during the

ischemic episode with palmitate, the tissue level of ATP could
fall below the level required for the maintenance of normal
cytosolic Ca^{2+} concentration.

Another possible explanation of our data is that these
alterations in calcium homeostasis are the result of membrane
damage due to accumulation of fatty acids and of their
intermediates in the myocardium. The reduced supply of oxygen
in the myocardial cell decreases β-oxidation rate (48), with a
consequent accumulation of long-chain acyl derivatives (8, 9).
These intermediates accumulate into the matrix space mostly as
long-chain acyl CoA and into the cytosol as long-chain acyl
carnitine. These acyl esters have detergent properties which
may alter several membrane functions and inhibit the Na^+-K^+
ATPase. The finding of an increased CPK release in the hearts
made ischemic with palmitate suggests an altered sarcolemmal
permeability. Under ischemic conditions, FFA toxicity may also
be related to the presence in the cell of FFA that are not
activated because of the reduced rate of β-oxidation (49, 50).
However the time course of the accumulation of nonesterified FA
in ischemic myocardium is slow, and these accumulate only as a
late event after 60 minutes of ischemia (51).

The possibility that the alteration of calcium homeostasis
induced by palmitate is due to an increased release of Ca^{2+}
from the sarcoplasmic reticulum is the most unlikely explanation
as it has been shown that palmitic acid enhances calcium
sequestration and not calcium release by sarcoplasmic reticulum
vesicles (50).

Whatever the mechanism involved, reperfusion of the ischemic
hearts when energy reserves are depleted and mitochondria
already overloaded with calcium, results in a massive,
respiration-linked uptake of Ca^{2+} and its irreversible
sequestration into mitochondria as Ca^{2+}-phosphate (52). When
palmitate was used as substrate, tissue and mitochondrial
calcium were three to four fold increased after 30 minutes of
reperfusion. This would impair the mitochondrial respiratory
function and the capacity to produce ATP so that a vicious
circle is probably established preventing restoration of the
already depleted energy reserves.

These deleterious effects of palmitate are completely
overcome by the addition of glucose in the ischemic perfusate
(Figure 6). There is not a simple explanation for this effect
of glucose. It could be related to an inhibition of fatty acid
uptake in general, as the myocardial cell prefers glucose as
carbon substrate during ischemia (53), or it could be due to an
increased rate of anaerobic glycolysis and oxidative

phosphorylation with a consequent reduction of ATP loss. Thus, sufficient ATP could remain available during the early stages of ischemia to maintain membrane ultrastructure and Ca^{2+} homeostasis. Under these circumstances, cytosolic calcium would not increase and mitochondria would not become overloaded with calcium, while resting tension would not rise.

In conclusion, many factors that may influence the severity of ischemic damage should be taken into account in studies that assess the effect of therapy on experimental myocardial ischemia or infarction. Different substrate availability can be achieved in the open chest, anesthetized dog, and such variation could account for some of the variation among animals and conflicting reports from different laboratories. Furthermore, as a two-fold increase in serum free fatty acids has been observed in patients suffering acute myocardial infarction (54), experiments designed to study the changes during acute ischemia and their possible clinical implications must consider the role of FFA as the ischemic substrate.

ACKNOWLEDGEMENTS

This work was partially supported by the Italian CNR grant CT 81.00379.04.

REFERENCES

1. Waters, D.D., Da Luz, P., Wyatt, H.L., Swan, J.C., & Forrester, J.S. (1977): Am. J. Cardiol. 39: 537.
2. Opie, L.H. (1980): Am. Heart J. 100: 355.
3. Hearse, D.J., Opie, L.H., Katzeff, I.E., Lubbe, W.F., Van Der Welf, T.J., Persach, M., & Boulle, G. (1977): Am. J. Cardiol. 40: 176.
4. Katz, A.M., & Messineo, F.C. (1981): Circ. Res. 48: 1.
5. Neely, J.R., & Feuvray, D. (1981): Am. J. Pathol. 102: 282.
6. Opie, L.H., & Bicknell, O.L. (1979): Cardiovasc. Res. 13: 693.
7. Vik-Mo, H., & Mjos, O.D. (1983): IN Myocardial Ischemia and Protection (ed) H. Refoum, P. Jynge, & O.P. Mjos, Churchill Livingstone, London, p. 35.
8. Liedtke, A.J. (1978): Circ. Res. 43: 652.
9. Lochner, A., Kotze, J.C.N., Benade, A.J.S., & Gevers, W. (1978): J. Mol. Cell. Cardiol. 10: 857.
10. Feuvray, D., & Plovet, J. (1981): Circ. Res. 48: 740.
11. Langendorff, O. (1895): Pflugers Archiv. 61: 291.

12. Krebs, H.A., & Henseleit, K. (1932): Hoppe-Seyler's Zeit.
    fur Physiol. Chem. 210: 33.
13. Ferrari, R., Williams, A., & Di Lisa, F. (1982): IN
    Advances in Studies on Heart Metabolism (eds) C.M.
    Caldarera, & P. Harris, Clueb, Bologna, p. 245.
14. Oram, J., Benntch, S.L., & Neely, J.R. (1973): J. Biol.
    Chem. 248: 5299.
15. Ducombe, W.G. (1964): Clin. Chim. Acta 9: 122.
16. Nayler, W.G., Ferrari, R., & Williams, A. (1980): Am. J.
    Cardiol. 46: 242.
17. Ferrari, R., Di Lisa, F., Raddino, R., & Visioli, O.
    (1982): J. Mol. Cell. Cardiol. 14: 737.
18. Bradford, M. (1978): Anal. Biochem. 72: 243.
19. Lamprecht, W., & Trautschold, E. (1974): IN Methodes of
    Enzymatic Analysis (ed) H.U. Bergmeyer, Academic Press, New
    York, p. 2101.
20. Wollenberger, A., Ristau, O., & Scoffa, G. (1960): Pflugers
    Archiv. 270: 399.
21. Oliver, I.T.A. (1955): Biochem. J. 61: 116.
22. Nayler, W.G., Poole-Wilson, P.A., & Williams, A. (1979): J.
    Mol. Cell. Cardiol. 11: 683.
23. Watts, J.A., Charles, O.K., & Lanoue, K.F. (1980): Am. J.
    Physiol. 238: H909.
24. Jennings, R.B., & Reimer, K.A. (1981): Am. J. Pathol. 102:
    241.
25. Langer, G.A. (1974): IN The Mammalian Myocardium (eds)
    G.A. Langer & A.J. Brady, J. Wiley and Sons Inc., New York,
    p. 193.
26. Dobson, J.G., & Mayer, S.E. (1973): Circ. Res. 33: 412.
27. Berne, R.M., & Rubio, R. (1974): Circ. Res. 23: 109.
28. Wood, J.M., Hutchings, A.E., & Brachfeld, N. (1972): J.
    Mol. Cell. Cardiol. 4: 97.
29. Larner, J. (1978): Circ. Res. 38 (Suppl. 1): 2.
30. Nayler, W.G. (1981): Am. J. Pathol. 102: 262.
31. Hearse, D.J., Garlick, P.B., & Humphrey, S.M. (1976): Am.
    J. Cardiol. 39: 286.
32. Rovetto, M.J., Lamberton, W.F., & Neely, J.R. (1975): Circ.
    Res. 37: 42.
33. Ferrari, R., Williams, A.J., & Nayler, W.G. (1979): J. Mol.
    Cell. Cardiol. 11: 13.
34. Ferrari, R., Di Lisa, F., Raddino, R., Curello, S., Ceconi,
    C., & Visioli, O. (1983): J. Mol. Cell. Cardiol. 15: 6.
35. Hearse, D.J. (1977): J. Mol. Cell. Cardiol. 9: 607.
36. Williams, A.J., Crie, J.S., & Ferrari, R. (1980):
    Circulation 62: 177.
37. Meerson, F.Z., Kagan, V.E., Yu, P., Kozlov, L.M., Belkina,
    U., & Arkhipenko, I. (1982): Basic Res. Cardiol. 17: 465.
38. Nicholis, D., & Crompton, M. (1980): FEBS Lett. 11: 261.
39. Lehninger, A.L. (1974): Circ. Res. 35: 83.

40. Neely, J.R., Whitmer, J.T., & Rovetto, M.Y. (1975): Circ. Res. 37: 733.
41. Smith, M.W., Collon, Y., Kaing, M., & Trump, B.F. (1980): Biochim. Biophys. Acta 618: 1992.
42. Henry, P.D., Schuchleid, R., Davis, J., Weiss, E.S., & Sobel, B.E. (1977): Am. J. Physiol. 233: H677.
43. Parr, D.R., Wimhurst, J.M., & Harris, E.J. (1973): Cardiovasc. Res. 9: 366.
44. McCormarck, J.G., & Denton, R.M. (1980): Biochem. J. 190: 5.
45. Denton, R.M., McCormarck, J.G., & Edgell, N.J. (1980): Biochem. J. 190: 107.
46. Shug, A.L., Shrago, E., Bittar, V., Folts, J.D., & Koke, J.R. (1975): Am. J. Physiol. 228: 689.
47. Shrago, E., Shug, A.L., Sul, H., Bittar, V., & Folts, J.D. (1970): Circ. Res. 38: 1.
48. Whitmer, J.T., Wenger, J.I., Rovetto, M.J., & Neely, J.R. (1978): J. Biol. Chem. 253: 430.
49. Adams, R.J., Cohen, W., Gupte, S., Johnson, J.D., Wallik, E., Wang, T., & Schwartz, A. (1979): J. Biol. Chem. 254: 12404.
50. Messineo, F.C., Pinto, P.B., & Katz, A.M. (1980): J. Mol. Cell. Cardiol. 12: 725.
51. Van der Vusse, G.J., Roemen, T.H.N., Prinzen, W.F., Comans, W.A., & Reneman, R.S. (1982): Circ. Res. 50: 538.
52. Jennings, R.B., Ganote, C.E. (1976): Circ. Res. 38: 80.
53. Idell-Wenger, J.A., & Neely, J.R. (1978): IN Disturbances in lipid and lipoprotein metabolism (eds) J.M. Dietschy, A.M. Giotto, & J.A. Ontko, American Physiological Society, Baltimore.
54. Oliver, M.F., Kurier, V.A., & Greenwood, T.W. (1968): Lancet i: 710.

FACTORS THAT INFLUENCE MYOCARDIAL LEVELS OF LONG-CHAIN ACYL CoA

AND ACYL CARNITINE

J. R. Neely and K. H. McDonough*

Department of Physiology
The Milton S. Hershey Medical Center
Hershey, PA 17033

*Department of Physiology
Louisiana State University Medical Center
New Orleans, LA 70112

High levels of fatty acids frequently have been found to be
detrimental to ischemic myocardium (for review see 1). The
mechanism of these effects is not understood but several
possibilities exist. First, it seems very clear that fatty
acids increase myocardial oxygen consumption when compared to
carbohydrates (2, 3). The theoretical increase in oxygen
consumption if the heart were using 100% lipid compared to 100%
carbohydrate is about 13%. However, increases in oxygen
consumption at constant workload caused by high levels of fatty
acids range from 20 to 50% (2, 3). Obviously, this increase in
oxygen consumption under conditions of limited oxygen supply,
such as ischemia, may place the heart in a negative energy
balance and precipitate a compensatory reduction in function.

A second possible mechanism of the fatty acid effects may
relate to accumulation in the tissue of either free fatty acids
or their long-chain acyl esters of CoA and carnitine (4). Under
normal aerobic conditions, long-chain acyl CoA and carnitine do
not accumulate to any significant extent even when abnormally
high levels of exogenous fatty acids are present (3). This
results from the fact that normal control of fatty acid
oxidation residues within the citric acid cycle at one end of
the pathway and at production of acyl CoA and carnitine on the

other end (3, 5). The cell contains a limited supply of CoA and
carnitine, and, when excess fatty acids are available, their
oxidation is limited by the activity of the citric acid cycle.
This, in turn, causes the conversion of CoA and carnitine to
their acetyl esters, and the limited supply of free CoA and
carnitine in the cytosol does not allow production of excessive
long-chain acyl CoA and carnitine. However, under oxygen
deficient conditions, β-oxidation becomes limited due to high
mitochondrial levels of NADH and $FADH_2$ (6). This prevents the
conversion of CoA and carnitine to their acetyl esters and
allows production and accumulation of high levels of their
long-chain acyl esters (6, 7).

Whether these acyl esters are responsible for increased
oxygen consumption and the reported alterations in mechanical
and electrical activity of the heart under oxygen deficient
conditions is not known. It is clear that both acyl CoA and
acyl carnitine affect the activity of several isolated enzyme
systems (for review see 1). It is also clear that both of the
acyl esters have detergent properties which could
non-specifically alter several membrane functions. In this
regard, the heart contains from 10 to 20 times more carnitine
than CoA and acyl esters of carnitine accumulate during ischemia
to a much larger extent than acyl CoA (6). Thus, any detergent
effect would more likely result from acyl carnitine than acyl
CoA.

It is difficult to demonstrate in the intact tissue that
these compounds have any detrimental effects. Associations
between accumulated acyl CoA and carnitine and altered
electrical (2, 3), and mechanical (9) activities as well as
histological evidence of mitochondrial destruction (10) have
been reported, but direct evidence for a cause and effect
relationship has not been obtained.

The purpose of the present paper is to review the conditions
that result in increased levels of acyl CoA and acyl carnitine
in rat hearts and to report some attempts to relate high tissue
levels of these compounds to altered metabolic and mechanical
activity.

Hearts from male Sprague-Dawley rats (250-250 g) were used.
Hearts were removed from rats anesthetized with sodium
pentobarbitol and were perfused by either the Langendorff or
working heart techniques with a Krebs-Henseleit bicarbonate
buffer containing either 11 mM glucose or glucose plus palmitate
bound to 3% bovine serum albumin and equilibrated with 95%
O_2:5% CO_2. Ischemia was induced either by lowering the
aortic perfusion pressure in Langendorff hearts or by use of a

one-way valve in the aortic outflow tube (11). At the end of
perfusion, hearts used for determining tissue levels of
metabolites were frozen with aluminum clamps cooled in liquid
nitrogen and tissue levels of long-chain acyl CoA and carnitine
were determined as described earlier (6). Diabetes was induced
by injection of animals with 60 mg alloxan/kg body weight and
the hearts were removed 48 hours later.

RESULTS AND DISCUSSION

     Several conditions result in altered levels of acyl CoA and
carnitine in the heart. Fasting (Table 1) caused a small
increase in long-chain acyl CoA (FACoA) and about a three-fold
increase in long-chain acyl carnitine (FACarn). It is also
clear that the levels of these acyl esters are dependent on the
exogenous supply of fatty acids. Hearts from fasted rats had
elevated FACoA at a perfusate palmitate concentration of 1.2 mM
but not at 0.4 mM. However, FACarn was higher at both fatty
acid concentrations. Diabetes (Table 1) resulted in a rise in
both FACoA and FACarn. Presumably, the increase in FACoA and
FACarn in hearts from fasted and diabetic animals results from
exposure of the heart to higher circulating levels of serum
fatty acid in vivo and, in the perfused heart, to increased
endogenous triglycerides. However, it is important to point out
that although the levels of acyl CoA and carnitine esters vary
considerably under aerobic conditions in response to changes in
hormone and substrate supply, their levels remain far below
those found under ischemic conditions.

     Ischemia (Table 1) resulted in higher levels of both FACoA
and FACarn even in hearts receiving no exogenous fatty acid.
Apparently the fatty acid was supplied by lipolysis of
endogenous lipids. Addition of exogenous palmitate resulted in
a small increase in acyl CoA and a large rise in acyl
carnitine. The level of acyl carnitine, but not acyl CoA, could
be increased further by addition of more palmitate or continued
perfusion under ischemic conditions with palmitate present.

     Rat cardiac muscle contains about 550 nmoles/g dry tissue of
CoA. The highest level of FACoA observed under ischemic
conditions represents 52% of this total. The normal cellular
distribution of CoA in heart is 90-95% mitochondrial and 5-10%
cytosolic. The concentration of total CoA in the cytosol would
be about 27-55 nmoles distributed in 1.8 ml or from 15 to 30
μM. This is the maximum FACoA concentration that could be
attained if all the CoA were converted to the acyl ester. Most
likely, the total FACoA will be less than total CoA under all
conditions. Since FACoA binds to lipid membranes and proteins

Table 1. Effects of fasting, diabetes, and supply of substrate and oxygen on tissue levels of long-chain acyl CoA and long-chain acyl carnitine in perfused rat hearts

Condition		Perfusate Palmitate (mM)	Perfusion time (min)	FACoA	FACarn
				(nmoles/g dry)	
Fed		0	40	80 ± 7	90 ± 4
Fasted		0	40	105 ± 6	303 ± 14
		0.4	40	93 ± 7	638 ± 47
		1.2	40	179 ± 4	872 ± 143
Fed		0	10	92 ± 2	130 ± 13
Diabetic		0	10	167 ± 10	277 ± 79
Fed	ischemic	0	10	147 ± 10	740 ± 142
	ischemic	0.4	10	240 ± 29	2424 ± 137
	ischemic	1.2	10	284 ± 10	3078 ± 143
	ischemic	1.2	45	288 ± 10	3533 ± 188

Hearts were removed from animals either fed, fasted overnight, or made diabetic for 48 hrs and perfused by the Langendorff technique for times indicated. The perfusate contained either 11 mM glucose or glucose plus palmitate bound to 3% bovine serum albumin at the concentration indicated. FACoA=long-chain acyl CoA. FACarn=long-chain acyl carnitine.

and is only slightly soluble in water, its effective
concentration in the cell is unknown. The above values serve
only to identify the total available. This total could,
however, be concentrated in one area, for example on
mitochondrial membranes, resulting in a very high local
concentration. The mitochondria contain from 422 to 495 nmoles
of CoA distributed in 280 mg of mitochondrial protein or about
280 microliters of matrix space. Thus, the concentration of
total CoA in the matrix space would be about 1.5 to 1.8 mM. The
FACoA concentration of mitochondria under ischemic conditions
could be 50 to 60% of this.

From a concentration standpoint, acyl carnitine is far more
dominant than acyl CoA. Rat heart contains about 6 μmoles of
total carnitine per g dry tissue of which 95% is cytosolic.
Thus, the concentration in the cytosol would be about 3 mM. The
highest level of FACarn observed in ischemic hearts (Table 1)
was about 3.5 μmoles/g dry. This could result in a cytosolic
FACarn concentration of about 1.8 mM, some 100 to 200 times the
maximum FACoA concentration in this cellular space.

Levels of acyl CoA and acyl carnitine do not increase under
all conditions of oxygen deficiency (12). Hearts perfused under
conditions of ischemia (coronary flow rates ranging from 1-5
ml/min) or hypoxic and anoxic conditions had high levels of the
acyl esters but zero coronary flow failed to increase acyl
carnitine and produced only a small increase in acyl CoA.
Likewise, incubation of cardiac muscle at 37° C resulted in
decreased levels of acyl CoA and carnitine. The failure of zero
coronary flow to raise the acyl esters is surprising since low
flow with no exogenous fatty acid present did result in elevated
tissue levels (Table 1). This flow dependence of acyl esters
may be related to tissue levels of lactate. High concentrations
of lactate inhibit fatty acid oxidation and reduce tissue levels
of acyl carnitine (13). Thus, at zero or very low coronary
flows where tissue lactate cannot be washed out, inhibition of
acyl carnitine production by lactate may prevent accumulation of
the ester.

Although high concentrations of exogenous fatty acids have
been shown to depress mechanical function in ischemic swine
hearts (9) and isolated hypoxic rat hearts (14), it has been
difficult to demonstrate an effect of a high fatty acid/albumin
ratio on the function of perfused rat hearts either during
ischemia or with reperfusion following ischemia. Hearts
perfused for 30 min with a coronary flow of 0.4 ml/min recovered
35% of their preischemic developed pressure after 30 min of
reperfusion when glucose was the only exogenous substrate
provided (Table 2). Hearts receiving 1.2 mM palmitate bound to

Table 2. Recovery of reperfused ischemic hearts: effects of fatty acid and tissue levels of long-chain acyl CoA and carnitine

Perfusate Palmitate (mM)	Reperfusion time (min)	ATP	C.P.	FACoA	FACarn	Recovery %
		μmoles/g dry		nmoles/g dry		
0	0	2.6 ± .05	3.9 ± .11	120 ± 18	136 ± 12	
	30	6.5 ± .29	24 ± 1.4	96 ± 1.7	83 ± 16	35 ± 6
1.2	0	2.7 ± .11	4.0 ± .14	235 ± 10	1398 ± 154	
	30	7.1 ± .22	27 ± .22	123 ± 2	200 ± 15	43 ± 6

Hearts were perfused as a Langendorff preparation with a coronary flow of 12 ml/min for 10 min with Krebs bicarbonate buffer containing 11 mM glucose, 3% bovine serum albumin and 1.2 mM palmitate were indicated. Ventricular pressure was measured from an intraventricular catheter inserted via the mitral valve. Coronary flow was reduced to 0.4 ml/min by lowering the aortic perfusion pressure and the ischemic perfusion was continued for 45 min in each group. One group of hearts receiving only glucose and one group receiving both glucose and palmitate were frozen at the end of the ischemic perfusion. Another group with each substrate was reperfused with a coronary flow of 12 ml/min and recovery of tissue metabolites and mechanical function determined after 30 min. Recovery of mechanical function is expressed as percent of the initial preischemic ventricular developed pressure. The data are means ± S.E. for 6 hearts in each group.

3% albumin recovered 43% of their preischemic function. This
recovery of mechanical function occurred even though the hearts
had been exposed to high levels of acyl CoA and acyl carnitine
during the 30 min of low flow ischemia (0 time values in Table
2). The acyl CoA and carnitine levels decreased during
reperfusion but exposure to the high levels during ischemia did
not alter the ability of the heart to resynthesize ATP and CP or
to regain mechanical function with reperfusion.

      Accumulation of acyl CoA and acyl carnitine may have
metabolic effects that are not immediately translated into
altered mechanical activity. For example, increased tissue
levels of triglycerides occur in ischemic hearts and in hearts
of diabetic animals (15). This increased esterification of
fatty acids may result from a high cytosolic level of acyl CoA
in each case. Acyl CoA not only serves as substrate for
esterification to triglycerides but also inhibits triglyceride
lipase activity (16, 17). Table 3 shows the effects of
palmityl-CoA on neutral lipase activity in rat heart
homogenate. Palmityl-CoA was an effective inhibitor of lipase
activity. The concentration required to significantly reduce
lipolysis was 100 M when no protein was added other than that
present in the tissue homogenate. In the absence of added BSA,
lipase activity was reduced to 83 and 33% of control by 100 and
200 µM palmityl-CoA, respectively. This effect of acyl CoA
could be partially prevented by adding 39 µM BSA. Lipolytic
activity was reduced to 93 and 57% of control at 100 and 200 µM
acyl CoA, respectively. With the higher concentration of BSA,
lipase activity was only reduced to 93 and 79% of control,
respectively. The increase in activity with 78 µM BSA was 95%
when no acyl CoA was added, 117% with 100 µM acyl CoA, and 34%
with 200 µM acyl CoA. Thus, albumin not only increased lipase
activity in the absence of acyl CoA, it also reduced acyl CoA
inhibition. This reduction of acyl CoA inhibition probably
resulted from acyl CoA binding to albumin. On the other hand,
palmityl-carnitine at very high concentrations was only slightly
inhibitory compared to palmityl-CoA (Figure 1). Palmitate was
an even weaker inhibitor than palmityl-carnitine. The lowest
concentration of palmityl-CoA to inhibit was 100 µM, but it took
four times as much palmityl-carnitine and thirteen times as much
palmitate to produce the same degree of inhibition. Thus,
palmityl-CoA was a much more effective inhibitor of lipase than
either the free acid or the acyl carnitine ester.

      It is interesting that addition of 100 µM palmityl-CoA
caused a 20% inhibition, whereas 150 µM resulted in a 63%
inhibition (Figure 1). This large jump in percent inhibition
with inhibitor concentration indicates that most of the
palmityl-CoA present at 100 µM was bound to the 14 mg of tissue

Table 3. Effects of palmityl-CoA and serum albumin on lipase
         activity

Palmityl-CoA	Lipase Activity (μmoles/g/min)		
M	0 BSA	39 M BSA	78 M BSA
0	0.42 ± .01	0.69 ± .03	0.82 ± .03
50	0.40 ± .02		
100	0.35 ± .01	0.64 ± .02	0.76 ± .02
150	0.18 ± .01		
200	0.14 ± .01	0.39 ± .03	0.54 ± .02
250	0.09 ± .01		
300	0.06 ± 0.1		

Samples of tissue homogenates (about 14 mg protein) were incubated
for 20 min with the concentrations of palmityl-CoA and bovine serum
albumin (BSA) indicated. The concentrations of albumin used, 39 and
78 μM represent about 12 and 24 mg protein, respectively. The rates
of glycerol release were linear for the 20 min incubations. Lipase
activity is expressed as moles glycerol release/g wet tissue/min.
The data represent the mean ± S.E.M. for 6 tissue homogenates.

proteins present in the homogenate. Inhibition of lipase was
proportional to concentration of palmityl-CoA only at
concentrations above 100 μM. Including 39 μM BSA completely
removed the inhibition of 100 μM acyl CoA and greatly reduced
the effect of 200 μM acyl CoA (Table 3). Increasing the
concentration of BSA to 78 μM almost eliminated the inhibition
at 200 μM palmityl-CoA. These data indicate that binding of
acyl CoA to protein effectively prevents inhibition of lipase
activity. Also, since 39 μM BSA (about 12 mg protein) prevented
most of the inhibition that occurred at acyl CoA concentrations
between 100 and 200 μM, most of the acyl CoA present at
concentrations below 100 μM was probably bound to the 14 mg of
tissue protein present.

    If this effect of palmityl-CoA has any relevance to events
in the intact tissue, the inhibitory concentration must be near
that found in the cytosolic space. Palmityl-CoA seemed to exert
its most effective control at concentrations between 100 and
150 μM, much too high for the concentration that might be
present in the cytosol. The concentrations used in the assay
are, however, over-estimates of the actual effective
concentrations present since the activity of palmityl-CoA

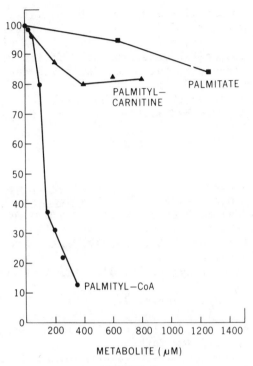

FIGURE 1

Inhibition of triglyceride hydrolysis by palmityl-coenzyme A, palmityl-carnitine and palmitate bound to 3% albumin. This incubation buffer consisted of 1 ml of Ediol (dialyzed against 50 mM Hepes and diluted 1:1 with 50 mM Hepes pH 7.0), 1 mM KCN, rotenone (100 μg/g heart tissue), Hepes pH 7.0, 0.06 grams of heart tissue and the indicated concentrations of metabolites in a total volume of 4.21 ml. The effect of palmityl-carnitine upon lipase activity was measured in the presence of 39 μM BSA. Palmitic acid was bound to 3% albumin. The effect of palmityl-CoA is with no added protein. Since the rate of lipolysis was elevated by albumin, the data for each concentration of metabolite are presented as percent of control determined at the same protein concentration, but without added metabolite.

hydrolase (18) present in the rat heart homogenate reduced the palmityl-CoA by 20 min to only 45-50% of that added initially (data not shown) and binding of acyl CoA to tissue proteins could be expected to reduce the concentration even further.

This inhibition of lipase activity by palmityl-coenzyme A may be an important part of increased triglycerides in ischemic and diabetic hearts. The effect of palmityl-CoA did not appear to be due to a nonspecific detergent-like action resulting from its amphipathic structure, but more likely was due to a specific interaction of palmityl-CoA with the enzyme. This conclusion is based on the observation that palmityl-carnitine which is also an amphipathic compound had little effect on lipase activity.

REFERENCES

1. Katz, A.M., & Messineo, F.C. (1981): Circ. Res. 48: 1.
2. Vik-Mo, H., & Mjos, O.D. (1983): IN Myocardial Ischemia and Protection (eds) H. Refoum, P. Jynge. & O.D. Mjos, Churchill Livingstone, London, p. 35.
3. Oram. J.F., Bennetch, S.L., & Neely, J.R. (1973): J. Biol. Chem. 248: 5299.
4. Neely, J.R., & Feuvray, D. (1981): Am. J. Pathol. 102: 282.
5. Idell-Wenger, J.A., & Neely, J.R. (1977): IN Pathophysiology and Therapeutics of Myocardial Ischemia (eds) A.M. Lefer, G.J. Kellcher. & M.J. Rovetto, Spectrum Publications, Inc., New York, p. 227.
6. Whitmer, J.T., Wenger, J.I., Rovetto, M.J., & Neely, J.R. (1978): J. Biol. Chem. 253: 4305.
7. Whitmer, J.T., Rovetto, M.J., & Neely. J.R. (1974): Fed. Proc. 33: 364.
8. Shug, A.L., Shrago, E., & Bittar, N. (1975): Am. J. Physiol. 228: 689.
9. Liedtke, A.J., Nellis, S., & Neely, J.R. (1978): Circ. Res. 43: 652.
10. Feuvray, D. (1983): IN Myocardial Ischemia and Protection (eds) H. Refoum, P. Jynge, & O.D. Mjos, Churchill Livingstone, London, p. 45.
11. Neely. J.R., Rovetto, M.J., Whitmer, J.T., & Morgan, H.E. (1973): Am. J. Physiol. 225: 651.
12. Neely, J.R., Garber, D., McDonough, K., & Idell-Wenger, J. (1979): Perspectives in Cardiovascular Research, Ischemic Myocardium and Antiangina Drugs, Vol 3, (eds) M.M. Winbury, & Y. Abiko, Raven Press, New York, p. 225.
13. Bielefeld, D.R., Vary, T.C., & Neely. J.R. (1983): Fed. Proc. 42: 1258
14. Henderson, A.H., Craig, R.J., Gorlin, R., & Sonnenblick, E.H. (1970): Cardiovasc. Res. 4: 466.

15. Denton, R.M., & Randle, P.J. (1967): Biochem. J. <u>104</u>: 416.
16. McDonough, K.H., Costello, M.E., & Neely, J.R. (1979): Fed. Proc. <u>38</u>: 894.
17. Severson, D.L., & Hurley, B. (1982): J. Mol. Cell. Cardiol. <u>14</u>: 467.
18. Lui, M.S., & Kako, K.J. (1975): J. Mol. Cell. Cardiol. <u>7</u>: 577.

ARE TISSUE NON-ESTERIFIED FATTY ACIDS (NEFA) INVOLVED IN

THE IMPAIRMENT OF BIOCHEMICAL AND MECHANICAL PROCESSES

DURING ACUTE REGIONAL ISCHEMIA IN THE HEART

G.J. van der Vusse, F.W. Prinzen, and R.S. Reneman

Department of Physiology
University of Limburg
P. O. Box 616
6200 MD, Maastricht, The Netherlands

After extraction from capillary blood by myocardial tissue,
non-esterified fatty acids (NEFA) can either be oxidized to
deliver energy for electromechanical processes, taken up in
fatty acid stores as triacylglycerides, or incorporated in
membrane structures as glycerophospholipids. Beside these
useful roles of NEFA for myocardial function, detrimental
effects of these fatty acids have been described. Raised plasma
levels of NEFA have been suggested to induce or facilitate
arrhythmias in patients with myocardial infarction (1) or to
extend the infarcted area (2). In vitro experiments with
isolated enzymes and subcellular fractions have shown that NEFA
can inhibit enzyme activities and mitochondrial energy
production (for reviews see 3, 4).

An extensive literature survey (4, 5) revealed that the
content of NEFA in normoxic myocardial tissue of the dog, an
animal commonly used in experimental models to study changes in
myocardial fatty acid metabolism due to ischemia, varied greatly
from study to study (see Table 1). In most of the reports, high
NEFA values were found that were hardly compatible with life,
considering the concentrations of NEFA known to inhibit
enzymatic activity and mitochondrial function.

Table 1. Content of NEFA in normoxic dog myocardium.

Amount (nmol·g^{-1})	References	Method
29	Van der Vusse et al. (6)	II
56	Hunneman & Schweickhardt (5)	II
500	Masters & Glaviano (7)	I
912	Weishaar et al. (8)	II
1210	Weishaar et al. (9)	II
2780	Suzuki et al. (10)	III
3570	Suzuki et al. (11)	III
4390	Oscai (12)	I
5900	Ahmed et al. (13)	I
8800	Regan et al. (14)	I
8900	Regan et al. (15)	I
9600	Regan et al. (16)	III
10800	Haider et al. (17)	I
12000	Regan et al. (18)	III
14950	Andrieu et al. (19)	III
17850	Sakurai (20)	III
21950	Liu & Spitzer (21)	III

I Titration; II Gas-liquid chromatography; III Spectrophotometry

The first aim of our experimental study was to determine the content of NEFA in normoxic myocardial tissue of the dog, and to explore possible pitfalls in the determination of these substances. Routinely, a gas-liquid chromatographic assay system was used in order to discriminate between the various fatty acids present in this lipid class.

Messineo and coworkers (22) and Feuvray and Plouet (23) suggested that accumulation of NEFA in ischemic myocardial tissue can be held responsible for the loss of mechanical function. Cowan and Vaughan Williams (24) hypothesized that increased NEFA levels were involved in the acceleration of glycogen breakdown in ischemic cardiac tissue. Besides, reduction of myocardial high-energy phosphate stores might be caused by NEFA stimulated uncoupling of myocardial mitochondria. This process may occur since Pressman and Lardy (25) and Borst and coworkers (26) found that fatty acids can effectively enhance mitochondrial ATPase activity in vitro.

The second aim of our investigations was to assess the time course of the accumulation of NEFA in ischemic myocardial tissue in order to determine whether the increase of myocardial tissue

content of these fatty acids preceeds the changes in biochemical
and mechanical processes during ischemia, which would be a
prerequisite for a causal relationship.

EXPERIMENTAL METHODS

The experiments were performed on 57 open-chest dogs,
premedicated intramuscularly with 10 mg fluanisone and 200 µg
fentanylcitrate per kg body weight. Anesthesia was induced
intravenously with sodium pentobarbital (10 mg/kg body weight)
and, after endotracheal intubation, was maintained with nitrous
oxide in oxygen (60/40, vol/vol) in combination with a
continuous infusion of sodium pentobarbital (2 mg/kg per hr).
The animals were artificially ventilated with a positive
pressure respirator (Pulmonat). Body temperature was kept
constant at 37.5° C. After incision of the chest, the
pericardium was opened over the antero-lateral aspect of the
heart. Regional myocardial ischemia was induced by stenosis of
the left anterior interventricular artery using an inflatable
silastic cuff. The mean coronary artery pressure distal to the
stenosis was about 3.0 kPa and was kept constant with an
autoregulating feedback system (27).

Insertion of catheters for hemodynamical measurements and
for collection of blood have been described in detail before
(27). Regional myocardial blood flow was measured with
radioactively labeled microspheres (28). Regional myocardial
shortening was assessed according to Arts and Reneman (29).
Transmural biopsies for lipid analysis, and for determination of
ATP, creatine phosphate and glycogen were taken from the
ischemic and normoxic area at time intervals indicated in the
text. Fifteen dogs served as controls (cuff remained deflated
throughout the experiment). The experiment was terminated after
taking the biopsies at a given time interval after induction of
ischemia. Lactate, potassium and inorganic phosphate in the
arterial and local venous blood (the vein, draining the ischemia
area) were measured with a Technicon auto-analyzer. Tissue ATP,
creatine phosphate and glycogen were measured in freeze-dried
tissue specimen with a fluorometric method as previously
described (30).

Extraction and determination of myocardial lipids have been
described in detail previously (27). Routinely, after storage
of the biopsies at -80° C, aliquots of deeply frozen tissue
(150-300 mg) were pulverized in an aluminum mortar with a
stainless steel pestle, previously cooled in liquid nitrogen.
The tissue powder was transferred to test tubes cooled with
liquid nitrogen. The test tubes were placed at -21° C and the
tissue powder was wetted with 2 ml of methanol at -21° C. The

content of the test tubes was allowed to warm to room
temperature and was subsequently weighed. Chloroform was added
until a mixture of chloroform and methanol of 2:1 vol/vol was
obtained. The anti-oxidant butylated hydroxytoluene (0.01%) was
present in the methanol and chloroform. Subsequently, a mixture
of heptadecanoic acid, cholesteryl heptadecanoate, and
triheptadecanoine was added to the extraction mixture to correct
for losses during the assay procedure. NEFA, triacylglycerol,
cholesteryl esters, and total phospholipids were isolated from
the extracts by thin- layer chromatography using TLC plates
coated with Silica gel F 254 (Merck, FRG). The lipid spots were
predeveloped with chloroform: methanol: H_2O: acetic acid
(10:10:1:1 vol/vol) until the liquid front had reached a level 1
cm above the site of application of these spots. Hexane:
diethyl ether: acetic acid (24:5:0.3 vol/vol) was used as
developing solvent. The lipid spots were made visible with
Rhodamine G, scrapped from the plate and transferred into test
tubes, containing 0.5 ml BF_3-methanol solution (7% BF_3).
The fatty acid moiety of the various lipid classes was
methylated at 20° C for 15 minutes (NEFA), at 100° C for 30
minutes (triacylglycerol), and at 100° C for 45 minutes
(cholesteryl esters and phospholipids). The methyl esters were
extracted from the methylating mixture with pentane. After
evaporation of the pentane under a stream of N_2 at 37° C,
the methyl esters originating from NEFA, triacylglycerol, and
phospholipids were dissolved in trimethyl pentane, containing
appropriate amounts of methyl pentadecanoate as internal
standard. The methyl esters of the cholesteryl esters were
rechromatographed on silica gel plates to remove the
anti-oxidant butylated hydroxytoluene.

RESULTS

    In normoxic left ventricular tissue the median values for
NEFA content in the inner, middle and outer layers were 30, 26
and 33 nmol per gram wet weight, respectively (Table 2). In
this table the relative fatty acid composition is also given.
Palmitic and stearic acids were the main constituents of the
NEFA class. The median values of the triacylglycerol content in
the inner, middle and outer layers of the left ventricular wall
were found to be 5.7, 5.5 and 14.1 µmol triacylglycerol fatty
acids per gram of tissue, respectively. Since in most animals
traces of fat could be observed macroscopically at the
epicardial surface, the gradient in triacylglycerol does not
necessarily reflect differences in the content in the myocytes
in the various layers. Cholesteryl esters were present in the
range from 180 to 430 nmol in either layer, whereas the amount

of fatty acids incorporated in the glycerophospholipid class was found to be approximately 35 μmol per gram of tissue. These data indicate that less than 0.1% of myocardial fatty acids are present in the non-esterified form. Since the content of NEFA in myocardial tissue appeared to be very low, special attention was paid to the following factors, which could artefactually increase this content:

1. Blank values. All solvents used in this study were high purity analytical grade. Contamination by finger prints, tobacco smoke, laboratory greases, etc. were excluded as much as possible (31). Despite these precautions a blank value of 3.3 ± 1.3 nmol NEFA per assay was found. This implies that the blank value represents about 25% of the amount of NEFA measured when the extract of 300 mg of tissue was used for the assay.

2. Reproducibility of the assay. The mean intra-assay coefficient of variation for myristic, palmitic, palmitoleic, stearic, oleic, linoleic and arachidonic acid was found to be 20.1, 6.1, 16.2, 6.0, 5.5, 4.8 and 27.1%, respectively. For total NEFA this coefficient was 2.3%.

3. Storage of frozen tissue. The frozen biopsies were routinely stored at -80° C for 4 to 8 weeks for further analysis. Storage at -20° C resulted in a highly increased amount of NEFA: 1085 ± 28 nmol per gram (n=4). In this situation the relative fatty acid composition for myristic, palmitic, palmitoleic, steric, oleic, linoleic and arachidonic acids was 0.9, 7.2, 3.7, 6.6, 33.7, 28.3 and 19.6%, respectively.

4. Storage of fresh biopsies at room temperature. Storage of tissue, freshly taken from the heart, in physiological saline at room temperature did not change the NEFA content when the time duration was restricted to 3 min. This finding indicates that manipulations that require time, such as cutting the biopsies in transmural sections can be done without significantly changing the NEFA level.

5. Homogenization and extraction procedure. Deeply frozen biopsies were routinely powdered at the temperature of liquid N_2 and extraction of the tissue powder was started at -21° C (see Methods). When the biopsies were homogenized in a methanol: chloroform mixture with

Table 2. Content of NEFA in the various layers of the left
ventricular wall of normoxic dog hearts (a) and the
relative fatty acid composition in one of these layers
(b). (Median values and 95% confidence limits.)

a. Total NEFA content

Layer	NEFA ($nmol \cdot g^{-1}$ wet weight)
Inner	30 (25–36)
Middle	26 (22–32)
Outer	33 (28–41)

b. Relative fatty acid composition (middle layer)

Fatty acid	Percentage of total NEFA
Myristic acid	0.4 (0 – 3.6)
Palmitic acid	29.8 (26.1–35.6)
Palmitoleic acid	10.6 (6.7–12.3)
Stearic acid	28.2 (16.6–39.8)
Oleic acid	14.2 (11.8–22.5)
Linoleic acid	8.8 (2.2–17.3)
Arachidonic acid	5.0 (0 – 8.9)

an ultra turrex blender a significantly higher NEFA
value was found: 86 $\pm$ 45 nmol per gram (n=8). This
increase was mainly caused by an elevated level of
oleic acid, which suggest autolysis of triacylglycerol
during thawing of the frozen tissue (6). The
efficiency of the extraction procedure was tested by
injection of a small volume of chloroform containing
[14]C-oleic acid into myocardial biopsies (n=6), just
prior to freeze-clamping of the tissue (32). Tissue
was powdered as described before and the recovery of
both endogenously present NEFA and ^{14}C-oleic acid was
measured. After the first extraction step 86.7 $\pm$ 8.4%
of endogenous NEFA was recovered, 12.4 $\pm$ 8.7% after the
second step, and 0.9 $\pm$ 0.4% after the third step.
Subsequent extraction steps revealed that no NEFA was
left in the tissue residue. Since 86.8 $\pm$ 10.8% of
[14]C-oleic acid was recovered after the first
extraction step, we may conclude that the extraction of
endogenous NEFA is adequate in the present method.

6. Specificity of the assay method. The assay system
described in the method section has generally been

accepted as highly specific for the determination of
fatty acids. Firstly, the thin-layer chromatographic
conditions used result in a complete separation of NEFA
from the other lipid class present in myocardial
tissue. Secondly, the methylating conditions used for
the NEFA fraction are very mild. NEFA will be readily
methylated whereas esterified fatty acids will not be
transmethylated. Thirdly, the gas-liquid
chromatographic conditions used are especially adapted
to the assay of methylated fatty acids. Besides,
casual contaminations will become readily visible on
the chromatographs.

We have compared a colorimetric assay for NEFA in
biological material according to Laurell and Tibbling
(33) with the GLC assay routinely used in our
laboratory. Direct colorimetric determination of NEFA
in the chloroform-methanol-hexane extract of myocardial
tissue resulted in extremely high NEFA values varying
from 5000 to 9000 nmol per gram tissue. However, when
the extract was chromatographed using thin-layer
chromatography and the NEFA spots were analyzed
colorimetrically we found a NEFA content of 15-31 nmol
per gram. These findings clearly indicate that
substances present in the original extract leads to
erroneously high NEFA values. These substances are
most likely phospholipids since addition of these
lipids to a standard mixture of NEFA readily lead to an
increased "NEFA" concentration when assayed
colorimetrically without a TLC step.

After stenosis of the left anterior interventricular
coronary artery, regional shortening ceased within 30 seconds.
Shortening in the circumferential and base-to-apex direction
were close to zero after 10 min (Table 3). This situation did
not change further in the affected region during the following
110 min. Blood flow in the ischemia area rapidly decreased
after induction of ischemia. In the outer layers a reduction of
40% could be measured, whereas flow in the inner layers fell to
20% after 10 min and 13% after 120 min of ischemia (Table 3).
Release of lactate, inorganic phosphate and potassium started
within one minute after the onset of ischemia and reached
maximal values (based on arterio-local venous differences) after
10 min. Thereafter the magnitude of the release gradually
diminished (Figure 1).

The contents of ATP, creatine phosphate and glycogen are
significantly reduced in the inner layer of the ischemic region
after 10, 60 and 120 min of ischemia. The fall in content of

Table 3. The values of myocardial mechanics, blood flow, and metabolism in the area perfused by the left anterior interventricular coronary artery during normoxia and ischemia.

Parameter	normoxia	ischemia (time in min)		
		10	60	120
Shortening (%)[a]				
Circumferential	5.2	0.2*	0.2*	0.0*
	3.9–7.3	(−0.3)–0.6	(−0.06)–0.3	(−1.1)–0.0
Base-to-apex	4.8	0.4*	−0.4*	−0.8*
	2.4–6.0	(−0.06)–1.0	(−0.5)–0.0	(−1.7)–0.0
Blood flow (ml.min^{-1}.g^{-1})[a]				
Inner layer	0.76	0.15*	0.13*	0.10*
	0.64–0.88	0.12–0.22	0.07–0.19	0.04–0.18
Outer layer	0.83	0.30*	0.34*	0.35*
	0.73–0.95	0.25–0.41	0.22–0.41	0.18–0.59
ATP (μmol.g^{-1} dry weight)[b]				
Inner layer	17	13*	6*	5*
	12–19	10–15	4–12	3–13
Outer layer	21	13	10*	11*
	13–26	11–16	6–16	5–15
Creatine phosphate (μmol.g^{-1} dry weight)[b]				
Inner layer	37	16*	11*	18*
	29–53	10–35	9–23	12–22
Outer layer	41	20*	15*	29*
	26–54	10–30	10–22	12–36
Glycogen (μmol.glucose g^{-1} dry weight)[b]				
Inner layer	150	100*	80*	60*
	130–180	45–165	40–170	35–120
Outer layer	170	130	90*	100*
	105–205	45–160	70–145	60–165
NEFA (nmol.g^{-1} wet weight)[b]				
Inner layer	28	33	64*	112*
	21–43	20–63	44–92	77–189
Outer layer	28	25	93*	54*
	22–45	18–81	57–137	47–61

Data refer to median values and 95% confidence limits; * significantly
different from normoxic values ($p < 0.05$); a: using the dog as its own
control; b: normoxic values as derived from control dogs.

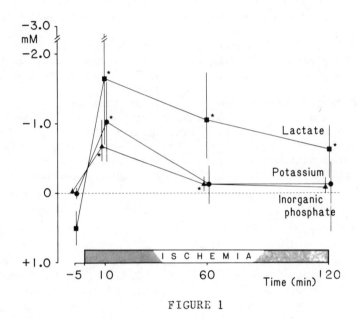

FIGURE 1

Arterio-local venous differences of lactate, potassium and
inorganic phosphate before and during myocardial ischemia.
Ischemia is induced at time 0 min. Median values and 95%
confidence limits are shown.
*Significantly different from pre-ischemic values (time - 5
min).

these substances in the outer layers reached the level of
significance at 60 and 120 min. The content of creatine
phosphate was already significantly reduced in the outer layer
after 10 min of ischemia (Table 3).

In contrast, the content of total NEFA did not change after
10 min neither in the inner nor in the outer layer of the
ischemic region (Table 3). Thereafter, the NEFA content
gradually increased in the inner (Table 3) and middle layers
during the following 110 min of ischemia (data not shown). The
changes in the outer layer, however, displayed a biphasic
pattern. The increase was highest after 60 min of ischemia.

In general, the increased content of NEFA during ischemia
was caused by higher contents of each individual fatty acid.
The fatty acids with the highest relative increase in the inner
layers after 120 min were arachidonic and linoleic acids (5.3
and 5.2-fold increase, respectively). In contrast, after 60 min
of ischemia a deviating pattern of relative NEFA increase was
observed in the outer layer. Linoleic acid showed the most
pronounced increase (6.0-fold). The content of NEFA in the
normoxic area of these regional ischemic hearts was not
significantly different from the control hearts (data not
shown).

DISCUSSION

Our experimental findings indicate that NEFA content in
normoxic dog myocardium is low (in the order of 30 nmol per gram
tissue) and represents less than 0.1% of the total fatty acids
present. These values are considerably lower than those
published by the majority of the authors listed in Table 1.
Beside differences in animal preparation, such as feeding
conditions and type of anesthesia used, differences in
methodology and specificity of the assay method of NEFA are
likely to be responsible for the overestimation of the NEFA
content in myocardial tissue, as has been pointed out in the
results section.

It has been emphasized that the present data refer to values
measured in tissue specimens containing myocardial cells,
interstitial fluid and trapped intravascular blood. On the
basis of the experiments of Rose and Goresky (34) we previously
calculated that the intracellular NEFA content is in the order
of 10 nmol per gram wet weight (27). Fractionation studies
performed by Masters and Glaviano (7) suggest that the bulk of
NEFA is localized in the cytoplasmic fraction. From a rough

estimation we may conclude that the total sarcoplasmic NEFA
concentration will be on the order of 15 $\mu mol \cdot l^{-1}$. This
value, however, relates to both protein bound and free NEFA.
Although specific NEFA binding proteins have been described for
myocardial tissue (35-37) no detailed information about binding
properties of these proteins has been reported. For this
reason, no attempt can be made to calculate the exact free NEFA
concentration in myocardial cells, except that it is likely to
be far below 15 $\mu mol \cdot l^{-1}$.

Ramadoss and coworkers (38) have found that 35 $\mu mol \cdot l^{-1}$
palmitate can produce 50% inhibition of phosphofructokinase, a
key enzyme in the glycolytic pathway. Glucokinase and
hexokinase were inactivated by NEFA at considerably higher
concentrations (39). Uncoupling of mitochondrial ATP
production, i.e. activation of ATPase, can be caused by 100
$\mu mol \cdot l^{-1}$ oleate (26). Hence, on the basis of the present
findings, there is no reason to assume that NEFA are a threat
for the heart under normoxic conditions. The intracellular NEFA
content is very limited and far below the concentrations known
to inhibit cytoplasmic and mitochondrial processes in vitro.
The question as to whether intracellular NEFA are involved in
the impairment of biochemical and mechanical processes during
the acute phase of ischemia of the heart remains to be
answered. Although a limited number of investigators have
reported that the content of NEFA increases in ischemic
myocardial tissue (8-11, 27), no attempt was made to investigate
the time course of the changes in myocardial NEFA content in
comparison with the metabolic and mechanical changes due to
shortage of oxygen. One may expect that in the case of a
detrimental effect of NEFA on myocardial function during the
initial phase of ischemia, the increase in tissue content of
these fatty acids would preceed cessation of myocardial
mechanical activity and derangements in cardiac metabolism.

The transition of aerobic to anaerobic metabolism is clearly
indicated by the reduction of myocardial glycogen and the
release of lactate into the veins draining the ischemic area.
This transition occurs within 10 minutes after the onset of
ischemia. Besides, the loss of tissue inorganic phosphate, most
likely due to utilization of creatine phosphate for
energy-requiring processes, is maximal in the same period.
Release of potassium ions due to disturbances at the level of
membrane bound Na^+/K^+ ATPase (40) or to a higher potassium
conductance (41) is also substantially present during the
initial phase of ischemia. The induction of ischemia resulted
in a rapid deterioration of myocardial shortening both in the
circumferential and in the base-to-apex direction.

Since tissue NEFA were not significantly increased during the first 10 min of ischemia, it is not feasible that these lipids are responsible for the impairment of myocardial contraction as has been suggested by Messineo and coworkers (22). Moreover, the accelerated degradation of glycogen (as suggested by 24), the decrease of myocardial ATP content (as would be expected from the NEFA induced mitochondrial uncoupling, shown in vitro by Borst and colleagues, 26) and the possible impairment of Na^+/K^+ ATPase (to occur in vitro, shown by Lamers and Hulsmann, 42) cannot be ascribed to accumulation of NEFA during the initial phase of oxygen deprivation. Whether the increased amounts of NEFA during prolonged ischemia are noxious for the myocardium remains subject to further investigation.

ACKNOWLEDGEMENTS

We are indebted to Marie Louise Coenen for her help in preparing the manuscript and to Theo Roemen and Will Coumans for their skillful technical assistance. These investigations were supported by the Foundation for Medical Research (FUNGO), which is subsidized by the Netherlands Organization of Pure Research (ZWO).

REFERENCES

1. Oliver, M.F., Kurien, V.A., & Greenwood, T.W. (1968): Lancet 1: 710.
2. Opie, L.H., Tansey, M., & Kennelly, B.M. (1977): Lancet 2: 890.
3. Katz, A.M., & Messineo, F.C. (1981): Circ. Res. 48: 1.
4. Van der Vusse, G.J. (1983): J. Drug Res. 8: 1579.
5. Hunneman, D.H., & Schweickhardt, C. (1982): J. Mol. Cell. Cardiol. 14: 339.
6. Van der Vusse, G.J., Roemen, T.H.M., & Reneman, R.S. (1980): Biochim. Biophys. Acta 617: 347.
7. Masters, T.N., & Glaviano, V.V. (1972): J. Pharmacol. Exp. Ther. 182: 246.
8. Weishaar, R., Ashikawa, K., & Bing, B.J. (1979): Am. J. Cardiol. 43: 1137.
9. Weishaar, R., Sarma, J.S.M., Maruyama, Y., Fisher, R., & Bing, R.J. (1977): Cardiology 62: 2.
10. Suzuki, Y., Kamikawa, T., & Yamazaki, N. (1981): Jap. Heart J. 22: 377.
11. Suzuki, Y., Kamikawa, T., Kobayashi, A., Masumura, Y., & Yamazaki, N. (1981): Jap. Circ. J. 45: 687.
12. Oscai, L.B. (1979): Can. J. Physiol. Pharmacol. 57: 485.

13. Ahmed, S.S., Lee, C.H., Oldewurtel, H.A., & Regan, T.J. (1978): J. Clin. Invest. <u>61</u>: 1123.
14. Regan, T.J., Passannante, A.J., Oldewurtel, H.A., Burke, W.M., & Ettinger, P.O. (1972): J. Appl. Physiol. <u>33</u>: 325.
15. Regan, T.J., Khan, M.I., Ettinger, P.O., Haider, B., Lyons, M.M., & Oldewurtel, H.A. (1974): J. Clin. Invest. <u>54</u>: 740.
16. Regan, T.J., Wu, C.F., Yeh, C.K., Oldewurtel, H.A., & Haider, B. (1981): Circ. Res. <u>49</u>: 1268.
17. Haider, B., Achmed, S.S., Moschos, C.B., Oldewurtel, H.A., & Regan, T.J. (1977): Circ. Res. <u>40</u>: 577.
18. Regan, T.J., Markov, A., Khan, M.I., Jesrani, M.U., Oldewurtel, H.A., & Ettinger, P.O. (1972): Rec. Adv. Stud. Cardiac Struct. Metab. <u>1</u>: 656.
19. Andrieu, J.L., Vial, C., Font, B., Goldschmidt, D., Lievre, M., & Faucon, G. (1979): Arch. Int. Pharmacodyn. Therap. <u>237</u>: 330.
20. Sakurai, I. (1977): Acta Pathol. Japan <u>27</u>: 587.
21. Liu, M.-S., & Spitzer, J.J. (1977): Circ. Shock <u>4</u>: 191.
22. Messineo, F.C., Pinto, P.B., & Katz, A.M. (1980): J. Mol. Cell. Cardiol. <u>12</u>: 725.
23. Feuvray, D., & Plouet, J. (1981): Circ. Res. <u>48</u>: 740.
24. Cowan, J.C., & Vaughan Williams, E.M. (1980): J. Mol. Cell. Cardiol. <u>12</u>: 347.
25. Pressman, B.C., & Lardy, H.A. (1956): Biochim. Biophys. Acta <u>21</u>: 458.
26. Borst, P., Loos, J.A., Christ, E.J., & Slater, E.C. (1962): Biochim. Biophys. Acta <u>62</u>: 509.
27. Van der Vusse, G.J., Roemen, T.H.M., Prinzen, F.W., Coumans, W.A., & Reneman, R.S. (1982): Circ. Res. <u>50</u>: 538.
28. Prinzen, F.W., Van der Vusse, G.J., & Reneman, R.S. (1981): Basic Res. Cardiol. <u>76</u>: 431.
29. Arts, T., & Reneman, R.S. (1980): Am. J. Physiol. <u>239</u>: H432.
30. Van der Vusse, G.J., Coumans, W.A., Van der Veen, F.H., Drake, A.J., Flameng, W., & Suy, R. (1983): Vasc. Surg. In press.
31. Christie, W.W. (1973): IN <u>Lipid Analysis</u>, Pergamon Press, Oxford, p. 30.
32. Van der Vusse, G.J., Roemen, T.H.M., Prinzen, F.W., & Reneman, R.S. (1981): Basic Res. Cardiol. <u>76</u>: 389.
33. Laurell, S., & Tibbling, G. (1966): Clin. Chim. Acta <u>16</u>: 57.
34. Rose, C.P., & Goresky, C.A. (1977): Circ. Res. <u>41</u>: 534.
35. Mishkin, S., Stein, L., Gatmaitan, Z., & Arias, I.M. (1972): Biochem. Biophys. Res. Commun. <u>47</u>: 997.
36. Ockner, R.K., Manning, J.A., Poppenhausen, R.B., & Ho, W.K.L. (1972): Science <u>177</u>: 56.
37. Gloster, J., & Harris, P. (1977): Biochem. Biophys. Res. Commun. <u>74</u>: 506.
38. Ramadoss, C.S., Uyeda, K., & Johnston, J.M. (1976): J. Biol. Chem. <u>251</u>: 98.

39. Lea, M.A., & Weber, G. (1968): J. Biol. Chem. 243: 1096.
40. Owen, P., Thomas, M., Young, V., & Opie, L.H. (1970): Am.
    J. Cardiol. 25: 562.
41. Rau, E.E., & Langer, G.A. (1978): Am. J. Physiol. 235:
    H537.
42. Lamers, J.M.J., & Hulsmann, W.C. (1977): J. Mol. Cell.
    Cardiol. 9: 343.

EFFECTS OF MYOCARDIAL ISCHEMIA AND LONG CHAIN ACYL CoA

ON MITOCHONDRIAL ADENINE NUCLEOTIDE TRANSLOCATOR

D. J. Paulson and A. L. Shug

Metabolic Research Lab
William S. Middleton Memorial Veterans Hospital and
Department of Neurology
University of Wisconsin
Madison, Wisconsin USA

The synthesis of ATP occurs predominantly within mitochondria through the process of oxidative phosphorylation, and the consumption of ATP occurs in the cytosol through a variety of energy-consuming reactions (1). These processes are separated by the inner mitochondrial membrane, but are linked through a specific transport protein, adenine nucleotide translocator, which transfers ATP out of the mitochondria in exchange for cytosolic ADP (2). This transport protein is specific for ATP and ADP only; AMP, GTP and GDP are not transported (3). The magnesium complexes of ATP and ADP are also inactive (4). The rate of adenine nucleotide transport is very rapid and requires short time intervals and low temperatures or specialized sophisticated equipment to measure transport kinetics (5, 6). In beef heart mitochondria, the extrapolated rate of adenine nucleotide translocater at 37° is 1800 μmoles/g protein (6). The transport of ATP and ADP is not an energy-consuming process (4). It will occur in uncoupled mitochondria but then ADP and ATP are translocated in both directions. In energized states, there is a preferential uptake of ADP and efflux of ATP. It has been proposed that this preference is derived from the mitochondrial membrane potential and the charge difference between ADP^{-3} and ATP^{-4}. Because the matrix is negatively charged as compared to the cytosol, ADP^{-3} is preferentially taken up and ATP^{-4} is released (4).

185

Another explanation for the asymmetrical transport of external
ATP and ADP is that the adenine nucleotide translocator protein
has different affinities for ADP and ATP depending upon the
energy state of the mitochondria (7).

Much debate has dealt with the role of adenine nucleotide
translocator in controlling mitochondrial respiration (4,
7-11). Several investigators showed that the extramitochondrial
ATP/ADP ratio exceeds the intramitochondrial ratio by a
substantial amount (4, 7). This result was interpreted as
evidence that the adenine nucleotide translocator was
rate-limiting for the overall process of oxidative
phosphorylation (4, 7). Others have proposed that the rate of
respiration is controlled by the extramitochondrial phosphate
potential, the intramitochondrial redox state, the activity of
oxygen and the cytochrome c oxidase (9-11). A recent study by
Groen et al. (8) determined inhibitor titration curves on
mitochondrial respiration at several different steps in
oxidative phosphorylation. They found that in the resting state
of respiration, nearly all control was exerted by the passive
permeability of the mitochondrial inner membrane to protons. In
the active states, control was distributed among different steps
including adenine nucleotide translocator and cytochrome c
oxidase. Thus, they concluded that it was impossible to speak
of a rate-limiting step of oxidative phosphorylation.

It has been suggested that the adenine nucleotide
translocator is functionally coupled to the mitochondrial
creatine kinase (12-21). In the scheme shown in Figure 1, the
ATP produced by oxidative phosphorylation is transported out of
the mitochondrial matrix by the adenine nucleotide translocator
in exchange for ADP. This ATP is preferentially used to
phosphorylate creatine by the mitochondrial creatine kinase.
The ADP formed through this reaction is then available for
exchange transport and further synthesis of ATP. This process
maintains a constant supply of ADP for mitochondrial (state 3)
respiration. The creatine-phosphate produced through these
reactions is transported to the myofibrils, sarcoplasmic
reticulum and sarcolemmal membranes where it is used by the
cytosolic isoenzyme of creatine kinase to form ATP. Thus
creatine-phosphate is used to transport energy from the
mitochondria to the various energy-consuming processes of the
cytosol (12).

Several studies (13-21) from different laboratories have
supported the above concept but others have challenged it (22,
23); therefore, it remains controversial. Evidence in support
of the functional coupling of the adenine nucleotide
translocator to mitochondrial creatine kinase is described

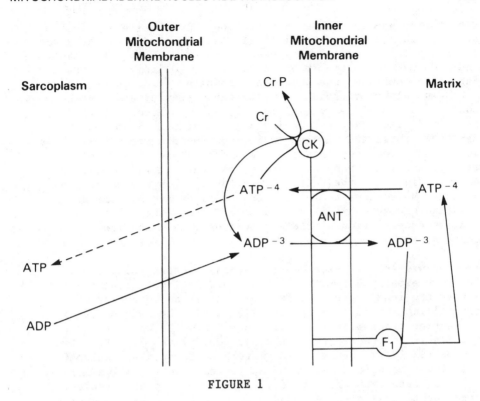

FIGURE 1

General scheme of mitochondrial adenine nucleotide translocator
(ANT) and its coupling to creatine kinase (CK).

briefly below. For detailed information the reader is referred
to the individual studies. Histochemical stains have located
mitochondrial creatine kinase on the exterior surface of the
inner mitochondrial membrane (13). Studies by Jacobus and
Lehninger (14) and Yang et al. (15) have shown that ATP
generated in the mitochondrial matrix is more effectively used
for creatine phosphate synthesis than ATP in the surrounding
medium. The membrane-bound creatine kinase is able to produce a
2.3-fold higher rate of creatine-phosphate formation than the
soluble enzyme (16), has a lower K_m for ATP, and is less
sensitive to feedback inhibition by creatine-phosphate (17).
Other studies have shown that the molar content of creatine
kinase sites is approximately equal to that of adenine
nucleotide translocator (16). Atractyloside, a competitive
inhibitor of adenine nucleotide translocator has also been shown
to inhibit mitochondrial synthesis of creatine-phosphate, but
the inhibition was reduced when the ADP responsible for

respiration was generated by mitochondrial creatine kinase (18, 19). A kinetic mathematical model has suggested that there was an intimate interaction between mitochondrial creatine kinase and adenine nucleotide translocator (20). Oligomycin titration data also confirmed the functional coupling (21). Others have not been able to reproduce some of these results and have challenged the above hypothesis (22, 23). A recent study has presented evidence which denies a close coupling between creatine kinase and adenine nucleotide translocator (24). This study found the coupling could be observed when the outer mitochondrial membrane was intact, but when it was removed by trypsin digestion the coupling was lost. Thus the connection between the adenine nucleotide translocator and mitochondrial creatine kinase is indirect and results from the compartmentalization of these processes within the inner membrane space.

Because ADP-ATP exchange is largely electrogenic, i.e., ADP^{-3} is exchanged for ATP^{-4}, the electrical potential across the inner mitochondrial membrane is an important factor controlling the rate of exchange (3, 25). The rate of adenine nucleotide translocator has also been shown to be affected by the levels of transportable nucleotide (26) and ATP/ADP ratio of the matrix (27). Depletion of mitochondria adenine nucleotide will lower transport rates and an increase in the ATP/ADP ratio will activate exchange (26-28). The rate of adenine nucleotide translocator has also been shown to be affected by endogenous inhibitors, long-chain acyl CoA esters (29, 30).

The inhibition of the adenine nucleotide translocator by long- chain acyl CoA derivatives has been shown in isolated mitochondria (29-32) and in sonicated vesicles (33-35), but the physiologic importance of this reaction has been questioned (4, 36, 37). The purpose of the present study is to assess how myocardial ischemia affects long-chain acyl CoA levels and to determine what effect, if any, these esters would have on the adenine nucleotide translocator. To accomplish this goal the effects of global ischemia on the levels of long-chain acyl CoA, both in whole tissue and mitochondria, were investigated in the isolated perfused rat heart. Adenine nucleotide translocator activity was determined by quantitatively measuring the uptake of ^{14}C-labelled ATP by isolated mitochondria.

METHODS

Heart Perfusion. Male rats (Sprague-Dawley, 225-250 g) were anesthetized with 40 mg/kg of sodium pentobarbital and the heart excised and mounted on the isolated working heart perfusion apparatus (38). Hearts were perfused initially for 10 min in a nonrecirculating retrograde fashion and then switched to a recirculating working mode with a left atrial filling pressure of 10 cm H_2O and afterload of 85 cm H_2O. The perfusion medium was a modified Krebs-Henseleit bicarbonate buffer gassed with 95% O_2 and 5% CO_2 and containing 1.2 mM palmitate, 5.5 mM glucose, and 2 mU/ml insulin. After a 10-min equilibration period, low-flow ischemia was induced by clamping the aortic line and restricting left atrial flow, utilizing a bypass line from a reservoir located 100 cm H_2O above the heart. The rate of flow was set by a micrometer caliper so that a 90% reduction in coronary flow (1.2 ml/min) was achieved. The 100 cm of H_2O hydrostatic pressure column to the left atrial line was used to maintain a constant level of coronary flow during the ischemic period. Ischemia was induced after the initial 10 min of perfusion and maintained for 30, 60, or 90 min.

Isolation of Mitochondria. Control and ischemic hearts were placed in ice-cold extraction medium (250 mM sucrose; 4 mM Tris, pH 7.4; 1 mM EGTA; and 0.2% fatty acid free bovine serum albumin). It was then rinsed several times, blotted dry, weighed, and minced in ice-cold isolation medium. The tissue was homogenized with a Potter-Elvejhem homogenizer and centrifuged for 25 sec in a Damon IEC centrifuge at 15,000 x g. The supernatant was poured through cheesecloth and centrifuged at 15,000 x g for 3 min. The resulting mitochondrial pellet was resuspended in extraction medium (containing no bovine serum albumin) so that the final protein concentration equaled 10 mg/ml.

Assays. Mitochondrial adenine nucleotide levels were determined by the methods of Adams (39) and Stanley and Williams (40) from neutralized perchloric acid extracts. Long-chain acyl CoA esters were measured from the acid-insoluble fraction using the method of Veloso and Veech (41). Protein was assayed using the Biuret method (42).

Adenine Nucleotide Translocator Assay. Rates of adenine nucleotide transport into isolated rat heart mitochondria were determined by measuring the slower forward transport of ATP-([^{14}C]U) at 2° C using the carboxyatractyloside inhibitor stop technique (28). The assay began by adding 0.5 mg of mitochondria to a 0.5 ml reaction mix containing 35 mM Tris, pH 7.4; 0.88 mM EDTA, pH 7.4; 88 mM KCl; 5 mM ruthenium red; 1 μCi ATP-([^{14}C]U); and 250 μM unlabeled ATP. The reaction was run for 10 seconds and terminated by addition of 1 micromole of carboxyatractyloside. Carboxyatractyloside-sensitive counts were obtained by subtracting the counts in blanks containing carboxyatractyloside prior to mitochondrial addition.

Immediately following the assay, the reaction mixture plus
mitochondria were pipetted into a microfuge tube containing
0.25 ml of silicone oil (density, 1.01-1.02 g/ml) and
centrifuged. The reaction mixture was aspirated off the top,
the tube was rinsed, and the bottom containing the mitochondria
was cut off and incubated with soluene until the tissue was
digested. The radioactivity found in the soluene extract was
counted. Results were expressed in nmoles/mg mitochondrial
protein/min.

RESULTS AND DISCUSSION

Effects of Ischemia on Long-Chain Acyl Coenzyme A

    The inhibition of β-oxidation and the buildup of long-chain
acyl CoA esters begins within minutes after the onset of
myocardial ischemia (43, 44) (Figure 2). Long-chain acyl
coenzyme A esters remain elevated throughout the entire ischemic
period. Since 90% of the tissue coenzyme A was reported to be
located within the mitochondrial matrix (45), it is generally
believed that the accumulation of long-chain acyl coenzyme A
occurs predominantly in this compartment. However, in Figure 2
we found that if mitochondria were isolated from ischemic
hearts, very little accumulation of long-chain acyl CoA esters
was found. Idell-Wenger et al. (45) found similar results and
suggested that the accumulated long-chain acyl coenzyme A esters
within the mitochondrial matrix were oxidized during the
isolation procedure. To prevent this oxidation they added 1 mM
KCN to the isolation medium which then should preserve the in
vivo levels of mitochondrial long-chain acyl CoA. This
procedure resulted in a substantial increase in long-chain acyl
CoA in mitochondria isolated from ischemic hearts (45) and it
was concluded that the accumulation of these esters therefore
occurs predominantly in this compartment. In agreement with
these results we found that adding 10^{-4} M KCN to the isolation
medium caused an increase in long-chain acyl coenzyme A in
ischemic mitochondria but it also produced an accumulation of
long-chain acyl coenzyme A in non-ischemic mitochondria (Table
1). In addition, it caused a decrease in the levels of ATP and
ADP and increased AMP in mitochondria isolated from both
ischemic and non-ischemic tissue. These results indicate that
addition of KCN to the isolation medium does not maintain the in
vivo levels of mitochondrial long-chain acyl coenzyme A, or
adenine nucleotide. Since both the levels of long-chain acyl
CoA (29-35) and adenine nucleotide (25-28) will affect the rate
of adenine nucleotide translocator, it is impossible to
determine accurately with these techniques the in vivo effects
of ischemia on this transport protein. Figure 3 shows that the
activity of adenine nucleotide translocator is decreased in both
ischemic and non-ischemic mitochondria isolated with 10^{-4} M

KCN in isolation media. No significant differences were
observed between mitochondria isolated from ischemic and
nonischemia hearts.

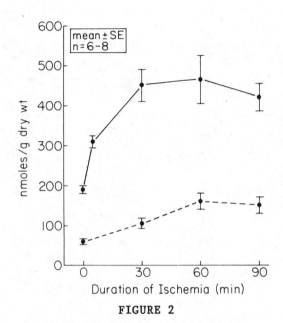

FIGURE 2

Effects of myocardial ischemia of varying durations on tissue
(●——●) and mitochondria (●---●) levels of long-chain acyl CoA.

Because of the difficulties of isolating from ischemic heart
mitochondria that maintain their in vivo state, we are forced to
extrapolate from in vitro experiments. Presumably, because 90%
of the total tissue CoA is found in the mitochondrial matrix
(45), the majority of the buildup of long-chain acyl CoA should
be in this compartment, but it is unknown how much occurs in the
intermembrane space or cytosol.

Table 1.

Mitochondria	KCN (M)	Long Chain Acyl CoA	ATP	ADP	AMP
			(nmoles/mg mitochondrial protein)		
Non-ischemic	0	0.22 ± 0.03	3.2 ± 0.3	5.5 ± 0.3	3.1 ± 0.4
Non-ischemic	10^{-4}	0.73 ± 0.05	0.9 ± 0.1	4.2 ± 0.3	8.7 ± 0.4
Ischemic	0	0.37 ± 0.04	3.2 ± 0.2	3.4 ± 0.2	1.6 ± 0.2
Ischemic	10^{-4}	1.02 ± 0.04	1.4 ± 0.1	4.7 ± 0.4	4.9 ± 0.6

Mitochondria from non-ischemic and 20 min. ishcemic hearts were isolated with media containing 0 or 10^{-4}M KCN.

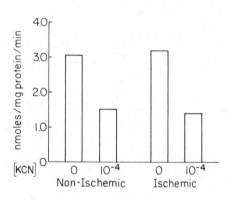

FIGURE 3

Adenine nucleotide translocator activity in mitochondria isolated from nonischemic and 30-min ischemic hearts with and without 10^{-4} M KCN in the extraction medium.

Effects of Long-Chain CoA on the Adenine Nucleotide Translocator

Several studies have shown that addition of long-chain acyl CoA to isolated mitochondria produces an inhibition of adenine nucleotide translocator activity (29-32). This inhibition occurs at concentrations well below the critical micelle level, 30 μM (46). This is illustrated in Figure 4. The effect of 5 μM palmityl CoA incubation at 22° C on the rate of ^{14}C-ATP transport in isolated rat heart mitochondria is shown. The K_i for long-chain acyl CoA inhibition has been reported to be as low as 0.5 μM (29-32) but it will vary with the concentration of mitochondria (36). The inhibition shown in Figure 4 can be reversed by adding 500 μM L- carnitine to the incubation medium (29, 30). Presumably addition of L-carnitine results in the conversion of the palmityl CoA to palmitylcarnitine through the enzyme palmitylcarnitine transferase I, as shown in Figure 5

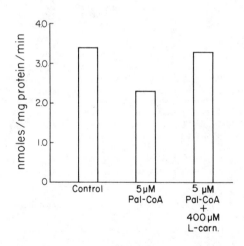

FIGURE 4

Inhibition of mitochondrial adenine nucleotide translocator by 5 μM cytosolic palmityl CoA and its reversal by 400 μM L-carnitine.

(47). Palmitylcarnitine has no direct effect on the adenine
nucleotide translocator activity (29, 30). This transport
protein is also inhibited from the outside site by
atractyloside, a competitive inhibitor (48), and
carboxyatractyloside, noncompetitive inhibitor (49).
Bongkregric acid will inhibit from the matrix site (4, 7).

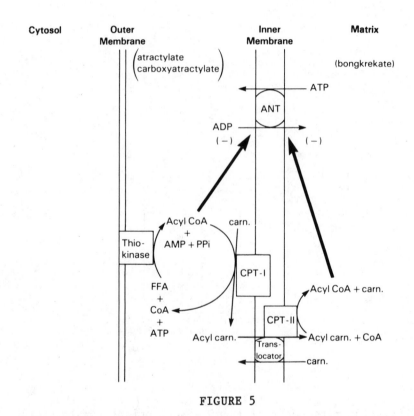

FIGURE 5

Localization and interaction of the carnitine-linked enzymes
with mitochondrial adenine nucleotide translocator.

The competitive inhibitory effect of cytosolic long-chain acyl coenzyme A on the mitochondrial adenine nucleotide translocator has been well established, but the metabolic significance of these findings in vivo has remained controversial (4, 7, 28-37). It has been suggested that the high concentration of cytoplasmic transportable nucleotides, and the coupling of the adenine nucleotide translocator to mitochondrial creatine kinase prevents the competitive inhibition of the adenine nucleotide translocator by cytosolic long-chain acyl CoA (4, 36). Under normal rapid respiring mitochondria, this coupling of mitochondrial creatine kinase to the adenine nucleotide translocator and the rapid oxidation of activated fatty acids probably prevents the inhibition by cytosolic long-chain acyl CoA. But under ischemic conditions the lack of oxygen will slow mitochondrial respiration and the link between the adenine nucleotide translocator and creatine kinase is probably disrupted. Under these conditions, long-chain acyl CoA may inhibit the adenine nucleotide translocator from the cytosolic site.

It has also been suggested that inhibition of adenine nucleotide translocator by cytosolic long-chain acyl CoA esters is prevented by binding of these esters to cellular proteins. La Noue et al. (36) showed that the K_i for cytoplasmic long-chain acyl CoA inhibition of adenine nucleotide transport increases dramatically with the mitochondrial protein concentration. Because the cellular mitochondria content is high, the effective K_i concentration for long-chain acyl CoA inhibition is much greater than the extrapolated levels found in the cytoplasmic compartment. However, this information does not take into account two considerations. First, long-chain acyl CoA esters are synthesized on the outer mitochondria membrane (50) and must be released into the inner membrane space to be taken up for β-oxidation by mitochondria; therefore when calculating the effective inhibitory concentration of long-chain acyl CoA, it is more important to consider the concentration within the inner membrane space than the entire cytoplasm. The second consideration is that the external long-chain acyl CoA has a K_i of 0.5 µM for inhibition of adenine nucleotide translocator in isolated mitochondria (29, 30) and a K_m of 10 µM for palmitylcarnitine transferase I (50). If the binding of cellular proteins to long-chain acyl CoA prevents inhibition of adenine nucleotide translocator, then such binding should also prevent oxidation of long-chain fatty acids. This is unlikely because the preferred fuel of the heart (51) is fatty acids. Therefore, we believe it is possible for long-chain acyl coenzyme A esters to inhibit the adenine nucleotide translocator from the cytosolic side. The fact that several studies have shown that the administration of L-carnitine to ischemic hearts will decrease long-chain acyl coenzyme A (52-54) supports this conclusion.

Another objection raised against the inhibitory effects of long-chain acyl coenzyme A esters is that the inhibition is relatively nonspecific in that they inhibit a number of transport processes, e.g., malate, citrate, and phosphate (37, 55). However, the K_i values for these transport processes are 20 to 80 times greater than the K_i for adenine nucleotide translocator. Other studies have shown a site-specific interaction of palmityl-CoA with the purified adenine nucleotide translocator protein (56).

The inhibition of adenine nucleotide translocator by mitochondrial matrix long-chain acyl CoA has also been challenged. The main objection was that the mitochondrial matrix contain relatively low levels of CoA (1 mM) as compared to adenine nucleotides (10 mM) (36). Therefore, long-chain acyl coenzyme A esters would have to compete with a much larger adenine nucleotide pool to inhibit the adenine nucleotide translocator. Because of this competition and the binding of long-chain acyl CoA to matrix proteins it was considered unlikely that long-chain acyl coenzyme A could inhibit the adenine nucleotide translocator from the matrix side. There are a number of flaws in this argument. First of all, not all adenine nucleotides compete for the binding with the long-chain acyl CoA ester (4, 7). Only the free forms of ATP and ADP (not the Mg- complexes) are transportable, as discussed previously (4). In addition, much of the adenine nucleotides are also bound to matrix proteins. Thus, competition of ATP and long-chain acyl coenzyme A is probably much lower than 10 to 1.

Studies in inverted sonicated mitochondrial vesicles have shown that palmityl coenzyme A is an effective inhibitor of adenine nucleotide transport from the matrix site and that the inhibition was of the mixed type (33-35). However, a recent study by La Noue et al. (36) was unable to demonstrate inhibition of adenine nucleotide translocator by matrix long-chain acyl coenzyme A in intact mitochondria. This study used a nonquantitative assay for adenine nucleotide translocator that coupled the transport of ATP out of mitochondria to the synthesis of glucose-6-phosphate. Palmityl coenzyme A was increased in the mitochondrial matrix by incubating the mitochondria with palmitylcarnitine and it was found that this treatment had no effect on glucose-6-phosphate formation. This finding was interpreted as evidence that the matrix long-chain acyl CoA has no effect on adenine nucleotide translocator. We believe this conclusion is not valid because the production of glucose-6- phosphate is not an assay for adenine nucleotide

translocator. It does not measure initial reaction kinetics nor
is it quantitative. A number of factors such as the interaction
of adenine nucleotide translocator with creatine kinase,
feedback inhibition, leakage of nucleotides, could affect
glucose-6-phosphate production.

Because of these criticisms, we have reexamined the effect
of matrix long-chain acyl coenzyme A on adenine nucleotide
translocator in intact mitochondria. We used a quanitative
assay that takes advantage of the slower forward transport of
ATP-([^{14}C]U) at 2° using the carboxyatractyloside inhibition
stop technique. The reaction followed first-order rate kinetics
for 10 to 15 seconds and was linear with protein concentration.
The 10-second time point and an external ATP concentration of
250 µM was used in Figure 6 to measure activity of the adenine
nucleotide translocator. When mitochondria were incubated with
60 µM palmitylcarnitine at 22° C for 15 min the levels of
matrix long-chain acyl CoA were increased from 0.08 to 0.73
nmoles/mg mitochondrial protein, while total transportable
nucleotides (ATP and ADP) were not affected. The velocity of
[^{14}C] ATP transport was severely inhibited. Figure 7 shows
that the increase in mitochondrial long-chain acyl CoA produced
by palmitylcarnitine incubation was actually less than the
extrapolated amount of matrix long-chain acyl CoA caused by
myocardial ischemia (1.14 nmoles/mg mitochondrial protein;
assuming that 90% of the accumulation of long-chain acyl CoA
occurs in the mitochondrial matrix and there are 53 mg
mitochondrial protein per gram wet weight). In other
experiments (not shown), the normal endogenous levels of
long-chain acyl CoA were decreased from 0.18 to 0.06 nmoles/mg
by adding 10 µM K$_3$Fe[CN]$_6$ and this reduction stimulated
adenine nucleotide translocator activity. Figure 8 shows that
adenine nucleotide activity was also inhibited by decreasing the
mitochondrial levels of transportable nucleotides. The
transportable nucleotides were decreased from 7.6 to 2.4
nmoles/mg by incubating mitochondria with 10^{-4} M KCN. When
these mitochondria were also incubated with 60 µM
palmitylcarnitine, the matrix levels of long-chain acyl CoA were
increased from 0.20 to 0.64 nmoles/mg and adenine nucleotide
translocator activity was further inhibited (Figure 8). These
data clearly demonstrate that accumulation of long-chain acyl
CoA within the mitochondrial matrix does indeed inhibit adenine
nucleotide translocator. Although it was not possible to
directly measure rates of adenine nucleotide translocator from
ischemic mitochondria because of the difficulty of isolating
mitochondria that maintain their in vivo condition, we believe
that the data presented here strongly suggest that the
accumulation of long-chain acyl CoA during myocardial ischemia
inhibits adenine nucleotide translocator.

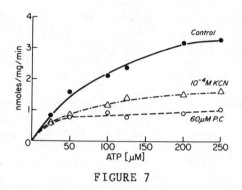

FIGURE 7

A comparison of the levels of mitochondrial long-chain acyl CoA
produced by palmitylcarnitine incubation and by 30 min of
ischemia (extrapolated from Figure 4, assuming 90% of the
accumulation was in the mitochondrial matrix and there are 53 mg
mitochondrial protein/g wet wt).

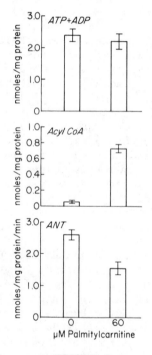

FIGURE 6

Effects of 60 μM palmitylcarnitine incubation at 22° C for 15
min on the levels of mitochondrial transportable nucleotides
(ATP and ADP), long-chain acyl CoA and the activity of adenine
nucleotide translocator.

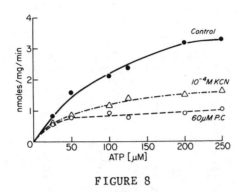

FIGURE 8

Mitochondria were depleted of their transportable nucleotides by incubation with 10^{-4} M KCN. Matrix levels of long-chain acyl CoA were increased by incubating these mitochondria with 60 μM palmityl- carnitine and the activity of adenine nucleotide translocator was measured over a wide range of external ATP concentrations (10-250 μM).

Although we have extrapolated from in vitro experiments that it is possible for the accumulation of long-chain acyl CoA during myocardial ischemia to inhibit the adenine nucleotide translocator, there still remain many questions that need to be addressed. For instance, what is the metabolic consequence of adenine nucleotide translocator inhibition during myocardial ischemia. Is this inhibition necessarily harmful or is it a normal mechanism for controlling mitochondrial function? The levels of long-chain acyl CoA are affected by a number of different metabolic conditions: fasting (57), diabetes (58), and hibernation (59). We would expect that an accumulation of long-chain acyl CoA during these different states would also inhibit adenine nucleotide translocator. One could speculate that long-chain acyl CoA may be an endogenous regulator of mitochondrial function through its effect on adenine nucleotide translocator. Thus, long-chain acyl CoA esters may help to regulate mitochondrial respiration, calcium transport, and ATP/ADP ratio.

ACKNOWLEDGEMENTS

This work was supported in part by the Research Service of the Veterans Administration and NIH grant HL-17736.

REFERENCES

1. Lehninger, A.L. (1972): Biochemistry, Worth, New York.
2. Klingenberg, M. (1976): IN The Enzymes of Biological Membranes: Membrane Transport, Vol. 3, (ed.) M. Anthony, Plenum Press, New York, p. 363.
3. Pfaff, E., & Klingenberg, M. (1968): Eur. J. Biochem. 6: 66.
4. Klingenberg, M., & Heldt, H.W. (1982): IN Metabolic Compartmentation, (ed.) H. Sies, Academic Press, London, p. 101.
5. Heldt, H.W., & Klingenberg, M. (1968): Eur. J. Biochem. 4: 1.
6. Klingenberg, M., Grebe, K., & Appel, M. (1982): Eur. J. Biochem. 126: 263.
7. Vignais, P.V. (1976): Biochim. Biophys. Acta 456: 1.
8. Groen, A.K., Wanders, R.J.A., Westerhoff, H.V., Van der Meer, R., & Tager, J.M. (1982): J. Biol. Chem. 257: 2754.
9. Wilson, D.F., Nelson, D., & Erecinska, M. (1982): FEBS Lett. 143: 228.
10. Wilson, D.F., & Owen, C. (1973): Biochem. Biophys. Res. Commun. 53: 326.
11. Van der Meer, R., Westerhoff, H.V., & Van Dam, K. (1980): Biochim. Biophys. Acta 591: 488.
12. Bessman, S.P., & Geiger, P.J. (1981): Science 211: 448.
13. Jacobs, H., Heldt, H.W., & Klingenberg, M. (1964): Biochem. Biophys. Res. Commun. 16: 516.
14. Jacobus, W.E., & Lehninger, A.L. (1973): J. Biol. Chem. 248: 4803.
15. Yang, W.C.T., Geiger, P.J., Bessman, S.P., & Borrebaek, B. (1977): Biochem. Biophys. Res. Commun. 76: 882.
16. Saks, V.A., Kupriyanov, V.V., Elizarova, G.V., & Jacobus, W.E. (1980): J. Biol. Chem. 255: 755.
17. Jacobus, W.E., & Saks, V.A. (1982): Arch. Biochem. Biophys. 219: 167.
18. Erickson-Viitanen, S., Viitanen, P., Geiger, P.J., Yang, W.C.T., & Bessman, S.P. (1982): J. Biol. Chem. 257: 14395.

19. Moreadith, R.W., & Jacobus, W.E. (1982): J. Biol. Chem. 257: 899.
20. Saks, V.A., Chernousova, G.B., Gukovsky, D.E., Smirnov, V.N., & Chazov, E.I. (1975): Eur. J. Biochem. 57: 273.
21. Saks, V.A., Lipina, N.V., Smirnov, V.N., & Chazov, E.I. (1976): Arch. Biochem. Biophys. 173: 34.
22. Altshuld, R.A., & Brierly, G.P. (1977): J. Mol. Cell. Cardiol. 9: 875.
23. Borrebaek, B. (1980): Arch. Biochem. Biophys. 203: 827.
24. Erickson-Viitanen, S., Geiger, P.J., Viitanen, P., & Bessman, S.P. (1982): J. Biol. Chem. 257: 14405.
25. Klingenberg, M., & Rottenberg, H. (1977): Eur. J. Biochem. 73: 125.
26. Pfaff, E., Heldt, H.W., & Klingenberg, M. (1969): Eur. J. Biochem. 10: 484.
27. Vignais, P.V., Vignais, P.M., Lauquin, G., & Morel, F. (1973): Biochimie (Paris) 55: 763.
28. Barbour, R.L., & Chan, S.H.P. (1981): J. Biol. Chem. 256: 1940.
29. Shug, A., Lerner, E., Elson, C., & Shrago, E. (1971): Biochem. Biophys. Res. Commun. 43: 557.
30. Pande, S.V., & Blanchaer, M.C. (1971): J. Biol. Chem. 246: 402.
31. Harris, R.A., Farmer, B., & Ozawa, T. (1972): Arch. Biochem. Biophys. 150: 199.
32. Barbour, R.L., & Chan, S.H.P. (1979): Biochem. Biophys. Res. Commun. 89: 1169.
33. Chua, B.H., & Shrago, E. (1977): J. Biol. Chem. 252: 6711.
34. Klingenberg, M. (1977): Eur. J. Biochem. 76: 553.
35. Lauquin, G.J.M., Villiers, C., Michejda, J.W., Hryniewiecka, L.V., & Vignais, P.V. (1977): Biochim. Biophys. Acta 460: 331.
36. La Noue, K.F., Watts, J.A., & Koch, C.D. (1981): Am. J. Physiol. 241: H663.
37. Morel, F., Lauquin, G., Lunardi, J., Duszynski, J., & Vignais, P.V. (1974): FEBS Lett. 39: 133.
38. Neely, J.R., Liebermeister, H., Battersby, E.J., & Morgan, H.E. (1967): Am. J. Physiol. 212: 804.
39. Adams, H. (1965): IN Methods of Enzymatic Analysis, (ed) H.H. Bergmeyer, Academic Press, New York, p. 573.
40. Stanley, P.E., & Williams, S.O. (1969): Anal. Biochem. 29: 381.
41. Veloso, D., & Veech, R.L. (1974): Anal. Biochem. 62: 449.
42. Keleti, G., & Lederer, W.H. (1974): IN Handbook of Micro-Methods for Biological Sciences, Van Niehand Reinhold, New York, p. 86.
43. Shug, A.L., Thomsen, J.D., Folts, J.D., Bittar, N., Klein, M.I., Koke, J.R., & Huth, P.J. (1978): Arch. Biochem. Biophys. 187: 25.

44. Whitmer, J.T., Idell-Wenger, J.A., Rovetto, M.J., & Neely, J.R. (1978): J. Biol. Chem. 253: 4305.
45. Idell-Wenger, J.A., Grotyohann, L.W., & Neely, J.R. (1978): J. Biol. Chem. 253: 4310.
46. Powell, G.L., Grothusen, J.R., Zimmerman, J.K., Evans, C.A., & Fish, W.W. (1981): J. Biol. Chem. 256: 12740.
47. Fritz, I.B., & Marquis, N.R. (1965): Proc. Natl. Acad. Sci. USA 54: 1226.
48. Heldt, H.W., Jacobs, H., & Klingenberg, M. (1965): Biochem. Biophys. Res. Commun. 18: 174.
49. Vignais, P.V., Vignais, P.M., & Defayl, G. (1973): Biochemistry 12: 1508.
50. Bremer, J., & Norum, K.R. (1967): J. Biol. Chem. 252: 1744.
51. Neely, J.R., & Morgan, H.E. (1974): Ann. Rev. Physiol. 36: 413.
52. Folts, J.D., Shug, A.L., Koke, J.R., & Bittar, N. (1978): Am. J. Cardiol. 41: 1209.
53. Liedtke, A.J., Nellis, S.H., & Whitesell, L.F. (1981): Circ. Res. 48: 859.
54. Suzuki, Y., Kamikawa, T., Kobayashi, A., Musumura, Y., & Yamazaki, N. (1981): Jap. Circ. J. 45: 687.
55. Halperin, M.L., Robinson, B.H., & Fritz, I.B. (1972): Proc. Natl. Acad. Sci. USA 69: 1003.
56. Woldegiorgis, G., Yousufzai, S.Y.K., & Shrago, E. (1982): J. Biol. Chem. 257: 14783.
57. Pearson, D.J., & Tubbs, R.K. (1967): Biochem. J. 105: 953.
58. Feuvray, D., Idell-Wenger, J.A., & Neely, J.R. (1979): Circ. Res. 44: 322.
59. Burlington, R.F., & Shug, A.L. (1981): Comp. Biochem. Physiol. 68: 431.

FATTY ACID AND CARNITINE-LINKED ABNORMALITIES

DURING ISCHEMIA AND CARDIOMYOPATHY

A. L. Shug and D. J. Paulson

Department of Neurology
University of Wisconsin and Veterans Hospital
Madison, Wisconsin USA

Myocardial ischemia, a condition whereby reduced perfusion provides an insufficient supply of oxygen to the heart, begins with potentially reversible metabolic and physiological changes which last about 20 minutes (1, 2). Many of these changes seem geared to protect the heart during periods of oxygen deficiency (3). Nevertheless, if perfusion is not restored within this period, irreversible changes in metabolism, structure and function occur, and ultimately the condition will lead to myocardial infarction and cellular death (1, 4, 5).

Table 1 lists some of the more important reversible alterations in metabolism that occur during the first few minutes of ischemia. Temporal studies have shown that the first measurable metabolic change to occur, after the initial O_2 insult, is a sharp decrease in the mitochondrial NAD/NADH ratio caused by decreased electron transport flux. This, in turn, affects coordination between the tricarboxylic acid cycle and related cytosolic enzymes (1, 4, 5). As a result, there is significant hydrogen accumulation and a decline in tissue pH (1, 4). These changes occur within a few seconds after the O_2 insult and are immediately followed by a decline in creatine phosphate (CP) and an increase in tissue levels of lactate and α-glyceralphosphate (α-GP). Simultaneously, there is a transient acceleration of glycolysis, accompanied by a utilization of cellular glycogen stores and a cessation of fatty acid oxidation (1, 4). Within the first 30 seconds, the

Table 1.   Temporal Sequence of Reversible Metabolic Change
During Early Myocardial Ischemia*

---

1. Decreased mitochondrial NAD/NADH ratio
2. Decreased tricarboxylic acid cycle flux
3. Decrease in pH
4. Decrease in creatine phosphate
5. Transient, increased glucose utilization and decrease in cellular glycogen
6. Increase in lactate levels
7. Increase in α-glycerophosphate
8. Decreased fatty acid oxidation
9. Increase in short-chain and long-chain acyl carnitine and hydroxylated fatty acids
10. Increased long-chain acyl CoA esters (LCACAE)/free carnitine ratio
11. Decreased mitochondrial adenine nucleotide translocator (ANT) activity
12. Affected area of the myocardium becomes cyanotic and cooler and depressed membrane potential changes (ECG) are noted after about 30 seconds. Heartbeat in ischemic zone ceases at about 1 minute.
13. Decrease in ATP and ADP, and increase in AMP

---

*The above alterations in metabolism occur during the first 30-60 seconds, with the exception of 13, which is more evident after about 2-5 minutes of ischemia.

affected area of the myocardium becomes cyanotic and cooler, and significant electrocardiographic changes are observed because of the depressed membrane potential (1).

Mitochondrial-creatine phosphokinase (M-CPK), an isoenzyme of cytosolic-creatine phosphokinase (C-CPK), is localized on the outer part of the inner mitochondrial membrane next to the adenine nucleotide translocator (ANT) (Figure 1) (6). ANT catalyzes an exclusive molecule-for-molecule exchange of ADP and ATP across the inner mitochondrial membrane, and in this manner links the enzymatic reactions of the mitochondrial cell compartment with that of the cytosol (7). As indicated in Figure 1, M-CPK catalyzes the reaction:
ATP + creatine (C) ⇌ ADP + CP in the forward direction. The ADP produced is then translocated into the mitochondria via ANT, thus stimulating respiration. The CP is stored in the cytosol and is later converted to ATP by C-CPK.

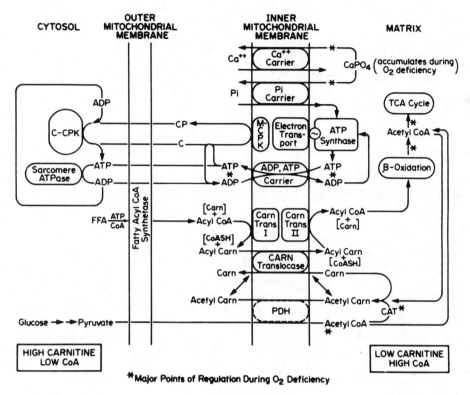

FIGURE 1

Mitochondrial regulation of carnitine-linked metabolism during ischemia.

In this manner, the joint action of M-CPK, ANT, C-CPK, and the sarcomere ATPase provides a continual supply of each substrate needed for the maintenance of State 3 respiration and muscle contraction (8). However, acidosis caused by the onset of ischemia inhibits cAMP-catalyzed phosphorylation of cardiac troponin-tropomyosin, thus explaining the rapid decrease in contractility regardless of tissue ATP levels (9). The drop in pH probably slows M-CPK formation of CP (6), and a variety of evidence indicates that the accumulation of long-chain acyl CoA esters (LCACAE) during this period of ischemia also inhibits ANT activity (10). Thus, the lowered pH and LCACAE inhibited ANT, break the metabolic link between ANT and M-CPK, and prevent CP formation.

It has been well established that long-chain fatty acids (FFA) are the preferred energy-yielding substrate of the myocardium (4), and because of this, carnitine plays a critical role in normal heart function. The manner in which carnitine $(CH_3)_3N^+CH_2CHOHCH_2COO^-$ facilitates FFA oxidation is illustrated in Figure 1. It should be noted that only the L-form of carnitine can be esterified in mammals, although both the D- and L-isomers may be transported across cellular and mitochondrial membranes (11). Esterification of FFA to the β-carbon of carnitine within the heart cell is required for their entry into the mitochondrion, where they are oxidized to carbon dioxide and water. After activation of FFA to the acyl CoA ester at the outer mitochondrial membrane, the necessary reactions are sequentially catalyzed by carnitine transferase I, carnitine translocase, and carnitine transferase II. The matrix-acyl CoA formed by the joint action of these enzymes is then ready to undergo β-oxidation, while the free carnitine produced is exchanged with long-chain acyl carnitine to continue the cyclic function of this carnitine-dependent fatty acyl CoA transport system (12). The formation of acetyl carnitine (see Figure 1) from acetyl CoA via matrix-localized carnitine acetyl transferase (CAT) may also play a vital role in mitochondrial energy production. It has been suggested that the function of CAT, which is found in relatively high amounts in heart tissue, is to equilibrate the mitochondrial acetyl CoA/CoA and acetyl carnitine/carnitine couples (13). Because acetyl carnitine or carnitine rapidly exchanges across the inner mitochondrial membrane, the entire cellular reservoir of carnitine is available for the maintenance of the acetylation state of the much smaller mitochondrial CoA pool. This function of CAT is of particular importance to the heart, because a single heart beat will consume more acetyl CoA than the total CoA content of mitochondria (14). In this manner, acetyl carnitine, a prime energy storage compound of the heart, and CAT play a critical role in the steady supply of energy required for myocardial contraction. The acyl-carrier function of carnitine illustrated in Figure 1 is required for FFA oxidation because the inner membrane of heart mitochondria is impermeable to LCACAE (12).

Congestive cardiomyopathy is a disease state of cardiac muscle characterized by poor myocardial contractility, compensatory ventricular hypertrophy and dilatation, often with complicating congestive heart failure and arrhythmias. In most cardiomyopathies, etiology is unknown and treatment nonspecific (15). Post-morten tissue samples have demonstrated myocardial fibrosis and occasional lipid deposition together with ultrastructural disarray of myofibrils, swelling, distortion, and disruption of subcellular organelles, including the mitochondria and sarcoplasmic reticulum (16). Lipid deposition

is commonly reported in hamster cardiomyopathy and fatty acid
oxidation is known be depressed (17). Carnitine deficiency has
been noted in animal models of cardiomyopathy since Wittels and
Bressler's report of depressed myocardial carnitine
concentrations in diphtheritic guinea pigs (18). The
concurrence and effects of various types of carnitine deficiency
in man have also been described (19), and recent studies
indicate that systematic carnitine deficiency may be a cause of
some forms of cardiomyopathy (20-22).

Changes in the tissue levels of free and esterified
carnitine have been reported during myocardial ischemia and
cardiomyopathy as well as a number of other diseases, although
some of these alterations could be accounted for by
interconversion between free and acyl carnitine rather than an
actual loss of the compound (23). Previous studies have shown
that the cellular loss of carnitine is accompanied by increased
synthesis of triglycerides and decreased fatty oxidation, and
addition of carnitine to such preparations reversed these
changes in metabolism (24). More recent investigations have
shown that the induction of myocardial ischemia or hypoxia
caused rapid and large changes in the relative tissue levels of
free and esterified carnitine (25). It was also noted during
these studies that repeated episodes of ischemia or anoxia, or
prolonged exposure to these conditions, resulted in the leakage
of free and acyl carnitine from the heart (23, 25). The
decrease in tissue levels of free carnitine accompanied
increases in acyl carnitine, LCACAE, and hydroxylated fatty
acids (23, 25, 26). These changes resulted in a very rapid
increase in the LCACAE/free carnitine ratio during the onset of
ischemia or hypoxia, which, in turn, was associated with the
inhibition of mitochondrial ANT activity (25, 27).

The aim of the present paper is to review the effects of
myocardial ischemia and cardiomyopathy upon fatty acid
carnitine-linked metabolism, and to consider the role these
early metabolic changes may play in damage to the myocardium.

METHODS AND MATERIALS

Canine Experiments. Adult mongrel dogs (10-20 kg) were
anesthetized with pentobarbital (30 mg/kg), intubated, and
placed on mechanical ventilation. The physiological
measurements and preparations used in the studies on the
open-chest dog model of myocardial ischemia were as previously
described (27). Ischemia was produced in these animals by a 70%
reduction of bloodflow in left anterior descending (LAD) branch
of the coronary artery. This produced an ST segment elevation

of greater than 2 mV which is indicative of ischemia (1). At
designated times, cardiac inflow and outflow were prevented by
clamping. Tissue representing the ischemic area (LAD bed) and
nonischemic area (circumflex bed) of the left ventricle was
rapidly excised, frozen in liquid nitrogen, and stored at -70°
C. The frozen tissues were extracted and analyzed within two
weeks.

Rat Studies. In the isolated perfused heart studies, rats
were anesthetized with 25 mg of sodium pentobarbital for 20-30
minutes after 150 units of sodium heparin were administered.
Hearts were quickly removed and mounted on the perfusion
apparatus essentially as described by Neely and Rovetto (28).
The perfusion medium was a modified Krebs-Henseleit bicarbonate
buffer (28), pH 7.4, which was equilibrated with $O_2:CO_2$
(95:5) at 37° C before use. The substrates glucose (11 mM)
and insulin (2 mµ/ml), and palmitate (1.2 mM) bound to 3%
albumin were perfused as indicated in the results. The
Langendorf of working heart preparations were as previously
described (28). Hypoxia was induced by perfusion with media
equilibrated with 95% N_2:5% CO_2. Global ischemia was
produced in the working isolated perfused rat heart preparations
by modification of the low cardiac output, high aortic
resistance method (28). The method involves the positioning of
a bypass on the left atrial (LA) line from the reservoir to the
LA cannula. A screw-clamp attached to the bypass allowed the
ischemic flow rate to be chosen prior to cannulation and when
turned in, was able to produce a $\leq$ 95% reduction in flow within
several seconds without manipulation of a pump (29). All hearts
were equilibrated by a preliminary 10 minute perfusion with
oxygenated buffer and glucose. At the end of the experiment the
hearts were freeze-clamped and stored at -70° C until
extraction for determination of the various metabolites. Male
rats (Spraque Dawley strain) weighing 180-220 g were used for
this study. Beef and rat heart mitochondria were prepared and
their respiratory activity determined as previously described
(10).

Cardiomyopathic and normal control hamsters were maintained
and bred in Dr. Lemanski's laboratory at the University of
Wisconsin. We have a breeding colony of cardiomyopathic
hamsters derived from stock (strain UM-X7.1) obtained from Dr.
Jasmin of the University of Toronto. By regulating the
light-dark cycle, all of the female hamsters (normal and
cardiomyopathic) have their estrus cycles synchronized, allowing
planned breeding for hamsters of known age.

Free carnitine was assayed by the method of Bohmer et al.
(30), while acetyl carnitine was determined by a slight

modification of the technique of Velosos and Veech (31).
Long-chain acetyl carnitine was extracted and converted to free
L-carnitine according to the method described by Oram et al.
(32) and carnitine was measured by the method of Bohmer et al.
(30). LCACAE were extracted from tissues according to the
procedure of Oram et al. (32) and determined by the enzymatic
cycling method of Veloso and Veech (31). Mitochondrial
preparations, ANT activity, ATP and CP levels were determined
essentially as previously described (10, 29, 33).

RESULTS AND DISCUSSION

It has been well established that fatty acid oxidation is
depressed during the onset of myocardial ischemia (4), and a
variety of studies have shown that it is β-oxidation which is
actually impaired, rather than the activation or transport
mechanisms (4). The suppression of fatty acid oxidation most
likely occurs at both the flavin and NAD points of entry into
the mitochondrial electron transport system. Because of this,
the accumulation of intermediates in the oxidation of fatty
acids, such as LCACAE, long- and short-chain acyl carnitine, and
β-hydroxy fatty acids (Table 1) have been shown to occur during
the early phase of ischemia (23, 25, 26). Related
investigations have shown that as LCACAE levels in the ischemic
myocardium increased, ANT activity declined (34). Table 2
summarizes the results of such experiments. Values for ATP and
CP, well known markers of early ischemia, have been included for
comparative purposes. As has been previously found, CP levels
dropped rapidly ($\leq$ 50%) within the first minute of ischemia,
while ATP values showed no significant change during this time.
Recent experiments (Figure 2) indicate that the rapid decline in
ATP and ADP that occurs later on during early ischemia is
localized in the myocardial cytosolic cell compartment. The
lowering of mitochondrial-ANT-exchangeable nucleotides
(ATP-ADP); however, seems to occur during the onset of the
irreversible phase of ischemia. This even may be temporarily
related to the increased mitochondrial LCACAE/free carnitine
ratio, and the resultant accumulation of matrix levels of
long-chain acyl carnitine (25, 29).

It should be noted that control, aerobic LCACAE values were
considerably higher in the isolated rat heart than in the open
chest dog, although the total amount of CoA in these tissues was
found to be quite similar (70 to 90 nmoles/gm wet wt.) (23).
The presence of elevated levels of LCACAE in control rat hearts
may be explained by the combined effects of high concentration
of FFA (1.2 mM palmitate) and the relatively low oxygen delivery
of the perfusate in the isolated working heart preparation.

Table 2. Effects of Ischemia upon LCACAE, ATP, CP and ANT Activity

Preparation	Treatment	Time (min)	LCACAE (nmol/g/ww)	ANT	ATP (µmol/g/ww)	CP (µmol/g/ww)
Rat	aerobic	20	31.6±1.7	5.27±0.45[a]	2.13±1.08	5.36±0.28
Rat[b]	Ischemic*	1	54.5±5.7[+]	-	1.94±0.16[+]	2.38±0.62[+]
Rat	ischemic	10	60.3±2.1[+]	2.01±0.2[a+]	1.55±0.09	1.40±0.28
Rat	ischemic	20	69.0±1.6[+]	1.30±0.44[a+]	1.05±0.03	1.37±0.40
Rat	hypoxic*	10	62.5±3.5[+]	2.31±0.54[a+]	0.74±16	0.56±0.23
Dog	control circumflex bed	60	17.5±4.9	17,500±760[c]	5.7 ±1.3	15.8±4.4
Dog	ischemic*	30	37.9±12.3[+]	8,100±530[c+]	2.1 ±0.12[+]	1.6±0.6[+]
Dog	ischemic LAD bed	60	75.1±20.4[+]	5,900±910[c+]	1.85 0.08[+]	1.5 0.9

[a]ANT activity nanamoles ADP transported 1 min/mg total protein.

[b]Rat using method of producing ischemia described under methods.

[c]DPM/min/0.1 mg mitochondria protein.

*Methods of producing ischemia or hypoxia where animals are described under methods.

[+]Indicates significant difference between groups at the p < 0.01 level.

N = 5-10 determination for each value given.

Values given are ± SEM.

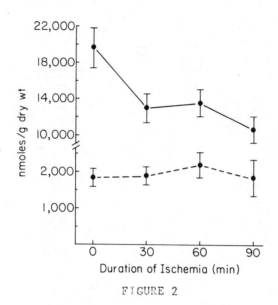

FIGURE 2

The effect of ischemia upon whole tissue and mitochondrial ATP and ADP levels.

The rate of LCACAE increase after the induction of ischemia in the rat heart was very rapid (Table 2), and similar findings have been noted in the open chest dog (10). Related studies indicate that ANT activity is reversibly inhibited after only a few minutes of ischemia (10). The more pronounced inhibition of ANT, observed after 10 minutes of ischemia or hypoxia, was accompanied by increased LCACAE levels. However, we have recently found that reoxygenation not only restores left ventricular contraction (dp/dt) to hearts treated by this protocol, but also returns LCACAE levels and ANT activity to control values. The demonstration of increased mitochondrial LCACAE levels, and inhibited ANT activity during the reversible phase of ischemia requires special techniques because of the oxidation of LCACAE which can occur during the isolation procedure (29, 33).

Thirty and sixty minutes of ischemia in the open chest dog caused the accumulation of LCACAE, and a corresponding inhibition of ANT activity (Table 2). The effects of reflow upon these parameters have not yet been tested in this model of myocardial ischemia. However, previous studies on mitochondria isolated from the ischemic LAD bed showed inhibited State 3 respiration, and ANT activity which was partially restored by the addition of carnitine (34). Mitochondria isolated from the LAD bed after 60 minutes of ischemia showed inhibition of both State 3 and State 4 respiration, and had very low respiratory activity in either State 3 or 4, which was unaffected by the addition of carnitine (35, 36). Recent observations indicate that irreversible damage occurred in the subendocardium after 120 minutes of ischemia in the open chest dog. This period of ischemia also adversely affected mitochondrial structure and the respiratory control ratio (State 3/State 4). These mitochondrial changes eliminated ANT activity and prevented possible beneficial effects from addition of carnitine (37).

Previous studies with isolated liver and heart mitochondria preparations showed that low concentrations of long-chain fatty acids inhibited the $ATP-^{32}P$ exchange reaction only when KCN was present (38). Later studies indicated that this may have been caused by the accumulation of LCACAE which, in turn, inhibited ANT and thus prevented the $ATP-^{32}P$ exchange (39). Recent experimentation (summarized in Figure 3) has shown that incubation of beef heart mitochondria with palmitate and KCN, which prevents O_2 uptake, does indeed cause the accumulation of palmitoyl CoA, which, in turn, results in a corresponding inhibition of ANT activity. In addition, it was found that the addition of L-carnitine to mitochondria incubated with palmitate and KCN prevented the accumulation of LCACAE, and reversed ANT inhibition. Because most of the CoA present in the beef heart mitochondria was converted to acyl CoA by incubation with palmitate and KCN, and since it is known that over 90% of the cellular CoA is located in the mitochondrial matrix (40), we have concluded that ANT was primarily inhibited at the matrix loci. More convincing evidence for this was the finding which has been recently presented (33).

Table 3 shows the effect of varying periods of ischemia or hypoxia upon carnitine tissue levels in rat and dog heart preparations. In the isolated rat heart rapidly induced severe ischemia ($\leq 95\%$ reduction in flow in 2 seconds) resulted in immediate alterations in free and acetyl carnitine, but did not significantly affect long-chain acyl carnitine levels. Twenty minutes of ischemia, which marked the onset of irreversible change, caused a slight loss of carnitine from the heart, mainly as the free or acetyl forms, but did not affect tissue levels of

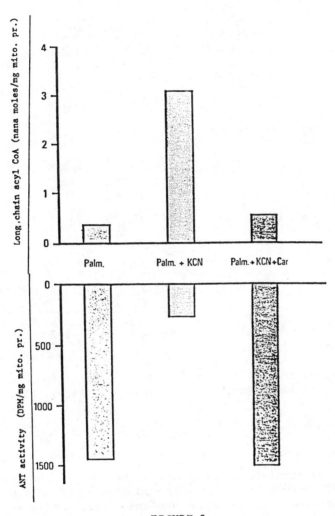

FIGURE 3

Reversal of LCACAE inhibited ANT activity by L-carnitine in isolated
bovine heart mitochondria. "Heavy" mitochondria in amounts of 10 to
50 mg/assay were incubated in the presence of 0.03 mM palmitate, 10
mM ATP, and 1 mM KCN (present when indicated) in a media as
previously described. Time of incubation was 5 minutes. At the end
of this period, the mitochondria were centrifuged and resuspended in
cold media with 1 mM KCN, and a small aliquot removed for ANT assay.
L-carnitine was present at 5 mM (when indicated).

Table 3. Tissue Levels of Carnitine During Ischemia

Preparation	Time Min	Free Carnitine nmol/g/ww	Acetyl Carnitine nmol/g/ww	L-C Acyl Carnitine nmol/g/ww	Total Carnitine nmol/g/ww
rat aerobic	20	359±34	153±17	224±18	736
rat ischem*	5	230±29[+]	259±26[+]	229±15	718
rat ischem	20	204±52[+]	178±19[+]	250±45	632[+]
rat hypox*	40	70±24[+]	71±11[+]	416±39[+]	557[+]
dog aerobic circum bed control	60	1023±130	178±57	113±46	1315
dog ischem*	30	676±169[+]	489±99[+]	221±31[+]	1386
dog ischem	60	378±48[+]	296±70[+]	237±59	911[+]

*Methods of producing ischemia or hypoxia in above animals are described under methods.

[+]Indicates significant different between groups at the $p > 0.05$ level. N = 5-10 determinations for each value cited. Values given are ± SEM.

long-chain acyl carnitine. In contrast, the hypoxic heart, which was not irreversibly damaged by 20 minutes of oxygen deficiency, showed a much greater decline in free and acetyl carnitine, while accumulating higher levels of long-chain acyl carnitine. The loss of carnitine was greater from the hypoxic heart. Long-chain acyl carnitine also accumulated in the ischemic dog heart and similar changes in free and acetyl carnitine were also noted. A considerable loss of carnitine was found after 60 minutes of ischemia, which marked the onset of irreversible damage. Recent experiments in the isolated perfused rat heart have shown much lower losses of carnitine during hypoxia or ischemia when values were expressed on a dry weight basis (36). The presence of insulin in the perfusion media seemed to retard the loss of carnitine (36). Nevertheless, the loss of carnitine from the isolated perfused rat heart during ischemia is much less than from the ischemic

Table 4. Cardiac Skeletal Muscle and Plasma Carnitine
          Concentrations in UM-X7.1 and Wild Strain Syrian
          Hamsters at 300 Days of Age.

A.   Carnitine Content - nmoles/gm wet weight

Age (days)	Group	Free	Short Chain Acyl	Long Chain Acyl	Total
300	Wild	228.9	331.6	120.4	680.9
	UM-X7.1	168.0	130.4	71.3	369.0

B.

Age (days)	Group	Skeletal Muscle nmoles/gm wet weight	Plasma μM
10	Wild	300.2	10.4
	UM-X7.1	248.3	9.9
50	Wild	444.6	27.8
	UM-X7.1	368.4	26.8
150	Wild	340.5	24.5
	UM-X7.1	466.0	27.0
300	Wild	268.9	40.3
	UM-X7.1	381.3	43.0

dog (Table 3), pig (45) or human heart (58). It is not certain
whether this is because of species difference, or changes
induced during the isolation of perfusion techniques. Recent
studies in the open chest dog have clearly shown that carnitine
is lost from both the reversibly (subepicardium) and
irreversibly (subendocardium) damaged heart after 3-hour
occlusion followed by 1-hour reperfusion (36, 37).

   Carnitine levels have been shown to be reduced in the
cardiomyopathic hamster heart (41). In Table 4 and Figure 4 we
show that carnitine values in the newborn normal (wild strain)
and cardiomyopathic (UM-X7.1) hamsters are similar, and rapidly
increase until about 50 days of age. After this time, there is
a considerable decrease in carnitine levels in strain UM-X7.1

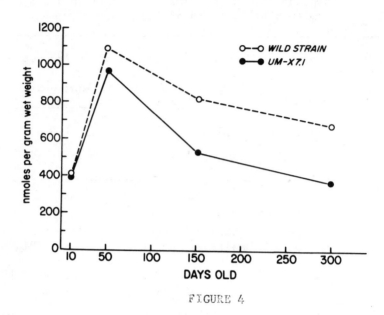

FIGURE 4

Total myocardial carnitine content in the wild strain and
UM-X7.1 hamsters as a function of age.

until at 300 days the wild strain hearts have about twice as
much carnitine as found in strain UM-X7.1. Skeletal muscle and
plasma levels remain the same for both strains during this
growth period. These results suggest that in the Syrian
cardiomyopathic hamster carnitine deficiency is caused by the
disease. These observations are in direct contrast to the human
forms of cardiomyopathy which appear to be caused by systemic
carnitine deficiency (20-22). In this disease the plasma
carnitine levels fall well below 10 nmoles/L, and skeletal
muscle (30 nmol/g/ww), and heart muscle (56.8 nmole/g/ww) were
found to be far below normal levels (21). It seems quite
certain that this type of usually fatal cardiomyopathy is caused
by carnitine deficiency, because treatment with only carnitine
completely restores the patient to normal (20-22). Recent
studies indicate that some forms of human cardiomyopathy
resemble the hamster disease in that carnitine levels appear to
decline in the heart secondarily to the onset of the disease
(42). In these patients, relatively high levels of carnitine

and acetyl carnitine are noted in the plasma and urine (42).   It is thought that carnitine may be leaked from the heart because of damage to the myocardial cell membrane transport system. Treatment of these patients with oral carnitine has also produced beneficial results (42).

Changes in some biochemical and physiological parameters during ischemia are shown in Table 5.   Induction of ischemia caused an immediate sharp rise in the LCACAE/free carnitine ratio, which was accompanied by a decline in left ventricular contraction (dp/dt), and ANT activity.   It is important to note that the exchangeable mitochondrial matrix nucleotides (EMMN) ATP and ADP did not change significantly during the 20 minute period of reversible ischemia.   Subtraction of total mitochondrial nucleotides from total frozen heart tissue levels gave nucleotide levels in the cytosolic compartment (Figure 2). These studies indicate that the level of nucleotides ATP and ADP drop rapidly in the cytosol during the reversible phase of ischemia, while mitochondrial levels remain unaffected.   Reflow partially restored cytosolic levels, but there was a loss in total cytosolic ATP, ADP and AMP of about 10 to 20% even though heart function was completely restored (29).   After a period of 30 minutes of ischemia, irreversible damage occurred and reflow did not restore dp/dt and did not lower or reverse the LCACAE/free carnitine levels or affect ANT activity (29).   These results indicate that a reversible LCACAE inhibition of ANT occurs early in ischemia, and may have a protective function by regulating O_2 consumption and maintaining its mitochondrial matrix ATP/ADP x P_i ratio.

The point at which elevated LCACAE/free carnitine ratios cease to be beneficial and become detrimental appears to correlate with the onset of the irreversible phase of ischemia (29).   Harmful effects of the LCACAE/free carnitine ratio during prolonged ischemia may be related to higher levels in the mitochondrial matrix, low carnitine tissue levels, and accumulated long-chain acyl carnitine (43).   Thus, a tissue deficiency of free carnitine, either by its leakage from the heart or by its esterification, will further increase the LCACAE/free carnitine ratio.   We have recently found that prolonged exposure of the isolated perfused rat heart to ischemia or hypoxia caused very high LCACAE/free carnitine ratios which were not readily reversed by reflow or reoxygenation (29).   Such high, irreversible LCACAE/free carnitine ratios would be particularly harmful because they could prevent mitochondrial O_2 uptake, regardless of flow or O_2 tissue levels.   Mitochondrial matrix CAT activity may also be inhibited which would jeopardize the maintenance of the acetyl CoA/acetyl carnitine in the mitochondrial contraction.

Table 5.   Changes in Biochemical and Physiological Correlates
           During Ischemia

Treatment	dp/dt mmHg/sec	LCACAE/Free Carnitine nmol/g	ANT nmol/g ADP trans/min/mg	EMMN* nmol/g wet wt.
20 min O_2	1673±135	0.09	5.30±0.37	280±5
5 min ischemia	200±24[+]	0.25[+]	2.49±0.18[+]	350±3
20 min ischemia	29±2[+]	0.34[+]	1.30±0.44[+]	270±1

*Exchangeable mitochondrial matrix nucleotides, ATP and ADP.

[+]Indicates significant differences between groups at the $p > 0.01$ level. N=10 determinations for each value cited.

The absence of free CoA and carnitine in the mitochondrial matrix could also prevent substrate oxidation regardless of oxygen availability. A number of other mitochondrial enzyme systems which are inhibited by LCACAE may also be affected (35). In addition, high matrix levels of LCACAE and long-chain acyl carnitine may cause lesions of the inner mitochondrial membrane by detergent action. Such lesions could allow calcium accumulation upon reflow, loss of adenine and pyridine nucleotides, and activation of membrane phospholipases, and thus signal the onset of irreversible tissue damage (37). These are some of the considerations which have led us to suggest that carnitine may protect the ischemic myocardium by lowering the LCACAE/free carnitine ratio (35).

As indicated in this presentation, and elsewhere (44-48), there is a considerable body of information that clearly demonstrates an important role of carnitine in the metabolism of the normal oxygen deficient and cardiomyopathic myocardium. Nevertheless, there remains a good deal of uncertainty regarding the mechanisms by which carnitine may protect the ischemic or carnitine-deficient heart (49). One of the reasons for this is the inability to demonstrate an effect of carnitine in the isolated perfused rat heart (49). The net uptake of carnitine in isolated rat heart preparations has not been observed; and indeed, a net increase in skeletal muscle has rarely been noted upon carnitine administration, despite apparent beneficial effects (19). Obviously, carnitine must, at sometime, be taken up by the heart and skeletal muscle, since it has been well established that these organs, which normally contain high levels of carnitine, lack the ability to synthesize this compound (50).

These seemingly contradictory observations may be partially explained by recent findings which show that carnitine enters the heart by an exchange-diffusion mechanism (51), which is quite similar to that of the mitochondrial carnitine translocator (52). This carnitine transport system appears to favor the exchange of extracellular L-carnitine for gamma-butyrobetaine (GBB), which is synthesized in heart and skeletal muscle (50). These studies support the view that net uptake of carnitine by the heart is dependent upon the rate of synthesis of GBB and its eventual exchange with L-carnitine. It should be mentioned, however, that unilateral transport of carnitine has been reported in isolated myocyte preparations (53). These results could have been caused by relatively large losses of carnitine encountered in the preparation of the myocytes, which in turn could induce the exchange diffusion system to function unilaterally (54). Although little is known about the control of GBB synthesis in heart tissue, the rate of net carnitine uptake in clinical (55) or animal systems (56) appears to be very low. It is suggested that carnitine levels in the normal heart are maintained largely by exchange between extracellular and intracellular carnitine. This is because recent studies have shown that treatment of rats with high levels of D-carnitine causes a tissue-specific depletion of L-carnitine from only heart and skeletal muscle (57). These findings, therefore, support the hypothesis that tissue carnitine levels are maintained in vivo primarily by the exchange carnitine transport system of the plasma membrane in heart and skeletal muscle. However, prolonged or repeated severe ischemic episodes can alter cell membrane permeability and cause carnitine to leak from the heart (Table 3). This defect may disturb the carnitine maintenance system, and eventually render the ischemic area of the heart carnitine deficient (58). As a result, the affected area will become abnormally dependent upon glucose oxidation, and show a greater susceptibility to ischemia because of the increased LCACAE/ free carnitine ratio and low cellular stores of acetyl carnitine (25).

The mechanisms of carnitine protection:

1. Elevate plasma levels of free carnitine. This could be of particular importance because carnitine plasma levels are normally far below that contained in heart tissue (23, 30). Raising plasma levels of carnitine to equal that of heart tissue could increase the exchange across the heart cell membrane of

free carnitine for intracellular long-chain acyl carnitine.
This action could decrease not only long-chain acyl carnitine
esters, but also acyl CoA and fatty acids as well by stimulation
of the reverse action of the acyl carnitine transferase system
(Figure 1). Lowering of tissue levels of fatty acids and acyl
esters of carnitine and CoA would benefit the heart because of
the well-known harmful effects of these substances (35, 39). In
addition, such high plasma levels of carnitine may allow
carnitine to enter the cell by simple diffusion if changes in
cell permeability permit.

The beneficial effects of L-carnitine treatment of
systemically carnitine deficient patients may also be related to
increased plasma levels coupled with very low tissue levels of
carnitine. This is because the initially prolonged presence of
low carnitine plasma levels results in the depletion of
carnitine from heart and skeletal muscles. The administration
of carnitine reverses the condition and causes an enormous
increase in plasma levels (22). This in turn may induce both
the cellular and mitochondrial carnitine exchange diffusion
systems to function unilaterally. The latter transport system
would continue to function until high intracellular levels
switch carnitine transport back to the normal exchange diffusion
system. These suggestions may also apply to patients with
ischemic heart disease if sufficient quantities of carnitine
have been lost from the heart.

2. Reverse LCACAE inhibition of mitochondrial ANT
activity. Carnitine has been shown to reverse LCACAE inhibition
of ANT in isolated mitochondria (Figure 2), and similar effects
have been noted in animal models of ischemia (27). This action
of carnitine would be of great benefit to the ischemic
myocardium because it would permit the resumption of normal
respiratory activity, as well as calcium transport and other
important mitochondrial functions (35) after reflow or
reoxygenation has been established. Carnitine administration
can lower the LCACAE levels even in the total absence of O_2
uptake (Figure 2), and in this manner prevent the accumulation
of irreversibly high mitochondrial matrix LCACAE/free carnitine
ratios, which, in turn, inhibit ANT and prevent mitochondrial
oxygen consumption regardless of reoxygenation or reflow.

3. Improve fatty acid or glucose oxidation and acetyl
carnitine storage. Increased tissue levels of free carnitine
can stimulate fatty acid oxidation or glucose as indicated in
Figure 1, when oxygen is present. In addition, higher levels
will stimulate the formation of acetyl carnitine which may be
required for heart contraction and, in fact, for the recovery of
the heart from ischemia.

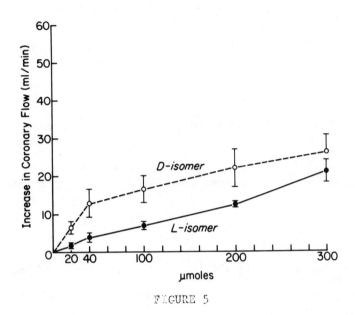

FIGURE 5

Effect of L- or D-carnitine upon coronary blood flow in the dog.

4. Increase in the synthesis of triglycerides (TG). TG formation takes place exclusively in the cytosolic cell compartment, while most of the LCACAE, necessary for its synthesis, is accumulated in the mitochondrial matrix (40, 60). During ischemia, when low tissue levels of O_2 prevent fatty acid oxidation, high levels of carnitine may facilitate the transfer of acyl groups from the mitochondria to the cytosol by reversing the acyl carnitine transport system (see Figure 1), and thus stimulating TG synthesis in the total absence of O_2. α-Glyceral phosphate, the other substrate required for TG formation, accumulates in the cytosol during ischemia (60), and so would not limit this action of carnitine. Increased synthesis of TG is considered beneficial to the ischemic heart because it would reduce harmful tissue levels of fatty acids, as well as long-chain acyl esters of carnitine and CoA.

5. Increase blood flow. Recent experiments in the open chest dog (Figure 5) have shown that both the L- and D-isomers of carnitine produce a dose-dependent increase in coronary flow. Such an effect could aid in supplying oxygen to ischemic tissues upon reflow.

ACKNOWLEDGEMENTS

These studies were supported by the Medical Research Service of the Veterans Administration and NIH Grant HL-17736. Special thanks go to Dr. Claudio Cavazza, Sigma Tau Chemical Co., Rome, Italy, for providing L-carnitine and D-carnitine used in these studies, and for his continued interest in our research program.

REFERENCES

1. Hillis, L.D., & Braunwald, E. (1977): N. Engl. J. Med. 296: 971.
2. Jennings, R.B., & Ganote, C.E. (1976): Circ. Res. 38 (Suppl. 1): I-80.
3. Katz, A.M. (1973): Am. J. Cardiol. 32: 46.
4. Neely, J.R., & Morgan, H.E. (1974): Ann. Rev. Physiol. 36: 413.
5. Jennings, R.B., Ganote, C.E., & Reimer, K.A. (1975): Am. J. Pathol. 81: 179.
6. Jacobus, W.E., & Lehninger, A.L. (1973): J. Biol. Chem. 248: 4803.
7. Pfaff, E., & Klingenberg, M. (1968): Eur. J. Biochem. 6: 66.
8. Bessman, S.P., & Geiger, P.J. (1968): Science 211: 448.
9. Stull, J.T., & Buss, J.E. (1977): J. Biol. Chem. 252: 851.
10. Shug, A.L., Koke, J.R., Folts, J.D., & Bittar, N. (1975): IN Recent Advances in Studies on Cardiac Structure and Metabolism, University Park Press, Baltimore, vol. 10, p. 365.
11. Huth, P.J., Thomsen, J.H., & Shug, A.L. (1978): Life Sci. 23: 715.
12. Bremer, J. (1977): TIBS 2: 207.
13. Tubbs, P.K., Ramsay, R.R., & Edwards, M.R. (1980): IN Carnitine Biosynthesis, Metabolism, and Functions, (eds) R.A. Frenkel and J.D. McGarry, Academic Press, New York, p. 207.
14. Neely, J.R., Denton, R.M., England, P.J., & Randle, P.J. (1972): Biochem. J. 128: 147.
15. Goodwin, J.F. (1974): Circulation 50: 210.

16. Olsen, E.G. (1975): Postgrad. Med. I **51**: 295.
17. Kako, K.J., Thornton, M.J., & Heggtveit, H.A. (1974): Circ. Res. **34**: 570.
18. Wittels, B., & Bressler, R. (1964): J. Clin. Invest. **43**: 630.
19. Engel, A.G. (1980): IN Carnitine Biosynthesis, Metabolism, and Functions, (eds) R.A. Frenkel and J.D. McGarry, Academic Press, New York, p. 271.
20. Chapoy, P.R., Angelini, C., Brown, W.J., Stiff, J.E., & Shug, A.L. (1980): N. Engl. J. Med. **303**: 1389.
21. Tripp, M.E., Katcher, M.L., Peters, H.A., Gilbert, E.F., Arya, S., Hodach, R.J., & Shug, A.L. (1981): N. Engl. J. Med. **305**: 385.
22. Waber, L.J., Valle, D., Neill, C., DiMauro, S., & Shug, A.L. (1982): J. Pediatr. **101**: 700.
23. Shug, A.L., Thomsen, J.D., Folts, J.D., Bittar, N., Klein, M.I., Koke, J.R., & Huth, P.J. (1978): Arch. Biochem. Biophys. **187**: 25.
24. Christiansen, R., Borrebaek, B., & Bremer, J. (1976): FEBS Lett. **62**: 313.
25. Shug, A.L., Huth, P.J., Hayes, B., Thomsen, J.H., Hall, P.V., Bittar, N., & Demling, R.J. (1980): IN Carnitine Biosynthesis, Metabolism and Functions, (eds) R.A. Frenkel and J.D. McGarry, Academic Press, New York, p. 321.
26. Moore, K.H., Radloff, J.F., Hull, F.E., & Sweeley, C.C. (1980): Am. J. Physiol. **239**: H257.
27. Folts, J.D., Shug, A.L., Koke, J.R., & Bittar, N. (1978): Am. J. Cardiol. **41**: 1209.
28. Neely, J.R., & Rovetto, J.M. (1975): IN Methods of Enzymology, (eds) B.W. O'Malley & J.G. Hartman, Academic Press, New York, Vol. 39, p. 43.
29. Hayes, B.E. (1980): Ph.D. Thesis, University of Wisconsin, Madison, Wisconsin.
30. Bohmer, T., Rydning, A., & Solberg, H.E. (1974): Clin. Chic. Acta **57**: 55.
31. Veloso, D., & Veech, R.L. (1974): Anal. Biochem. **62**: 449.
32. Oram, J.F., Wengner, I.I., & Neely, J.R. (1975): J. Biochem. **250**: 73.
33. Paulson, D.J., & Shug, A.L. (1982): Circulation **66**: 434.
34. Shug, A.L., Shrago, E., Bittar, N., Folts, J.D., & Koke, J.R. (1975): Am. J. Physiol. **228**: 689.
35. Shug, A.L. (1979): Texas Reports Biol. Med. **39**: 409.
36. Shug, A.L. personal observations.
37. Regitz, V., Paulson, D.J., Hodach, R.J., Little, S.E., Schaper, W., & Shug, A.L. (1984): Basic Res. Cardiol. **195**: In press.
38. Falcone, A.B., & Mao, R.L. (1965): Biochim. Biophys. Acta **105**: 233.
39. Shug, A.L., Lerner, E., Elson, C., & Shrago, E. (1971): Biochem. Biophys. Res. Commun. **43**: 557.

40. Idell-Wenger, J.A., Grotyohann, L.W., & Neely, J.R. (1978): J. Biol. Chem. 253: 4310.
41. Hoppel, C.L., Tandler, B., Parland, W., Turkaly, J.S., & Albers, L.D. (1981): J. Biol. Chem. 257: 1540.
42. Tripp, M.E., & Shug, A.L. (1983): J. Am. Coll. Cardiol. 1: 724.
43. Feuvray, D., & Plouet, J. (1981): Circ. Res. 48: 740.
44. Challoner, D.R., & Prals, H.J. (1972): J. Clin. Invest. 51: 2071.
45. Liedtke, A.J., Nellis, S.H., & Copenhaver, G. (1979): J. Clin. Invest. 64: 440.
46. Suzuki, J., Kamikawa, T., & Yamazaki, N. (1980): IN Carnitine Biosynthesis, Metabolism, and Functions, (eds.) R.A. Frenkel & J.D. McGarry, Academic Press, New York, p. 341.
47. Thomsen, J.H., Shug, A.L., Yap, V.U., Patel, A.K., Karras, T.J., & DeFelice, S.L. (1979): Am. J. Cardiol. 43: 300.
48. Cherci, A., Fonzo, R., Lai, C., Mercuro, G., & Corsi, M. (1978): Boll. Soc. Ital. Cardiol. 23: 71.
49. Neely, J.R., Garber, D., McDonough, K., & Idell-Wenger, J. (1979): IN Ischemic Myocardium and Antianginal Drugs, (eds) M.M. Winbury & Y. Abiko, Raven Press, New York, p. 225.
50. Bressler, R. (1970): IN Lipid Metabolism, (ed) S.J. Wakil, Academic Press, New York, p. 49.
51. Molstad, P. (1980): Biochim. Biophys. Acta 597: 166.
52. Pande, S.V., & Parvin, R. (1976): J. Biol. Chem. 251: 6683.
53. Bahl, J.J., Navin, T.R., & Bressler, R. (1980): IN Carnitine Biosynthesis, Metabolism, and Functions, (eds) R.A. Frenkel & J.D. McGarry, Academic Press, New York, p. 91.
54. Pande, S.V., & Parvin, R. (1980): J. Biol. Chem. 255: 2994.
55. Thomsen, J.H., personal communication.
56. Vary, T.C., & Neely, J.R. (1982): Am. J. Physiol. 242: H585.
57. Paulson, D.J., & Shug, A.L. (1981): Life Sci. 28: 2931.
58. Spagnoli, L.G., Corsi, M., Villaschi, S., Palmieri, G., & Maccari, F. (1982): Lancet June 19: 1419.
59. Katz, A.M., & Messineo, F.C. (1982): J. Mol. Cell. Cardiol. 14: 119.
60. Crass, M.F. (1979): IN Metabolic and Morphologic Correlates in Cardiovascular Function, (eds) M.F. Crass & L.A. Sordahl, University of Texas Medical Branch, Galveston, p. 439.

CONSEQUENCES OF FATTY ACID EXCESS IN ISCHEMIC MYOCARDIUM

AND EFFECTS OF THERAPEUTIC INTERVENTIONS

A. J. Liedtke and W. P. Miller

Cardiology Section
Department of Medicine
University of Wisconsin
Madison, Wisconsin

Suspicion that long-chain fatty acids may impair cardiac performance was first reported by Hoak and workers (1) who infused stearic acid bound to albumin into previously anticoagulated but otherwise normal dogs and ducks and noticed an increased prevalence of sudden death and heart failure. This same group in later studies reported that elevating serum free fatty acids in geese caused supraventricular tachycardia, ventricular ectopy, and sudden death and was associated histologically with several lesions including myocytic degeneration, destructive changes in myofibrils, and intramitochondrial inclusion particles (2). That this association was something more than just an isolated laboratory finding unique to experimental animals was next reported by Oliver and colleagues (3). In 200 patients suffering acute myocardial infarction, a twofold increase in serum free fatty acids was observed within the first 48 hours following the onset of pain. Patients with the highest increases in serum fatty acids had the highest prevalence of atrial and ventricular arrhythmias; ventricular tachycardia and fibrillation; second and third degree heart blocks; and total numbers of death. When an anti-lypolytic agent (5-fluoro-3-hydroxy-methylpyridine hydrochloride) was administered within 5 hours from the onset of symptoms, the numbers of patients with ventricular tachycardia were significantly reduced, provided that the elevated plasma levels of free fatty acids were successfully lowered and maintained in the normal range throughout the treatment period

225

(4). While the majority of this early work focussed primarily
on the correlation between fatty acid excess and disorders of
rhythm in aerobic and ischemic heart muscle, relatively little
emphasis was placed on determining the influence of fatty acids
on disorders in mechanical function. Such was the purpose of
these studies. This paper will review the effects of excess
fatty acids in the intact working swine heart preparation, a
model analogous to the human myocardium in many respects, and
survey the benefits of two therapies specifically designed to
modify and alter fatty acid metabolism. These data were in part
previously published (5-7).

MATERIALS AND METHODS

Swine of either sex, weighing 33.6 - 86.4 kg (average 48.6
kg) were studied following anesthesia with pentobarbital (35
mg/kg) and the establishment of controlled positive pressure
ventilation using 100% O_2. Frequent determinations of the
animals' arterial pH, PO_2, and PCO_2 were obtained throughout
each study to assure adequacy of ventilation and acid-base
balance.

Preparations and Instrumentation

A method was developed in open-chest swine to control and
regulate coronary perfusion in intact, working hearts.
Following bilateral thoracotomy and transternotomy and treatment
with heparin (3 mg/kg IV), one of two models for cardiac
perfusion were prepared. In the first, perfusion circuits were
constructed connecting a femoral artery with the main left and
right coronary arteries. The main left coronary artery was
perfused via a Gregg cannula inserted retrogradely through the
left subclavian artery, and the right coronary was perfused by a
cannula positioned near its origin. Flow was determined in each
system by adjusting the respective mean perfusion pressures to
slightly above average aortic pressure so as to compensate for
internal line resistances. In those studies requiring
independent adjustments in regional flow, a separate third
cannula was inserted high in the anterior descending artery.
Flows to each artery were controlled by separate low-flow Sarnes
perfusion pumps. For the purpose of sampling for metabolites
and oxygen across the myocardium, venous cannulas were passed
into the coronary sinus or anterior branch of the great cardiac
vein. The hemiazygos vein, which in swine drains directly into
the coronary sinus, was ligated.

In a second perfusion model similarly prepared in
open-chest, heparinized, anesthetized swine, a right heart

bypass arrangement was constructed connecting both vena cavae
and the pulmonary artery. The pulmonary artery was ligated just
proximal to the insertion of the bypass cannula. Cardiac output
was maintained by a Sarns modular pump. A reservoir inserted
proximal to the pump served as a priming chamber and was filled
with 1500 ml low molecular weight dextran. Flow rates were
adjusted to produce left ventricular systolic pressures of
between 90-100 mm Hg. Following these procedures, a right
ventriculotomy was performed and a drainage pump inserted to
collect coronary effluent blood. This was passed through a
blood oxygenator (O_2:CO_2 mixture of 97%:3% at 37.5° C) and
returned to the main left and right coronary arteries cannulated
as above. Coronary perfusion to each artery was again supported
by separate low-flow perfusion pumps. Sampling ports in the
arterial and venous tubing were used for obtaining arteriovenous
differences of oxygen and metabolites across the myocardium.

Additional cannulas were placed in the left ventricle and
distal aorta for measuring pressures. A high-fidelity,
manometer-tipped pressure device was advanced retrogradely from
an internal carotid artery to determine left ventricular
pressure. A Teflon tubing catheter connected to a P 23 db
pressure transducer was inserted into the descending aorta via
an internal mammary artery. Epicardial displacement transducers
(8) or mid-myocardial ultrasonic crystals were placed in the
perfusion distribution of the anterior descending artery for
measuring regional shortening. Signals from these instruments,
together with the electrocardiogram, were displayed on an
eight-channel Brush recorder and stored on a Digital Equipment
Corporation PDP 11/10 computer for later off-line analysis.

Data Analyses

Estimates of global left ventricular performance were
determined from measurements of heart rate, left ventricular
(LVP) and mean aortic pressures, and the maximum rate of left
ventricular isovolumetric pressure development (LV max dp/dt) at
normal and ischemic coronary flows. These were correlated with
regional measurements of epicardial or mid-myocardial
displacement in lengths (L) and an integrated index of work
obtained throughout a reconstructed cardiac cycle (work = $\int$LVP
dl/dt dt). Data were collected on-line at 10 minute intervals
during the experiments and reduced off-line. From each sampling
time 240 data points per cardiac cycle were obtained for 10
consecutive heart beats at held expiration to define an average
representative beat. Any cycle period which deviated by more
than two standard deviations from previous beats was excluded
from the averaging routine.

General metabolic function was evaluated from the rates of myocardial oxygen consumption. Myocardial oxygen consumption (MVO_2) was calculated from coronary flow rates, coronary perfusate hemoglobin (Hb) concentrations, and hemoglobin oxygen saturations according to the expressions:

$$MVO_2 \text{ (mmol/hr/g dry)} = 1.39 * \text{coronary flow rate}$$

$$\text{(ml/hr)} * \text{Hb conc (gm/100 ml)} * \text{arterial-venous } O_2$$

$$\text{sat } (\Delta\%)/22.4 \text{ (ml/mmol)} - \text{dry wt of heart (g)}$$

Serum was also obtained at 10 minute intervals to determine the total fatty acid content (μmol/ml) using the colorimetric procedure of Duncombe (9). Fatty acid specific activity (SA) was determined in dpm/ mol FFA following infusions of 70 μCi palmitate [$^{14}C(U)$] into the coronary circulation. By also obtaining the total blood volume (V) in the coronary circuit at the time of sampling (t) in the right heart bypass model, it was possible to solve for the total labeled palmitate in the perfusate $(DPM_p)_t = dpm_t * V_t$. By knowing the amount of labeled palmitate added to the circuit (A in dpm) in the preceding sampling interval (t-10), it was possible to calculate FFA uptake by the heart as: FFA uptake$_t$ (μmol FFA/hr/g dry) = $[(DPM_p)_{t-10} - (DPM_p)_t + A_{t-10}] * 60$ min/hr $\div$ SA_t $\div$ dry wt of heart (g dry). The palmitate added (A) was corrected for the small quantity of product (8-15%) lost extracorporeally in the syringe, tubing, and/or oxygenator.

In either perfusion model, fatty acid oxidation was estimated by measuring $^{14}CO_2$ production from [$^{14}C(U)$] palmitate according to the expression (10):

$$^{14}CO_2 \text{ production (}\mu\text{mol FFA/hr/g dry)} = \text{venous-arterial}$$

$$^{14}CO_2 \text{ (dpm/ml)} * \text{coronary flow (ml/hr)}/SA_{art}$$

$$\text{(dpm/}\mu\text{mol FFA)} * \text{dry wt of heart (g)}$$

When sampling for venous $^{14}CO_2$ in the regional perfusion model, the ratio of specific activities of palmitate in the vein and artery was used to correct for the dilution of venous counts that occurred from admixture of venous effluents from other adjacent circulations.

At the completion of the perfusion trials, transmural sections of left ventricular myocardium near the apex were immediately removed and frozen between blocks of aluminum cooled in liquid nitrogen. These tissue samples were analyzed for acid

soluble and long-chain acyl CoA and acid soluble and long-chain
acyl carnitine (5).

Experimental Protocol

The general plan of these studies was to evaluate the
effects of fatty acids on myocardial mechanical and metabolic
functions during aerobic and ischemic conditions and to test the
effects of two potential therapies: carnitine and oxfenicine.
Perfusion trials lasted either 70 or 90 min, the final 30 min of
which was always during a reduction of global or regional
coronary flow causing moderate ischemia. Augmented serum levels
of fatty acids were effected by infusions of heparin and 10%
emulsion of triacylglycerols (Intralipid) administered
systemically or by labeled and unlabeled palmitate administered
directly into the coronary perfusate. Infusions were begun
immediately at the start of the perfusion trials and continued
throughout the course of the trials to maintain serum fatty
acids at elevated values. Carnitine and oxfenicine were
administered at different periods throughout the trials
depending on the protocol. Lidocaine in 50-100 mg boluses were
given in all animals to avoid ventricular ectopic dysrhythmias.
Metabolic and mechanical information were collected at least
every 10 min throughout the perfusion trials, and tissue samples
were collected at the conclusion of the trials or sooner in the
case of unexpected animal death. The data were analyzed by
paired and unpaired Student t-tests or by two component, a
posteriori analysis of variance and Studentized Newman-Keuls
tests (11). Significance was defined for probability values of
less than 5%. Distribution of data, where listed, always
appears as the standard error of the mean.

RESULTS

In a first series of studies, the effects of excess fatty
acids on mechanical and metabolic functions were compared at
conditions of normal and mildly ischemic ($-39\Delta\%$) restrictions in
coronary flow. One group of hearts received no fatty acid
supplements; the other was treated with infusions of Intralipid
and heparin sufficient to raise serum fatty acids four-fold.
Total perfusion time was 90 min. Coronary flow was held at
aerobic levels for 60 min, then reduced to ischemic levels for
30 min. It can be seen from Table 1A and 1B that by 60 min
treatment with Intralipid, excess fatty acids had significantly
depressed left ventricular pressures, max dp/dt, and regional
work index. Myocardial oxygen consumption was increased in
treated hearts, commensurate with the influence of fatty acid

Table 1A.　Effects of Excess Fatty Acids on Mechanical Function in Aerobic and Ischemic Myocardium

	FFA μmol/ml	Cor.Flow$_a$ ml/min/gd	Δ%i %	Cor.Flow$_i$ ml/min/gd	LVP mmHg	Δ%a %	Δ%i %	max dp.dt mmHg	Δ%a %	Δ%i %	Δ%*RWa %	Δ%*RWi %
Group 1 n=10	0.34 ±.02	5.57 ±.33	-23	3.58 ±.20	107 ±5	-1	-21	3996 ±460	+2	-27	+44	-27
Group 2 n=8	1.49 ±.12	6.16 ±.48	-38	3.70 ±.37	108 ±5	-25	-44	3708 ±495	-23	-69	-70	-73
P	<.005	NS	<.05	NS	NS	<.05	<.01	NS	<.05	<.01	<.005	<.05

Table 1B.　Effects of Excess Fatty Acids on Metabolic Function in Aerobic and Ischemic Myocardium

	MVO$_2$ mmol/hr/gd	Δ%a %	Δ%i %	Fatty acyl CoA nmol/gd	Δ%i %	Total CoA nmol/gd	Δ%i %	Fatty acyl Carn. nmol/gd	Δ%i %	Total Carn nmol/gd	Δ%i %
Group 1 n=10	1.10 ±.06	-2	-23	70.1 ±6.5	+73	372.2 ±15.2	-3.4	20.6 9.8	+1745	4297.2 ±264.3	-6
Group 2 n=8	1.12 ±.10	+17	-38	-	(+) +149	-	(+) +7.4	-	(+) +3226	-	(+) -21
P	NS	<.05	<.05	-	<.005	-	NS	-	<.05	-	<.05

Abbreviations:　mean ± SEM values refer to data at initial perfusion; FFA = free fatty acids; Cor = coronary; subscript a refers to data following 60 min aerobic flows; subscript i refers to data following 30 min ischemia; Δ% = percent change as compared with the listed initial value; subscript RW = regional work index; * = initial value expressed as 100%; NS = not statistically different; CoA = coenzyme A; carn = carnitine; gd = gm of dry tissue; (+) = percent change with respect to aerobic values in hearts not supplemented with excess fatty acids; P = statistical comparisons between Groups 1 and 2 using non-paired Student t tests.

substrate on altering the P/O ratio or on stimulating
oxygen-wasting pathways (12). Following 30 min ischemia,
mechanical function was even further depressed in fatty
acid-treated hearts and oxygen consumption was reduced. These
findings were associated with appreciable increases in the
tissue contents of acyl CoA and acyl carnitine in ischemic
myocardium which were much greater in fatty acid-treated
hearts. Total tissue carnitine was also decreased significantly
in treated hearts, presumably from loss of acid-soluble
carnitine through sarcolemma no longer intact due to the
detergent-like actions of fatty acids on biological membranes
(13).

   Since carnitine is a critical co-factor in fatty acid
metabolism and since its depletion may compromise the acetyl
carnitine transferase mechanism for redistributing accumulations
of acyl CoA intracellularly (14), a next study was performed to
test the effects of repleting lost carnitine on myocardial
function. Two groups of animals were compared (n=22); group 2
received infusions of DL carnitine (100 mg/kg iv); both were
supplemented with excess fatty acids (Intralipid with heparin).
Perfusions were again 90 min with 60 min normal coronary flow
and 30 min mild ischemia (-40Δ% flow restriction). Table 2
lists the comparisons between groups. Serum carnitine values
were 8.5 and 1474 nmol/ml in groups 1 and 2, respectively.
Carnitine tissue stores were significantly increased in group 2
hearts over untreated hearts and were associated with
significant improvements in mechanical function both at normal
and ischemic coronary flows. Myocardial oxygen consumption was
less increased at aerobic flows in carnitine-treated hearts,
suggesting less availability of excess fatty acids to substrate
pathways in myocytes or blunting of the oxygen-wasting
pathways. Total tissue contents of long-chain acyl CoA were
significantly reduced in carnitine-treated hearts whereas
long-chain esters of carnitine were increased.

   The mechanism of carnitine therapy was pursued in a separate
study. The right heart bypass heart preparation was employed
here so labeled palmitate could be infused globally into the
heart muscle to define fatty acid uptake and rates of
oxidation. Twenty hearts (11 untreated, 9 treated with
L-carnitine) were perfused for 70 min. and rendered globally
ischemic (-41Δ% restriction in flow) for the final 30 min.
Serum carnitine values were 8.7 and 6687 nmol/ml, respectively,
in untreated and treated groups; serum fatty acids were
augmented to 0.76 μmol/ml in both groups (upper left panel,
Figure 1). Other metabolic events are shown in Figure 1. At
comparable levels of myocardial oxygen consumption, L-carnitine
treatment significantly decreased fatty acid uptake by 33% (P <
.05) during the middle portion of the perfusion trials (30-50
min perfusion) which included both normal and ischemic coronary

Table 2A

Effects of Carnitine Replacement on Mechanical Function in Fatty Acid-Treated Ischemic Hearts

	FFA	Cor Flow$_a$	Cor Flow$_i$	LVP	Δ%a	Δ%i	max dp/dt	Δ%a	Δ%i	Δ%*RWa	Δ%*RWi
	μmol/ml	ml/min/gd	ml/min/gd	mmHg	%	%	mmHg/sec	%	%	%	%
Group 1 n = 12	1.46 ±.11	6.06 ±.32	3.55 ±.25	108 ± 4	-15	-38	3765 352	-9	-53	-41	-64
Group 2 n = 10	1.35 ±.09	6.09 ±.68	3.69 ±.13	106 ± 3	-0.7	-14	4390 +465	-15	-31	-3	-36
P	NS	NS	NS	NS	NS	<.025	<.05	<.05	<.05	<.025	<.005

Table 2B

Effects of Carnitine Replacement on Metabolic Function in Fatty Acid-Treated Ischemic Hearts

	MVO$_2$	Δ%a	Δ%i	Fatty acyl CoA	Total CoA	Fatty acyl Carn	Total Carn
	nmol/hr/gd	%	%	nmol/gd	nmol/gd	nmol/gd	nmol/gd
Group 1 n = 12	1.05 ±.07	+25	-29	164 ± 9	371 +20	614 +88	3416 +185
Group 2 n = 10	0.91 ±.09	+2	-22	142 +5	372 +19	773 +87	4353 +425
P	NS	<.001	NS	<.025	NS	<.05	<.005

Abbreviations: identical to those in Table 1.

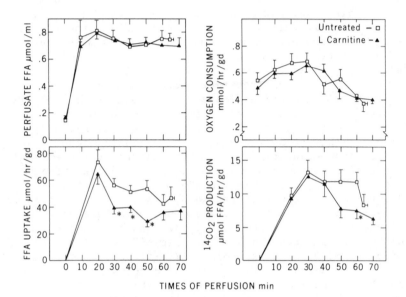

FIGURE 1

Metabolic responses in two heart groups supplemented with excess
fatty acids. Treatment with L-carnitine decreased fatty acid
uptake during the middle portion of the perfusion trials and
secondarily decreased the rate of fatty acid oxidation.
Coronary perfusion was held at normal levels from 0-30 min and
reduced globally to ischemic levels from 40-70 min.

flows. This was accompanied by a significant decline in
$^{14}CO_2$ production at 60 min perfusion in treated hearts.
These data confirm that carnitine prevents, in part, entry of
excess fatty acids into myocytes and substrate utilizing
pathways.

The impact of fatty acid excess on myocardial function was
also pursued from another standpoint. Oxfenicine, an agent
shown to stimulate the activity of pyruvate dehydrogenase and
secondarily glucose metabolism in heart muscle (15), was also
shown to inhibit palmitate oxidation in rat diaphragm (16). It
was reasoned that if this action also occurred in myocardium,
the intoxicating properties of excess fatty acids might be
attenuated. To test this, two groups of hearts (n=15) were
compared. Both groups received Intralipid with heparin
sufficient to raise serum free fatty acids three-fold (0.30 to
0.91 µmol/ml). Both received labeled palmitate selectively into
the perfusate of the left anterior descending coronary
circulation. Total perfusion time was 90 min; oxfenicine was
added (17-33 mg/kg) at 30 min perfusion; regional ischemia in
the anterior descending circulation was induced over the final
30 min perfusion by reducing flow 50%. As can be seen from the
results of the study listed in Table 3, $^{14}CO_2$ production
from labeled palmitate was decreased by 51% (P < .025) at normal
flows in oxfenicine-treated hearts and was even further reduced
during ischemia. Oxfenicine markedly decreased the levels of
long-chain acyl carnitine in both aerobic (478 $\pm$ 113 vs. 79 $\pm$ 22
nmol/g dry, P < .005) and ischemic (667 $\pm$ 92 vs. 260 $\pm$ 52 nmol/g
dry, P < .001) myocardium sampled at the conclusion of the
studies. These changes suggested an inhibition of enzyme
function with the drug at either the acyl CoA synthetase or acyl
carnitine transferase I steps. Oxfenicine improved mechanical
function during ischemia with lesser declines in left
ventricular pressure (P < .01) and max left ventricular dp/dt (P
< .025). Oxygen consumption was greater in treated hearts and
may have reflected enhanced pyruvate dehydrogenase activity and
greater glucose utilization in group 2 hearts. Thus, oxfenicine
inhibits fatty acid oxidation and improves mechanical function
in regionally ischemic hearts, possibly by lessening the
accumulation of intoxicating fatty acid intermediates and
promoting competitive substrate utilization with glucose.

DISCUSSION

The first portion of this report evaluated the early effects
of excess fatty acids on cardiac performance. Serum fatty acid
levels were increased only moderately to evaluate the early
threshold changes in function and metabolism. Both at control

Table 3A Effects of Oxfenicine on Mechanical Function in Fatty Acid Supplemented-Aerobic and Ischemic Hearts.

	FFA	Cor Flow$_a^\Phi$	Cor Flow$_i^\Phi$	LVP	$\Delta\%a$	$\Delta\%i$	max dp/dt	$\Delta\%a$	$\Delta\%i$	$\Delta\%*RWa$	$\Delta\%*RWi$
	μmol/ml	ml/min/gd	ml/min/gd	mmHg	%	%	mmHg/sec	%	%	%	%
Group 1 n = 7	0.93 +.02	5.14 +.52	2.51 +.28	97 +5	-4	-32	2638 +337	-4	-49	+2	-60
Group 2 n = 8	0.90 +.02	5.70 +.13	2.97 +.21	100 +3	0	-9	3032 +227	0	-37	+16	-37
P	NS	NS	NS	NS	NS	<.01	NS	NS	<.025	NS	NS

Table 3B Effects of Oxfenicine on Metabolic Function in Fatty Acid Supplemented-Aerobic and Ischemic Hearts.

	MVO$_2^\Phi$	$\Delta\%a^\Phi$	$\Delta\%i^\Phi$	$^{14}CO_2^\Phi$	$\Delta\%a^\Phi$	$\Delta\%i^\Phi$	acyl CoA$_a$	$\Delta\%i^\Phi$	acyl Carn$_a$	$\Delta\%i^\Phi$
	mmol/hr/gd	%	%	mol/hr/gd	%	%	nmol/gd	%	nmol/gd	%
Group 1 n = 7	1.04 +.07	+16	-49	22 +5	-5	-71	90 +20	+12	478 +113	+40
Group 2 n = 8	1.05 +.09	+31	-33	32 +7	-56	-95	79 7	+16	79 22	+229
P	NS	NS	<.001	NS	NS	<.005	NS	NS	<.005	<.001

Abbreviations as in Table 1. In this regionally perfused preparation only flows in the anterior descending circuit were reduced in ischemia. Data in the anterior descending circuit are denoted by Φ. Group 2 received 17-33 mg/kg oxfenicine.

and mildly ischemic coronary flows, excess fatty acids significantly depressed global and regional mechanical function. These changes were associated with a progressive build-up of long-chain fatty acyl CoA and carnitine derivatives in ischemic hearts and a loss of total tissue carnitine. In the second part of the report, studies were described which showed that suppression of fatty acid oxidation assisted ischemic heart muscle and improved cardiac function.

Experiments were conducted in swine hearts which were selected for their many similarities to man in cardiovascular function, anatomy and perfusion distribution of the coronary circulation. Mild, rather than severe, restrictions in coronary flow were chosen so that therapeutic modalities might have a better opportunity of demonstrating some improvements in cellular function. Exogenous fatty acids were augmented to levels previously observed clinically (17) and not to unduly excessive levels beyond the pathophysiological range as has been criticized by Rogers et al. (18).

Observations have long been held that fatty acids in excess are detrimental to cardiac function. Since the original animal and clinical reports by Hoak et al. (1, 2) and Oliver et al. (3), several investigations have been published supporting these findings (19-21), and the relationship has been the subject of recent reviews (13, 22).

Several mechanisms to account for these derangements have been proposed. Electrical arrhythmias are suggested to result from an interference by fatty acids on glycolytically derived ATP in the cytoplasm (23) or from biotoxic detergent effects on membranes enhanced by high molar ratios of FFA-albumin (20). Additionally, fatty acids have been shown to uncouple electron transport in mitochondria, impair oxidation (24, 25), and in excess concentrations promote swelling of biomembranes and leakage of intracellular contents. DeLeris et al. (21) in working rat hearts showed that adding excess fatty acids to the coronary perfusate led to a 5- to 10-fold increase in the release of LDH enzyme.

More recently, attention has shifted to an evaluation of the effects of selective fatty acid intermediates on interfering with intracellular enzyme function and membrane transport. Of major interest has been the role and influence of long-chain acyl CoA. Several workers using subcellular preparations of heart, brain, and liver (26-28) have demonstrated that palmityl acyl CoA is capable of inhibiting a variety of enzyme systems including palmityl acyl CoA:carnitine palmityl acyl transferase (K_i 3 μM), long-chain acyl CoA synthetase (K_i 5 μM), and Na^+, K^+-ATPase (K_i 80 μM) (29). As reported by Vignais

(30) and Shug et al. (31), the enzyme most sensitive to the
inhibitory effects of long-chain acyl CoA is adenine nucleotide
translocase (K_i 0.1-0.3 µM). As can be seen, decreases in
this translocase activity can occur at concentrations of the
ester well within the critical micelle level. Moreover, because
long-chain acyl CoA increases about 2-fold over aerobic values
during restrictions in coronary flow (32, 33), inhibition of
this enzyme by the ester has been further speculated to be an
early and important event in myocardial ischemia (31, 33). Such
interactions are reasoned to be even more pronounced in ischemic
hearts supplemented with excess fatty acids. In the present
data using swine hearts, similar increases in fatty acyl CoA
groups were noted at less severe levels of ischemia and were
accompanied by greater percentage increases in acyl carnitine.
With the addition of excess fatty acids in ischemic hearts,
there were even greater and near-linear increases in acyl
esters, particularly long-chain acyl carnitine. These data
support and confirm the association between fatty acid
intermediates and cardiac impairment and may reflect a causal
relationship.

Because an appreciable fraction of total carnitine was lost
to the ischemic cell, a therapeutic hypothesis was proposed to
replace this loss by pharmacological doses of DL- and
L-carnitine. Carnitine, a naturally occurring and actively
synthesized quaternary ammonium compound, is an essential
cofactor in the transfer of activated fatty acids from the
cytosol to mitochondrial matrix. It also functions to transfer
acetyl units between cytosol and mitochondria. This latter
transfer system has been postulated to modify and modulate the
acyl transferase reaction and serve as a buffer of matrix acetyl
CoA by storing excess acetyl units in the cytoplasm (14).
Carnitine, while not synthesized by the myocyte, is actively
taken up by the heart, particularly as the L-isomer, and is
concentrated against a plasma-cytosol gradient (34). The uptake
of carnitine by sarcolemma appears to result from active
selective transport which is saturable and slightly energy
dependent (35).

In experimentally induced heart failure resulting from
hypertrophy (36) and coronary ischemia (33, 37), carnitine is
lost from the myocytes as the acid soluble fraction. This loss
was also seen in the working, ischemic swine heart animal model
system. Early attempts at replacing carnitine in ischemic
hearts have been encouraging. Thomsen et al. (38) demonstrated
positive benefits with carnitine in patients with coronary
artery disease whose hearts were paced until angina occurred.
In this group, carnitine significantly increased the heart rate
blood pressure product, the pacing duration to angina, and

lactate extraction while decreasing left ventricular
end-diastolic pressure and ST-T wave abnormalities. Folts et
al. (39) in ischemic dog hearts documented that carnitine
increased electrophysiological changes, increased tissue stores
of high energy phosphates, and in harvested mitochondria
restored adenine nucleotide translocase activity. They also
concluded that carnitine possessed antidysrhythmic actions which
prevented the development of ventricular fibrillation.

The present data support and extend these findings and show
that both the DL- and L-isomers of carnitine preserve mechanical
function at no further cost to oxygen consumption during
ischemia. The influence of carnitine treatments was best seen
in those tudies using labeled palmitate tracer to study fatty
acid utilization and oxidation. The decrease in fatty acid
uptake and $^{14}CO_2$ production suggested a reduced availability
of excess fatty acids into the heart cell. Such effects on
fatty acid uptake were reported previously in isolated aerobic
hearts (40).

In swine hearts, carnitine therapy also decreased tissue
stores of long-chain acyl CoA after 30 min of ischemia. This
reduction in acyl CoA suggests a favorable redistribution of
product between cytosol and mitochondria and away from membrane
surfaces such that enzymatic activities were not as inhibited.
The increase in carnitine esters with carnitine treatment did
not appear to be of consequence. In vitro studies have shown
that palmityl carnitine is capable of inhibiting certain
enzymes, including Na^+, K^+- ATPase in the sarcolemma. The
reported K_i for this intermediate is 44-48 μM and the absence
of functional impairment with therapy noted in the in vivo swine
hearts suggests that intracellular concentrations did not reach
these levels.

In final studies, the impact of excess fatty acids on fatty
acid metabolism in ischemic hearts was modified by the
administration of oxfenicine. Contrasting the tissue levels of
carnitine intermediates between oxfenicine-treated and untreated
hearts suggested that the main locus of the drug's action was
either at the fatty acid activation step or at the acyl
carnitine transferase I reaction. This interference with
preferred substrate metabolism in treated heart muscle was not
associated with any decline in energy production or mechanical
function but rather an overall improvement in cardiac
performance. Oxfenicine caused reductions in long-chain esters
of both CoA and carnitine and lowered whole tissue contents of
the latter moiety to values below those associated with either
excess fatty acid treatments, myocardial ischemia, or both (5).
Such decreases could reasonably be argued to improve

derangements in cellular functions previously reported to occur with accumulation of this inhibitory intermediate. Other possibilities to explain benefits of oxfenicine include a favorable removal of oxygen-wasting pathways (12) associated with the presence of excess fatty acids or a stimulation of glucose metabolism through enhanced activity of pyruvate dehydrogenase (15, 16). Mild-to-moderate ischemia with retention of some coronary washout does not provoke an all-or-none type suppression of myocardial metabolism. Important elements of oxidative metabolism persist for some period of time despite reduced oxygen delivery. We have previously shown in swine hearts that 40-50 mM pyruvate was able to increase oxidative decarboxylation 5-fold during moderate global ischemia (41). Thus the notion that oxfenicine enhances carbohydrate oxidation in ischemic hearts fits nicely with these previous data. The added contribution of energy production from this alternate substrate would assist in maintaining critical subcellular processes and preserve contractile performance. Thus, these data indicate that a reduction in fatty acid intermediates accompanied by a presumed enhancement of glucose utilization collectively preserved function in working ischemic heart muscle.

ACKNOWLEDGEMENTS

    This work was supported by USPHS Grant 2 R01 HL21209.

REFERENCES

1. Hoak, J.C., Connor, W.E., Eckstein, J.W., & Warner, E.D. (1964): J. Lab. Clin. Med. 63: 791.
2. Hoak, J.C., Connor, W.E., & Warner, E.D. (1968): J. Clin. Invest. 47: 2701.
3. Oliver, M.F., Kurien, V.A., & Greenwood, T.W. (1968): Lancet 1: 710.
4. Rowe, M.J., Neilson, J.M.M., & Oliver, M.F. (1975): Lancet 1: 295.
5. Liedtke, A.J., Nellis, S.H., & Neely, J.R. (1978): Circ. Res. 43: 652.
6. Liedtke, A.J., Nellis, S.H., & Whitesell, L.F. (1981): Circ. Res. 48: 859.
7. Liedtke, A.J., & Nellis, S.H. (1979): J. Clin. Invest. 64: 440.
8. Nellis, S.H., & Liedtke, A.J. (1979): Am. J. Physiol. 236: H657.
9. Duncombe, W.G. (1963): Biochem. J. 88: 7.

10. Liedtke, A.J., Hughes, H.C., & Neely, J.R. (1975): Am. J. Physiol. <u>228</u>: 655.
11. Snedecor, G.W., & Cochran, W.G. (1972): <u>Statistical Methods</u>, The Iowa State University Press, Ames, Iowa.
12. Vik-Mo, H., & Mjøs, O.D. (1981): Am. J. Cardiol. <u>48</u>: 361.
13. Katz, A.M., & Messineo, F.C. (1981): Circ. Res. <u>48</u>: 1.
14. Hochachka, T.W., Neely, J.R., & Driedzic, W.R. (1977): Fed. Proc. <u>36</u>: 2009.
15. Higgins, A.J., Morville, M., Burges, R.A., & Blackburn, K.J. (1981): Biochem. Biophys. Res. Commun. <u>100</u>: 291.
16. Higgins, A.J., Morville, M., Burges, R.A., Gardiner, D.G., Page, M.G., & Blackburn, K.J. (1980): Life Sci. <u>27</u>: 963.
17. Mueller, H.S., & Ayres, S.M. (1978): Am. J. Cardiol. <u>42</u>: 363.
18. Rogers, W.J., McDaniel, H.G., Moraski, R.E., Rackley, C.E., & Russell, R.O., Jr. (1977): Am. J. Cardiol. <u>40</u>: 365.
19. Kjekshaus, J.K., & Mjøs, O.D. (1972): J. Clin. Invest. <u>51</u>: 1767.
20. Willebrands, A.F., Terwell, H.F., & Tasserson, S.J.A. (1973): J. Mol. Cell. Cardiol. <u>5</u>: 259.
21. DeLeris, A.E., Opie, L.H., & Lubbe, W.F. (1975): Nature <u>253</u>: 746.
22. Liedtke, A.J. (1981): Prog. Cardiovasc. Dis. <u>23</u>: 321.
23. Prasad, K., & MacLeod, B.P. (1969): Circ. Res. <u>24</u>: 939.
24. Pressman, B.C., & Lardy, H.A. (1956): Biochim. Biophys. Acta <u>21</u>: 548.
25. Hülsmann, W.C., Elliot, W.B., & Slater, E.C. (1960): Biochim. Biophys. Acta <u>39</u>: 267.
26. Wood, J.M., Bush, B., Pitts, B.J.R., & Schwartz, A. (1977): Biochem. Biophys. Res. Commun. <u>74</u>: 677.
27. Bremer, J., & Norum, K.R. (1967): J. Biol. Chem. <u>242</u>: 1744.
28. Oram, J.F., Wenger, J.I., & Neely, J.R. (1975): J. Biol. Chem. <u>250</u>: 73.
29. Lamers, J.M.J., & Hulsman, W.C. (1977): J. Mol. Cell. Cardiol. <u>9</u>: 343.
30. Vignais, P.V. (1976): Biochim. Biophys. Acta <u>456</u>: 1.
31. Shug, A.L., Shrago, E., Bittar, N., Folts, J.D., & Koke, J.R. (1975): Am. J. Physiol. <u>228</u>: 689.
32. Whitmer, J.T., Idell-Wenger, J.A., Rovetto, M.J., & Neely, J.R. (1978): J. Biol. Chem. <u>253</u>: 4305.
33. Shug, A.L., Thomsen, J.H., Folts, J.D., Bittar, N., Klein, M.I., Koke, J.R., & Huth, P.J. (1978): Arch. Biochem. Biophys. <u>187</u>: 25.
34. Böhmer, T., Eiklit, K., & Jonsen, J. (1977): Biochim. Biophys. Acta <u>465</u>: 627.
35. Bressler, R., Navin, T., & Bahl, J.J. (1979): Clin. Res. <u>27</u>: 501A.

36. Wittels, B., & Spann, J.F. (1968): J. Clin. Invest. 47:
    1787.
37. Schwartz, A., Wood, M.A., Allen, J.C., Bornet, E.P., Entman,
    M.L., Goldstein, M.A., Sordahl, L.A., Sucki, M., & Louis,
    R.M. (1973): Am. J. Cardiol. 32: 46.
38. Thomsen, J.A., Shug, A.L., Yap, V.U., Pattel, A.K., Karras,
    T.J., & DeFelice, S.L. (1979): Am. J. Cardiol. 43: 300.
39. Folts, J.D., Shug, A.L., Koke, J.R., & Bittar, N. (1978):
    Am. J. Cardiol. 41: 1209.
40. Rodis, S.L., D'Amata, P.H., Koch, E., & Vahouny, G.V.
    (1970): Proc. Soc. Exp. Biol. Med. 133: 973.
41. Liedtke, A.J., & Nellis, S.H. (1978): Circ. Res. 43: 189.

MEMBRANE PHOSPHOLIPID METABOLISM DURING MYOCARDIAL ISCHEMIA:

MECHANISMS OF ACCUMULATION OF UNESTERIFIED ARACHIDONATE

K. R. Chien, L. M. Buja, and J. T. Willerson

Department of Internal Medicine (Cardiovascular Division)
The University of Texas Health Science Center
5323 Harry Hines Boulevard
Dallas, TX   75235

Recent studies have suggested that alterations in membrane structure and function are causally related to the development of irreversible injury during myocardial ischemia (1-4). In an ischemic canine myocardial model, studies by Jennings et al. have demonstrated the presence of sarcolemmal membrane defects by electron microscopy which correlate with the time course of the onset of irreversible injury and the accumulation of tissue calcium (1). Studies in a perfused rabbit septal model (4) have correlated the decrease in myocardial contractile performance during ischemia with the development of increased sarcolemmal membrane cation permeability (4). Calcium blocking agents have been demonstrated to have protective effects on the development of irreversible injury in calcium accumulation during myocardial ischemia (5, 6). Acute myocardial infarction in man is characterized by leakage of cytosolic enzymes across the sarcolemmal membrane and into the intravascular space (7). In addition, the accumulation of technetium-99m pyrophosphate, a marker of a sarcolemmal membrane calcium permeability defect (8), is a sensitive marker of myocardial cell injury in clinical and animal studies (9). While it is becoming increasingly clear that alterations in the structure and calcium permeability properties of membranes are involved in the development of irreversible cell injury, the biochemical basis responsible for

these membrane changes is unknown (10). However, recent studies
in ischemic liver model have suggested that the degradation of
membrane phospholipids is causally related to the loss of cell
viability during ischemia (11-14). In this model, the
degradation of membrane phospholipids is related temporally to
the development of the membrane calcium permeability defect, a
several-fold increase in tissue calcium content, and the
development of irreversible damage in ischemically injured cells
(11). Pharmacologic inhibition of the phospholipid degradation
results in a protection against the alterations in calcium
homeostasis and the development of irreversible cell injury (11,
12).

Recently, these initial studies have been confirmed by other
investigators (15, 16). There are now several reports of
phospholipid degradation during ischemia in the kidney (17, 18),
brain (19), and myocardium (20-25). In ischemic canine
myocardium, there is a temporal and topographical correlation
between the accumulation of tissue calcium, the uptake of
technetium-99m pyrophosphate, and the development of an in vitro
sarcolemmal calcium permeability defect (8). Treatment of
sarcolemmal vesicles with an exogenous phospholipase results in
a marked increase in passive calcium permeability (8).
Sarcolemmal vesicles isolated from ischemic canine myocardium
display greater than 50% increase in passive calcium
permeability, as well as a 20% decrease in phosphatidylcholine
content (8). In addition, pretreatment with chlorpromazine has
been demonstrated to have protective effects in perfused heart
models of myocardial ischemia (4).

The exact biochemical mechanisms responsible for the loss of
membrane phospholipid during ischemia are not clear. However,
studies on the synthesis of prostaglandins in several cell types
have provided insight into the biochemical mechanisms
responsible for the release of arachidonate, a fatty acid found
almost entirely in membrane phospholipid. The initial
deacylation of arachidonate from phospholipid is due to the
activation of at least two distinct phospholipases. The
phospholipase A_2 activity releases fatty acyl groups from the
SN-2 position resulting in the subsequent formation of lysophospholipids and free fatty acids (26). The phospholipase C
activity cleaves the water soluble head group from
phospholipids, resulting in the accumulation of diacylglycerol
(27). Studies in platelets (27), amnion cells (28), and
Madin-Darby kidney cells (29, 30) have demonstrated that the
release of arachidonate by phospholipases during prostaglandin
synthesis is immediately followed by reacylation with other
fatty acid moieties. The net effect of this deacylation-
reacylation cycle is a release of free arachidonate with little

or no decrease in total phospholipid content. Thus, the net loss of total phospholipid from the membrane is dependent not only on the rate of deacylation by phospholipases, but also on the rate of reacylation. These results in non-myocardial cells may be relevant to the mechanisms of phospholipid degradation during myocardial ischemia. Myocardial cells contain phospholipase A and C activities (31, 32) as well as a lysophosphatidylcholine reacylase activity in cardiac membranes (33). In an ischemic canine model, Van der Vusse et al. (20) demonstrated that unesterified arachidonate can accumulate after 2 hours of myocardial ischemia. However, until recently, the time course of the accumulation of arachidonate and its temporal relationship to the depletion of membrane phospholipids was not known (34).

RESULTS AND DISCUSSION

Previous studies in canine myocardium have demonstrated that one hour of fixed LAD occlusion is sufficient to produce irreversible injury, accumulation of tissue calcium, and the development of sarcolemmal calcium permeability defect (8). However, there was no statistically significant decrease in total phospholipid content in the ischemic versus the corresponding nonischemic tissue at this time (8). Since it is now clear that there is over a 70% increase in free arachidonate content after 1 hour of ischemia in this model (34), the seeming discrepancy is most likely due to the inherent difficulty in detecting nmol/g wet weight quantities of membrane phospholipid degradation by simply measuring the total phospholipid content which is present in μmol/g wet weight amounts. Thus, increases in tissue free arachidonate may be a more sensitive indicator of phospholipid degradation during myocardial ischemia. Interestingly, the time course of the accumulation of arachidonate paralleled the time course of the irreversible injury which has been previously described in this model (3). Since ischemic liver displays over a 20% decrease of total phospholipid content after 1 hour of ischemia (11), the myocardium appears to have a lower rate and extent of phospholipid degradation during ischemia. If phospholipid degradation is contributing to the development of irreversible injury during myocardial ischemia, then myocardial cell membranes must be more vulnerable to the effects of phospholipid degradation than the liver cell. There are several potential mechanisms of arachidonic acid accumulation during myocardial ischemia. The most obvious possibility would be that the free acid accumulates secondary to increased uptake of arachidonate from the serum. However, this possibility is unlikely, since the myocardium extracts very little arachidonate from

extracellular sources under normoxic conditions (20).
Furthermore, Neely et al. (35) have demonstrated that fatty acid
uptake in general is inhibited during ischemia, as the
myocardial cell prefers glucose as a carbon substrate during
hypoxia.

The second possible mechanism of arachidonate accumulation
is simply due to the impaired beta oxidation of fatty acids
which occurs in ischemic myocardium. However, arachidonic acid
is not only poorly oxidized by myocardial cells, but also is an
extremely poor substrate for the carnitine acyl transferase
(36). Thus, under normal conditions, any free arachidonate
would be shunted away from oxidation and towards
esterification. In addition, it has recently been demonstrated
that myocardial cells contain a lysophosphatidylcholine
reacylase which has a 2.5-fold greater activity with
arachidonoyl CoA than with oleyl CoA (34).

The third possibility is that arachidonate accumulates
secondary to either an increased rate of deacylation or
decreased rate of reacylation from membrane phospholipids
(Figure 1) (36). Unlike other fatty acids in the myocardial
cell, over 98% of arachidonate is esterified in the SN-2
position of phospholipids. Myocardial cells contain an
endogenous membrane-bound phospholipase A_2 which will
deacylate arachidonate from phosphatidylcholine. The resulting
free arachidonate can then be activated to arachidonoyl CoA by
the acyl CoA synthetase and then reesterified by the
lysophosphatidylcholine reacylase (33) to resynthesize the
intact phosphatidylcholine molecule. This
deacylation-reacylation cycle closely controls the levels of
free arachidonate as well as the fatty acid composition of
myocardial membrane phospholipids. Since the myocardial cell
contains a 10-fold higher activity of lysophosphatidylcholine
reacylase and cytosolic lysophospholipase activity than
phospholipase activity, it would be expected that the generation
of lysophosphatidylcholine during ischemia would be transient
and that its accumulation would not be proportional to the
extent of phospholipid degradation during ischemia. If the
reacylation of arachidonate were inhibited, it would be expected
that the cytosolic lysophospholipase would deacylate the SN-1
fatty acid resulting in the production of free fatty acid and
glycerophosphoryl choline, and the depletion of phospholipid
from the myocardial membrane (Figure 1).

Recent studies in our laboratory examined the temporal
relationship of free arachidonate with the onset of phospholipid
depletion during fixed ligation of the left anterior descending
coronary artery in canine myocardium (34). Evidence of a
phospholipid deacylation-reacylation cycle was demonstrated by
analyzing the fatty acid composition of phosphatidylcholine, the

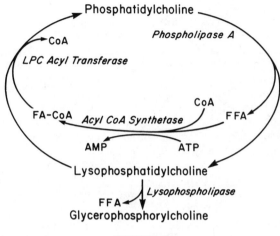

FIGURE 1

Phosphatidylcholine deacylation-reacylation cycle.

major phospholipid class which is depleted during prolonged
myocardial ischemia. To facilitate a rapid quantitative
analysis of fatty acid composition, a high pressure liquid
chromatography method was adapted for these studies. The
following results were demonstrated in ischemic canine
myocardium: (1) the accumulation of unesterified arachidonate
was minimal during 10-30 minutes of ischemia but was
significantly increased after prolonging the duration of
ischemia to 1-3 hours; (2) these increases in free arachidonate
preceded the development of significant decreases in total
phospholipid content; (3) the decrease in arachidonate content
of phosphatidyl choline is accompanied by similar decreases in
all of the fatty acyl moieties of phosphatidyl choline; (4) the
arachidonate content and fatty acid composition of
lysophosphatidyl choline and diacylglycerol are unchanged during
myocardial ischemia; (5) there is evidence of a
deacylation-reacylation cycle in phosphatidylcholine prior to
the accumulation of free arachidonate. These data suggest that
the accumulation of arachidonate may be a more sensitive measure
of phospholipid degradation than decreases in total phospholipid

content in ischemic myocardium. In addition, we postulated that
defective reacylation of arachidonate into phosphatidylcholine
may contribute to the net loss of membrane phospholipid during
myocardial ischemia.

The inhibition of reacylation of arachidonate may be
secondary to ATP depletion during myocardial ischemia. The
reacylation of arachidonate first requires the activation of
arachidonate to arachidonoyl CoA by the arachidonoyl CoA
synthetase (Figure 1). The demonstration by Jennings et al.
(37) that the depletion of high energy phosphates beyond a
certain critical level correlates with the onset of irreversible
injury, suggests that the inhibition of arachidonoyl CoA
synthetase activity might occur partially as a result of ATP
depletion. Although Neely et al. (35) have demonstrated that
total long-chain acyl CoA content is elevated during ischemia,
the cytosolic levels of CoA and arachidonoyl CoA content in
particular, are unknown. Since the biochemical basis of fatty
acyl CoA accumulation during ischemia is based on the inhibition
of beta oxidation, most of the increase is located in the
mitochondria. Preliminary studies in our laboratory have
demonstrated that arachidonoyl CoA is a poor substrate for the
carnitine acyl transferase. Thus, most of the arachidonoyl CoA
is probably localized in the cytosol. Measuring the level of
arachidonoyl CoA content in ischemic myocardium as a function of
the duration of ischemia, the time course of accumulation of
free arachidonate, and the ATP content of the cell will become
important in the evaluation of this hypothesis. If the
arachidonoyl CoA level is low at a time when the free
arachidonate level is high, this would provide direct evidence
of decreased arachidonate activation. If ATP depletion is
playing a role in this inhibition, the ATP level in the cell
should be near the Km of the arachidonoyl CoA synthetase.
Interestingly, the "critical" level of ATP in ischemic
myocardium, which has been demonstrated to be around 1-2 μmol/g
wet weight, corresponds to the Km of ATP of arachidonoyl CoA
synthetase for human platelets which is approximately 0.5-1.0 mM
(38). Alternatively, since the arachidonoyl CoA synthetase is a
membrane-bound enzyme, decreased activity could be secondary to
structural inhibition of the synthetase secondary to membrane
injury. Clearly, further characterization of the ATP
requirements and activity of the myocardial membrane
arachidonoyl CoA synthetase needs to be obtained during the
evolution of myocardial ischemia, up to and including the
development of irreversible cell injury.

REFERENCES

1. Herdson, P.B., Sommers, N.H., & Jennings, R.B. (1963): Am. J. Pathol. 45: 367.
2. Shen, A.C., & Jennings, R.B. (1972): Am. J. Pathol. 67: 417.
3. Burton, K.P., Hagler, H.K., Templeton, G.H., Willerson, J.T., & Buja, L.M. (1977): J. Clin. Invest. 60: 1289.
4. Burton, K.P., Hagler, H.K., Willerson, J.T., & Buja, L.M. (1981): Am. J. Physiol. 241: H714.
5. Henry, P.D., Shucheib, R., David, J., Weiss, E.S., & Sobel, B.E. (1977): Am. J. Physiol. 288: H677.
6. Nayler, W.G., Ferrari, R., & Williams, A. (1980): Am. J. Cardiol. 46: 242.
7. Hearse, D.J., & Humphrey, S.M. (1975): J. Mol. Cell. Cardiol. 1: 325.
8. Chien, K.R., Reeves, J.P., Buja, L.M., Bonte, F., Parkey, R.W., & Willerson, J.T. (1981): Circ. Res. 48: 711.
9. Willerson, J.T., Parkey, R.W., Bonte, F.J., Lewis, S.E., Corbett, J., & Buja, L.M. (1980): Sem. Nucl. Med. 10: 54.
10. Farber, J.L., Chien, K.R., & Mittnacht, S. (1981): Am. J. Pathol. 102: 271.
11. Chien, K.R., Abrams, J., Serroni, A., Martin, J.T., & Farber, J.T. (1978): J. Biol. Chem. 253: 4809.
12. Chien, K.R., Abrams, J., Pfau, R.G., & Farber, J.T. (1977): Am. J. Pathol. 88: 539.
13. Chien, K.R., & Farber, J.T. (1977): Arch. Biochem. Biophys. 180: 191.
14. Chien, K.R., Sherman, C., Mittnacht, S., & Farber, J.T. (1980): Arch. Biochem. Biophys. 205: 614.
15. Wattiaux, R., & Wattiaux-DeConinck, S. (1980): Biochem. Pharmacol. 29: 963.
16. Matsumoto, J., Tanaka, T., Gamo, M., Saito, K., & Honjo, I. (1981): Biochim. Biophys. Acta 664: 527.
17. Patel, Y., Stewart, J., Matthys, E., & Venkatacham, M.A. (1982): Clin. Res. 30: 541A.
18. Smith, M.W., Collan, Y., Kaling, M., & Trump, B.F. (1980): Biochim. Biophys. Acta 618: 192.
19. Bazan, N.G. (1970): Biochim. Biophys. Acta 218: 1.
20. Van der Vusse, G.I., Roeman, T.H.M., Prinzen, F.W., Coumans, W.A., & Reneman, R.S. (1982): Circ. Res. 50: 538.
21. Corr, P.B., Snyder, D.W., Lee, B.I., Gross, R.W., Keim, C.R., & Sobel, B.E. (1982): Am. J. Physiol. 243: H197.
22. Hsueh, W., Isaksan, P.C., & Needleman, P. (1977): Prostaglandins 13: 1073.
23. Vasdev, S.C., Kako, K.J., & Biro, G.P. (1979): J. Mol. Cell. Cardiol. 11: 1195.
24. Shaikh, N.A., & Downar, E. (1981): Circ. Res. 49: 316.

25. Chien, K.R., Pfau, R.G., & Farber, J.L. (1979): Am. J. Pathol. 97: 505.
26. Van den Bosch, H. (1974): Ann. Rev. Biochem. 43: 243.
27. Prescott, S.M., & Majerus, P.W. (1981): J. Biol. Chem. 256: 579.
28. Okita, J.R., MacDonald, P.C., & Johnston, J.M. (1982): J. Biol. Chem. 247: 14029.
29. Beaudry, G.A., King, L., Daniel, L.W., & Waite, M. (1982): J. Biol. Chem. 257: 10973.
30. Daniel, L.W., King, L., & Waite, M. (1981): J. Biol. Chem. 256: 12830.
31. Hostetler, K.Y., & Hall, L.B. (1980): Biochem. Biophys. Res. Commun. 96: 388.
32. Weglicki, W.B. (1980): IN Degradative processes in Heart and Skeletal Muscle (ed) K. Wildenthal, Elsevier/North Holland, Amsterdam, p. 377.
33. Gross, R.W., & Sobel, B.E. (1982): J. Biol. Chem. 257: 6702.
34. Chien, K.R., Han, A., Bush, L.R., Buja, L.M., & Willerson, J.T. (1983): Circ. Res. In press.
35. Idell-Wenger, J.A., & Neely, J.R. (1978): IN Disturbances in Lipid and Lipoprotein Metabolism (eds) J.M. Dietschy, A.M. Gotto, & J.A. Ontko, American Physiological Society, Baltimore, p. 269.
36. Chien, K.R. Unpublished observations.
37. Jennings, R.B., Hawkins, H.K., Lowe, J.E., Hill, M.L., Klotman, S., & Reimer, K.A. (1981): Am. J. Pathol. 82: 187.
38. Wilson, D.B., Prescott, S.M., & Majerus, P.W. (1982): J. Biol. Chem. 257: 3510.

PHOSPHOLIPASE AND ISCHEMIC DAMAGE: POSSIBILITIES OF

INTERVENTIONS

M. Chiariello, G. Ambrosio, M. Cappelli-Bigazzi,
G. Marone and M. Condorelli

Department of Internal Medicine
Second School of Medicine, University of Naples
Naples, Italy

It has been recently suggested that derangement of
phospholipid metabolism may represent one of the prominent
biochemical changes leading to the production of irreversible
injury during cellular ischemia (1-3). In the ischemic liver, a
close correlation was found between the development of
irreversible cell damage and the rate of degradation of
microsomal membrane phospholipids. More recently, an
accelerated phospholipid degradation was demonstrated also in
the ischemic myocardium (4).

Although several mechanisms have been suggested to
contribute to the development of irreversible cell injury during
ischemia, such as the accumulation of potentially damaging
concentration of long-chain acyl-CoA esters and acyl-carnitine
(5, 6), or the release of lysosomal enzymes (7), there is
increasing evidence that the activation of endogenous, membrane-
bound phospholipases may represent the most relevant mechanism
to explain the accelerated lipid degradation eventually leading
to the loss of the normal membrane function. It has been also
shown that pretreatment with chlorpromazine reduced in the
ischemic liver the phospholipid depletion and the extent of
cellular damage.

Although these considerations clarify to some extent the
pathogenesis of the irreversible injury in ischemia, several

questions bearing on the role of ischemia-induced phospholipase
activation still remain unanswered. What is the time-course of
phospholipid degradation during prolonged myocardial ischemia?
Can this course be permanently modified by a phospholipase
inhibitor given after the beginning of ischemia? Is
phospholipase inhibition able to prevent necrosis of jeopardized
ischemic cells and, therefore, reduce myocardial infarct size?
Is an intervention that reduces myocardial ischemia by improving
oxygen imbalance also capable of reducing the rate of
phospholipase activation?

TIME-COURSE OF PHOSPHOLIPID DEGRADATION

A large number of rats undergoing ligation of the left main
coronary artery were sacrificed at times ranging from 0 to 48
hours following the intervention. To monitor myocardial injury,
the total CPK activity of the left ventricle was assessed in the
supernatant of the homogenates. Furthermore, in the same
samples phospholipids were extracted from supernatants and their
concentrations measured as µg of inorganic phosphorus/mg of
protein. Left ventricular CPK activity fell dramatically
following 2 hours of ischemia, and decreased progressively
approaching a "plateau" 12 hours after coronary occlusion
(Figure 1). Simultaneously, a similar fall in myocardial
phospholipid concentration was found; it dropped to less than
50% of the control value 2 hours after the occlusion, and
remained at this low level throughout the study (Figure 2).

An additional group of rats also underwent coronary artery
occlusion and were treated after the intervention with
quinacrine, a powerful phospholipase inhibitor (8). They were
sacrificed at the same time intervals as the controls and left
ventricular CPK activity and phospholipid concentration were
measured.

During the first few hours CPK activity and phospholipid
concentration exhibited the same trend as in control-occluded
rats. However, 24 and 48 hours post-occlusion,
quinacrine-treated rats showed significantly higher myocardial
phospholipid content, as compared to controls (Figure 2).
Myocardial injury, as assessed by CPK depletion, also was
reduced during the late phase of the study in quinacrine-treated
rats (Figure 1). These data seem to demonstrate that the
degradation of myocardial phospholipid indeed occurs during the
first 2 hours of ischemia, and that this effect is still evident
48 hours following coronary occlusion. The simultaneous decline
in left ventricular CPK activity suggests the possibility of a
correlation between phospholipid degradation and degree of

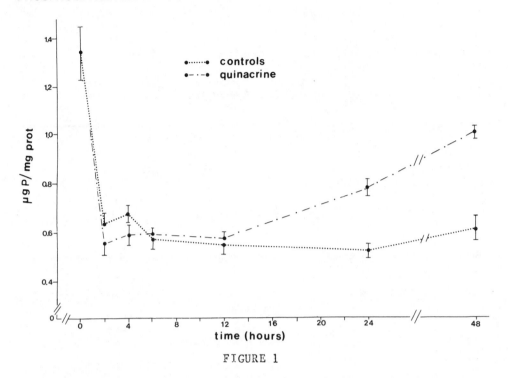

FIGURE 1

Time-course of myocardial phospholipid concentration (PL)
following coronary artery occlusion in control rats and in
animals treated with quinacrine (75 mg/kg t.i.d.,
subcutaneously). Note the different trend of the two lines from
12 to 48 hours. Each point represents the mean ± SEM of at
least 8 experiments.

myocardial injury. The treatment of the occluded rats with the
phospholipase inhibitor quinacrine significantly modified the
time-course of myocardial phospholipid concentration and CPK
depletion. The rise in left ventricular phospholipid content
and CPK activity observed from 12 hours post-occlusion seems to
indicate that phospholipase inhibition allows the ischemic
myocardium to resynthesize phospholipids, thus leading to a
preservation of ischemic cell viability.

EFFECTS OF PHOSPHOLIPASE INHIBITION ON INFARCT SIZE

The effect of phospholipase inhibition on infarct size was
assessed in the experimental animal at the time of peak
necrosis, i.e., 48 hours after coronary artery occlusion, and at
the completion of the scar formation, 21 days post-occlusion.
In the acute study rats were randomized into a control group
receiving coronary occlusion, a treated group that, following

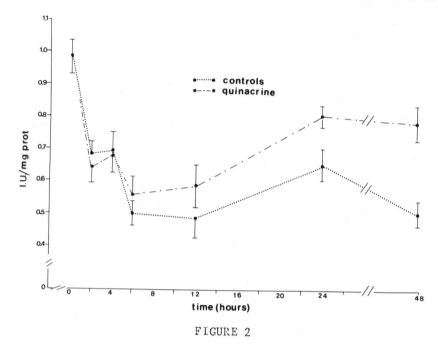

FIGURE 2

Time-course of left ventricular CPK activity following coronary
artery occlusion in control rats and in animals treated with
quinacrine (75 mg/kg t.i.d., subcutaneously). Each point
represents the mean ± SEM of at least 8 experiments.

occlusion was treated with quinacrine, and a sham-operated group
receiving the same surgical procedure as the others with the
exception that the suture passed around the coronary artery was
not tied. Forty-eight hours post-intervention all rats were
sacrificed and phospholipid content was measured in the
supernatant of left ventricular homogenate. In
quinacrine-treated rats, myocardial phospholipid content was
similar to that observed in sham-operated rats; in contrast, in
control occluded rats, left ventricular phospholipid
concentration was significantly lower (Figure 3). These results
confirm that phospholipase inhibition is able to restore the
normal myocardial phospholipid concentration 48 hours after the
induction of ischemia. In the same animals, quinacrine
administration was also able to induce a remarkable reduction in
the size of myocardial necrosis, as assessed by left ventricular
CPK depletion. Actually, left ventricular CPK activity in rats
treated with quinacrine was significantly higher than in control
occluded rats (Figure 4), and infarct size calculated as
previously described (9, 10) was 45.8 ± 5.7% of left ventricle
in control rats and only 15.1 ± 6.8% of left ventricle in
quinacrine treated rats, this representing a 67.0% reduction in

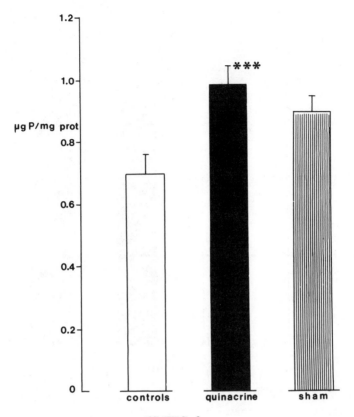

FIGURE 3

Myocardial phospholipid concentration (PL) measured 48 hours
after the surgical procedure in sham-operated rats, in animals
with control coronary artery occlusion, and in coronary occluded
rats treated with quinacrine (75 mg/kg t.i.d. subcutaneously).
Phospholipid concentration in quinacrine-treated rats was
signficantly higher than in controls. Numbers are expressed as
mean ± SEM.
***: different from controls, p < 0.001.

infarct size (Figure 5). The beneficial effects of
phospholipase inhibition were not confined to the acute phase of
the infarction, but were long-lasting. In fact, additional rats
divided into control-occluded, quinacrine-treated, and
sham-operated groups, were sacrificed 21 days post-occlusion,
when the repairing process was completed, and the size of
myocardial scar was assessed from the left ventricular hydroxyproline content. Since hydroxyproline is present in the
collagen in a fixed ratio, left ventricular collagen content was

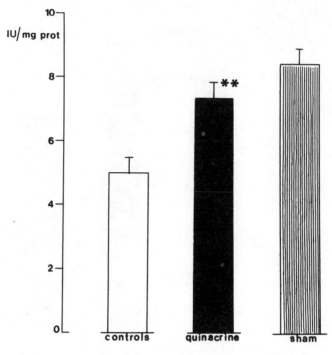

FIGURE 4

Left ventricular CPK activity measured 48 hours after the
surgical procedure in sham-operated rats, in animals with
control coronary artery occlusion, and in coronary occluded rats
treated with quinacrine (75 mg/kg t.i.d., subcutaneously).
Numbers are expressed as mean ± SEM.
**: different from controls, p < 0.01.

also calculated by multiplying hydroxyproline concentration by a
factor of 7.46 (11). Furthermore, hydroxyproline concentration
measured in the center of myocardial scar in 10 additional rats
that had undergone coronary occlusion three weeks earlier, was
found to average 12.01 ± 3.24 μg/mg of dry weight. By taking
this value and using the hydroxyproline concentration of
sham-operated rats for reference, the size of the scar was
calculated by a simple formula. In quinacrine- treated rats,
myocardial hydroxyproline and collagen concentration was
significantly less than in control rats, though higher than in

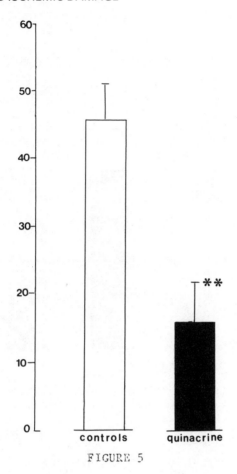

FIGURE 5

Infarct size (IS) calculated by CPK depletion 48 hours following
coronary artery occlusion in control and in quinacrine-treated
rats, expressed as % of the left ventricle (% LV). Numbers are
expressed as mean ± SEM.
**: Different from controls, p < 0.01.

sham-operated animals, this showing that the amount of scar was
smaller in treated rats (Figure 6). Infarct size calculated by
this method was also smaller in quinacrine-treated as compared
to control occluded rats, the reduction of 49.8% being
comparable to that observed in the acute study (Figure 7).

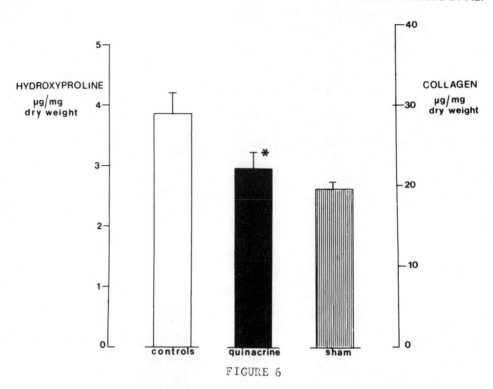

FIGURE 6

Left ventricular hydroxyproline and collagen content in
sham-operated, control occluded and quinacrine-treated rats 21
days after the surgical procedure. Treated rats received
quinacrine 75 mg/kg t.i.d., subcutaneously, for 48 hours
following coronary artery occlusion. Numbers are expressed as
mean ± SEM.
*: Different from controls, p < 0.02.

These results suggest that phospholipase inhibition by
interrupting one of the critical biochemical events induced by
ischemia may preserve the integrity and viability of ischemic
myocardial cells following coronary artery occlusion.

EFFECTS OF OXYGEN-SPARING INTERVENTIONS ON PHOSPHOLIPASE
ACTIVATION

It is well known that drugs that reduce myocardial oxygen
requirements may favorably influence survival of jeopardized
myocardial cells during acute ischemia. Beta-adrenergic
blocking drugs, which decrease myocardial oxygen consumption by
reducing heart rate and cardiac inotropism, were shown to

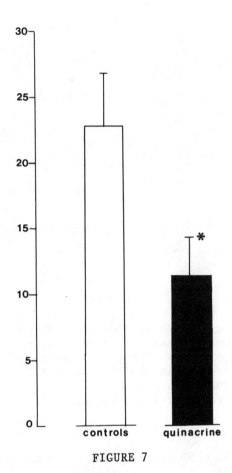

FIGURE 7

Infarct size (IS) calculated by left ventricular collagen
content and expressed as % of left ventricle (% LV) in control
occluded and quinacrine-treated rats, 21 days following coronary
artery occlusion. Numbers are expressed as mean ± SEM.
*: different from controls, p < 0.02.

protect ischemic myocardium after experimental coronary artery
occlusion (12). Since ischemia triggers myocardial
phospholipase activation, it is conceivable that a drug which
reduces the degree of tissue ischemia following coronary artery

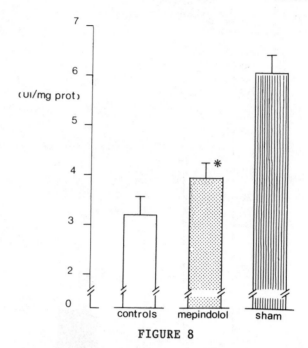

FIGURE 8

Left ventricular CPK activity measured 48 hours after the
surgical procedure in sham-operated, control occluded and
mepindolol treated rats. Treated animals, following coronary
occlusion received mepindolol 1 mg/kg t.i.d., subcutaneously.
Values are expressed as mean ± SEM.
*: different from controls, p < 0.05.

occlusion should also be capable of decreasing myocardial
phospholipid degradation. This possibility has been
investigated in rats with coronary artery occlusion. Following
ligation, a group of these animals was treated with mepindolol,
a newly developed beta-blocker reported to act mainly on heart
rate and to affect only slightly cardiac inotropism (13).
Forty-eight hours after the intervention rats were sacrificed
and phospholipid content and CPK activity were measured in the
supernatant of left ventricular homogenates. Left ventricular
CPK activity was significantly higher in mepindolol-treated rats
as compared to control- occluded animals, though lower than in
sham-operated rats (Figure 8). This result was paralleled by
the data of phospholipid assays. Ischemia-induced phospholipase

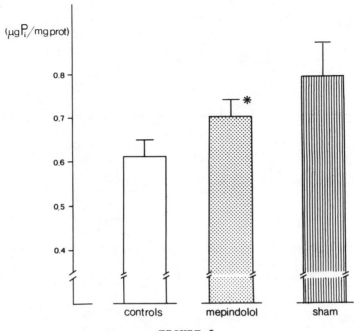

FIGURE 9

Myocardial phospholipid concentration measured 48 hours after the surgical procedure in sham-operated, control occluded and mepindolol-treated rats. Treated rats, following coronary artery occlusion, received meprindolol 1 mg/kg t.i.d., subcutaneously. Values are expressed as mean $\pm$ SEM. *: different from controls, $p < 0.05$.

activation produced a significant fall in myocardial phospholipid concentration in control occluded as compared to sham-operated animals; mepindolol treatment in coronary occluded rats resulted in a reduced left ventricular phospholipid degradation, in comparison to controls (Figure 9).

It cannot be ruled out, however, that mepindolol exerts this beneficial action on phospholipid degradation through a direct inhibition of myocardial phospholipase, since beta-blockers have been shown to prevent the in vitro activation of phospholipase A_2 from human platelets (14). Therefore, it can also be hypothesized that the protective effect of beta-blockers is

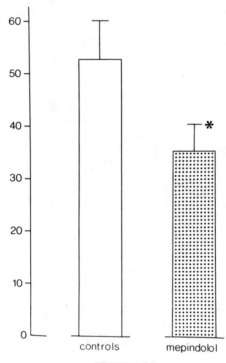

FIGURE 10

Infarct size (IS) expressed as percent of the left ventricle (%
LV) calculated by left ventricular CPK depletion 48 hours after
coronary artery ligation in control occluded and
mepindolol-treated rats. Treated rats received mepindolol 1
mg/kg t.i.d. subcutaneously, for 48 hours following coronary
artery occlusion. Values are expressed as mean ± SEM.
*: different from controls, p < 0.05.

partially mediated by the inhibition of myocardial
phospholipases. The beneficial effect of mepindolol was
demonstrated in our experience by the reduction in the treated
group of infarct size calculated by the CPK method 48 hours
after coronary artery occlusion (Figure 10). Moreover, the
protective action of the drug was not confined to the acute
phase of the infarction, but appeared to be long-lasting. In
fact, left ventricular hydroxyproline and collagen content in
rats treated with mepindolol 21 days post-occlusion, i.e., at
the completion of the healing process, was significantly smaller
as compared to animals with control coronary artery occlusions
(Figure 11). Therefore, the calculated size of the scar in

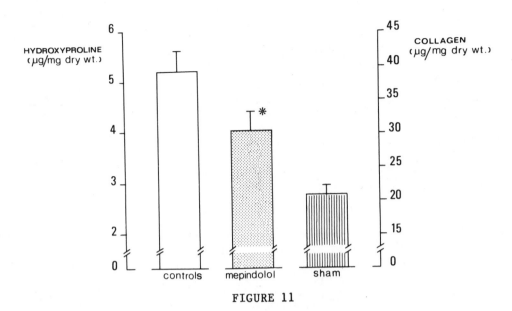

FIGURE 11

Left ventricular hydroxyproline and collagen content measured 21
days after the surgical procedure in rats with control coronary
occlusion, in coronary occluded rats treated with mepindolol and
in sham-operated rats. Treated animals received mepindolol 1
mg/kg t.i.d., subcutaneously, for 48 hours following coronary
artery occlusion. Values are expressed as mean ± SEM.
*: Different from controls, p > 0.05.

treated animals was also significantly smaller as compared to
controls (Figure 12).

In conclusion, these data seem to demonstrate that: a) the
degradation of myocardial phospholipids is a major event in the
development of cellular injury following coronary artery
occlusion in the rat; b) there is a temporal correlation between
left ventricular phospholipid degradation and CPK depletion,
considered as a marker of irreversible cell injury and necrosis;
c) phospholipase inhibition induced by quinacrine reduces
permanently the size of myocardial infarction, probably by
protecting the integrity and function of cell membranes; d) an
intervention, such as mepindolol, reducing myocardial ischemia

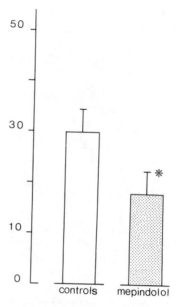

FIGURE 12

Infarct size (IS), expressed as percent of left ventricle (%
LV), calculated by collagen content 21 days after coronary
artery occlusion in control occluded and mepindolol-treated
rats. Treated animals received mepindolol 1 mg/kg t.i.d.,
subcutaneously, for 48 hours following coronary artery
occlusion. Values are expressed as mean ± SEM.
*: Different from controls, p < 0.05.

in coronary-occluded rats, also partially prevents myocardial
phospholipid degradation.

Although further experimental studies are required before
this information can be applied clinically, it indicates a
possible new approach in the treatment of acute myocardial
infarction directed to modify the biochemical events triggered
by ischemia, leading to irreversible cell injury.

REFERENCES

1. Chien, K.R., & Farber, J.L. (1977): Arch. Biochem. Biophys. 180: 191.
2. Chien, K.R., Abrams, J., Serroni, A., Martin, J.T., & Farber, J.L. (1978): J. Biol. Chem. 253: 4809.
3. Farber, J.L., Chien, K.R., & Mittnacht, S. Jr. (1981): Am. J. Pathol. 102: 271.
4. Chien, K.R., Reeves, J.P., Buja, L.M., Bonte, F., Parkey, R.W., & Willerson, J.T. (1981): Circ. Res. 48: 711.
5. Shug, A.L., Thomasen, J.H., Foltes, J.D., Bittar, N., Klein, M.I., Koke, J.R., & Huth. P.J. (1978): Arch. Biochem. Biophys. 187: 25.
6. Idell-Wenger. J.A., & Neely, J.R. (1978): IN Disturbances in Lipid and Lipoprotein Metabolism (eds) J.M. Dietschy, A.M. Gotto, Jr., & J.A. Ontko, Am. Physiol. Soc., Baltimore, p. 269.
7. Wildenthal. K., Decker, R.S., Poole, A.R., Griffin, E.E., & Dingle, J.T. (1978): Lab. Invest. 38: 656.
8. Juan, H. (1977): Naunyn-Schmiedeberg's Arch. Pharmacol. 301: 23.
9. Maclean, D., Fishbein, M.C., Braunwald, E., & Maroko, P.R. (1978): J. Clin. Invest. 61: 541.
10. Chiariello, M., Brevetti, G., De Rosa, G., Acunzo, R., Petillo, F., Rengo, F., & Condorelli. M. (1980): Am. J. Cardiol. 54: 766.
11. Neuman, R.E., & Logan, M.A. (1950): J. Biol. Chem. 184: 299.
12. Reiner, K.A., Rasmussen, M.M., & Jennings, R.B. (1973): Circ. Res. 33: 353.
13. Bonelli, G. (1978): J. Clin. Pharmacol. 16: 78.
14. Vanderhoek, J.Y., & Feinstein, M.B. (1979): Mol. Pharmacol. 16: 171.

CARDIAC PERFUSION, PAST AND PRESENT

R. J. Bing

Huntington Medical Research Institutes and
Huntington Memorial Hospital
100 Congress Street
Pasadena, CA   91105

HISTORICAL BACKGROUND

In its early phase cardiac metabolism was exclusively
concerned with the nutrition of the heart. The isolated
perfused organ appeared to be ideally suited for that purpose.
Most of this work has been admirably summarized in 1926 in "A
Text Book of Physiology" by Robert A. Tigerstedt, the discoverer
of the enzyme renin (1). One section of this book deals with
the "chemical conditions for the beating heart." Prominent
amongst the frequently quoted pioneers are Ludwig, Langendorff,
Kronecker, Howell, Martin, Greene, Gaskell, Bowditch. Clark,
Loewi, Locke, and particularly Ringer (1). Starling and Evans
play a predominant role in the investigation of the use of
organic material by the heart (2). In 1983 as we celebrate
Ringer´s centennial, the work of Ringer is particularly
pertinent. It is amusing to read that Ringer, investigating the
role of calcium in cardiac contraction was first misled by using
tap water for perfusion. Tap water, as he discovered later,
contained not only CaCl but also KCl which antagonized the
calcium effect (1). One year later Ringer discovered that the
arrested heart could be made to beat again by the addition of
calcium chloride. In 1883 he concluded that calcium is
essential for maintenance of cardiac contraction (1).

For obvious reasons the early experiments on the nutrition
of the heart muscle were carried out on hearts of cold-blooded
animals, particularly the frog. Perfusion of the heart of
warm-blooded animals was introduced in 1846 by Wild, a pupil of

the German physiologist, Ludwig (1). Wild used a live animal as the donor connecting the aorta of a dead animal to the carotid artery of a live donor. This led Martin and Applegarth from the Johns Hopkins Hospital in 1980 to develop the first "Langendorff" preparation by perfusing the aorta of an isolated heart from a reservoir (1). Without knowledge of their publication, Langendorff, five years later, described the same preparation which now bears his name (1).

Since this symposium is in part devoted to the role of lipids in relation to cardiac metabolism and function it is of interest to look at the early discoveries in this field. Tigerstedt quotes three authors, Camis in 1908, Gayda in 1911, and Loewi in 1914, who, by determining the respiratory quotient, discovered that "fat" was used by the heart (1). Starling and Evans found that the dog heart utilizes 0.68 gram fat (2). Clark in 1913 working on the perfused frog heart, discovered cardiac utilization of oleate and other free fatty acids (1).

I have dwelt on these early results because they determined the future course of cardiac metabolism. Determination of the nutrition of the human heart in situ was a direct and logical extension of their work (3). More recently the course of cardiac metabolism has been influenced by biochemistry and biophysics by separation of sub- cellular particles and organelles; this has made possible separate observations of the intermediary metabolism in mitochondria, sarcoplasmic reticulum and sarcolemma of the heart (4). But there is still much to be learned from observations on the isolated perfused mammalian heart. Renewed stimulation for the study of the isolated mammalian heart has come from the laboratory of Neely et al. (5). Their perfusion technique has been particularly useful in the under- standing of the regulation of glycolysis in the ischemic and anoxic myocardium (6). Using a supported working cardiac perfusion system, Neely and coworkers were able to define the mechanisms of glycolytic inhibition in the ischemic myocardium. Their findings have been confirmed and extended on the heart in situ by Kubler and Spiekermann (7) and by Opie (8).

Neely's perfusion studies were primarily carried out on the rat heart. This has limited the options for the study of glycolytic intermediates and glycolytic flux, excluding determinations of high energy phosphates, which necessitate specimens of greater weight. The use of perfluorochemicals has now made it possible to perfuse larger mammalian hearts using Neely's working heart preparation (9). The remainder of this discussion is concerned with hemodynamic and metabolic data on the different types of the failing rabbit heart perfused in vitro with Fluosol-43 (10). The effect of TA-064, a new positive inotropic agent, will be briefly mentioned (11). In addition, the paper deals with a new approach to the problem of coronary spasm, using the isolated heart perfused with Fluosol-43 oxygenated with a bubble oxygenator.

MATERIAL AND METHODS

Experimental Heart Failure

In principle the system of Neely was used (5). However, in order to assure adequate oxygenation, the hearts were perfused with Fluosol-43, fortified with Ca^{++}, Mg^{++}, $H_2PO_4^+$, $NaHCO_3$ and glucose in the same concentrations as contained in Krebs-Henseleit solution (12). Adequate oxygenation was achieved with a disposable blood bubble oxygenator (Bentley Laboratories, Inc.). Using this system, high values for O_2 tension entering the left atrium were obtained (average 550 mm Hg). Myocardial O_2 consumption was calculated from coronary blood flow and coronary arterio-venous O_2 difference, using an oxygen solubility constant value (K) of 0.94×10^{-4} ml O_2/ml solution/mm Hg PO_2 for Fluosol-43 (12). After preliminary retrograde perfusion in a Langendorff perfusion apparatus for 10 minutes the hearts were transferred quickly to a perfusion system which incorporated the features of Neely's supported heart preparation (5). The perfusion apparatus was modified to circulate a volume of only 250 ml of perfusion fluid, and the heart chamber was enlarged. Hemodynamic measurements consisted in determinations of cardiac output (CO), coronary flow (CF), myocardial O_2 consumption (MVO_2), left ventricular systolic pressure (LVSP), and end-diastolic pressure (LVEDP) and maximal rate of left ventricular pressure rise (dp/dt_{max}).
Biochemical determinations include cyclic-AMP and the following glycolytic intermediates: lactate (Lact), pyruvate (Pyr), alpha-glycerophosphate (-GP), dihydroxyacetone phosphate (DHAP) and fructose-1,6-diphosphate (F-1,6-DP), glucose-6-phosphate (G-6-P) and fructose-6-phosphate (F-6-P) (13). The myocardial redox state was monitored by comparing the ratio of lactate to pyruvate. Inhibition at the level of phosphofructokinase (PFK) was calculated as

$$\text{PFK Inhibition} = ([G-6-P] + [F-6-P]/[F-1,6-DP])$$

The levels of the high energy phosphates were measured in the remaining tissue powder: creatine phosphate (CP) and adenosine-5'-triphosphate (ATP), adenosine-5'-diphosphate (ADP) and adenosine-5'-monophosphate (AMP) (13).

Three types of heart failure of the isolated heart preparation were studied both by hemodynamics and biochemical means: (1) spontaneous failure, (2) sodium pentothal induced failure, (3) failure due to increased pre- and afterload.

In the first model the heart was permitted to fail spontaneously. This occurred primarily as a result of inadequate coronary perfusion and represents therefore global ischemia. In sodium pentothal induced failure, from 60 to 100 mg of this compound were administered via the aortic cannula, until left ventricular systolic pressure had decreased by 70%. Measurements were then carried out and frozen biopsies were obtained. In the third model, an increase in pre- and afterload resulted from elevation of the bubble trap chamber and from partially restricting aortic outflow. Once a steady state had been reached, hemodynamic observations were made and finally frozen biopsies were taken. When the effect of TA-064 was studied, it was injected directly into the tubing leading to the left atrium. The drug was first dissolved in an equimolar concentration of 0.05 Mol HCl on the day of the experiment; 0.1 mg/0.5 ml was used.

Coronary Artery Spasm

To visualize the coronary arteries color arteriograms were introduced. To accomplish this, Patent Blue dye (0.5 ml of 0.1% solution) was injected into the tubing leading to the left atrium. Immediately afterwards a Nikon F3 camera was activated. The camera was gated in such a manner that exposures were taken during the height of systole and the nadir of diastole. Slides were then developed and projected on a screen with a magnification of x50. To calculate the diameter of a vessel, a 2 cm scale was placed in the same plane as the heart. The inside diameter of the vessel was then determined with a caliper using the scale in the picture as a reference. Localized spasm of the arteries was produced directing a spary of 2 ml of histamine, at concentrations ranging from 10^{-6} to 2×10^{-2} M, directly at a visible coronary artery (usually the left anterior descending), using a 24-gauge needle attached to a 2 cc syringe. Dose response curves were then constructed relating the concentration of histamine to the total coronary vascular resistance. In the second set of experiments, generalized vasoconstriction was produced by injection of histamine (1 cc at concentrations of 10^{-6} to 2×10^{-2} M) directly into the left atrial cannula. The sequence of events followed the same pattern. Hemodynamic measurements were taken

after each injection. Large vessel resistance was calculated as
follows:

$$\text{Large vessel resistance} = 8\mu / \pi R_i \quad (4)$$

where μ, the viscosity, is a constant and R_i is the internal
radius (4), determined from the color arteriogram.

   Arteriolar resistance was calculated as:

   Arteriolar resistance = Mean aortic pressure mm Hg
        (mm Hg/ml/min)   coronary flow ml/min

When atherosclerosis was produced, animals were maintained for
from two to three months on 2% cholesterol, plus 2% coconut oil.

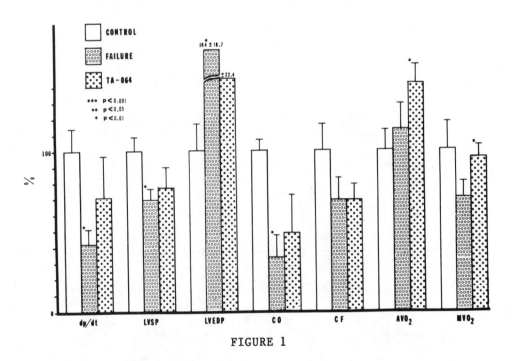

FIGURE 1

Hemodynamic effects of spontaneous myocardial failure. Global
ischemia is present (fall in coronary flow and myocardial oxygen
consumption). Significant hemodynamic manifestations of failure
are observed.

RESULTS AND DISCUSSION

Experimental Heart Failure

Figure 1 illustrates the hemodynamic results obtained in the
spontaneously failing heart. The marked decline in dp/dt_{max},
LVSP and CO are noticeable. LVEDP increased markedly. Of
special significance was the decline in coronary flow, not
adequately compensated for by an increase in A-V O_2
difference. This, therefore, represented global ischemia.
Ischemia was responsible for the decline in high energy
phosphates, the increase in lactate/pyruvate ratios, and
increased inhibition at the level of PFK (Figure 2).

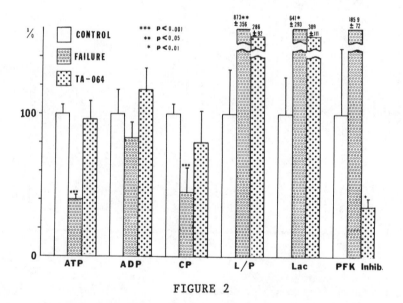

FIGURE 2

Cardiac metabolic effects of spontaneous myocardial failure.
There is a decline in ATP and CP. L/P ratio is elevated; there
is inhibition at the level of PFK.

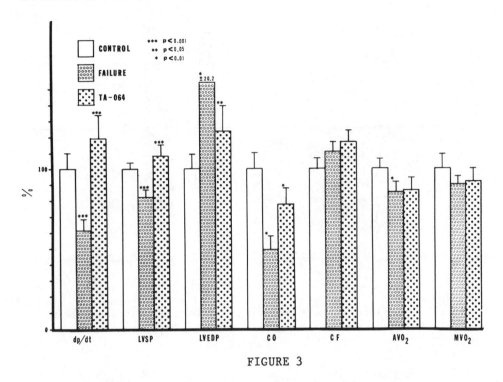

FIGURE 3

Sodium pentobarbital failure. There are significant
manifestations of myocardial failure, but coronary flow and
myocardial oxygen consumptions are not altered.

In contrast, in sodium pentothal induced failure, coronary
flow was not reduced, and was even slightly elevated (Figure
3). Myo- cardial O_2 consumption remained at its control
value. Myocardial insufficiency was present since dp/dt_{max},
and CO declined and left ventricular end-diastolic pressure rose
(Figure 3). There was no apparent decline in high energy
phosphate (Figure 4). Inhibition at the level of PFK
increased. The lactate/pyruvate ratio remained unchanged
(Figure 4). This type of failure, therefore, differs markedly
from spontaneous failure, primarily because of the absence of
myocardial ischemia. Wollenberger also found no change in high
energy phosphate in sodium pentothal-induced failure (14). Lane
and associates discovered that sodium pentothal depresses
cardiac contractility through inhibition of calcium uptake (15).

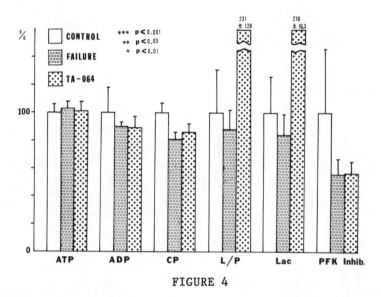

FIGURE 4

Cardiac metabolic effects of failure induced by sodium pentobarbital. The changes are not statistically significant.

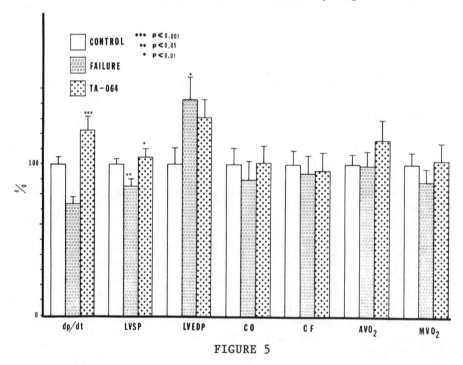

FIGURE 5

Hemodynamic effects of failure due to increased pre- and
afterload. Changes in left ventricular systolic pressure and
left ventricular end-diastolic pressure are noticed.

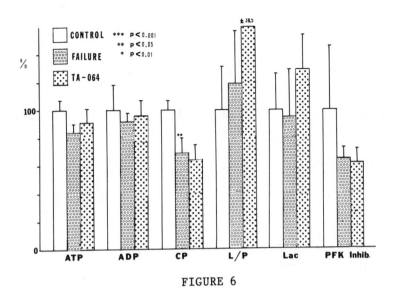

FIGURE 6

Cardiac metabolic effects of elevation of pre- and afterload.
There is a significant decline in creatine phosphate.
Phosphofructokinase activity is inhibited.

As shown in Figure 5, in failure resulting from increased
pre- and afterload, the decline in dp/dt$_{max}$, ventricular
systolic pressure and cardiac output was significant. Coronary
flow and myocardial oxygen consumption remained unchanged. As
shown in Figure 6, however, significant defects in creatine
phosphate, in L/P ratios and the degree of inhibition of PFK
were encountered. In many instances the addition of TA-064
corrected the hemodynamic and metabolic defects described above
(Figures 1 to 6). This compound also had marked positive
inotropic effects on patients with congestive heart failure
(11). In unpublished observations from this laboratory, the
action of TA-064 varied with the type of myocardial failure
(16).

The experiments described above demonstrate the value of the
supported, well-oxygenated perfused heart in the study of
myocardial failure. In clinical situations, there is also lack
of uniformity of the biochemical manifestations (17, 18). Here
too the common denominator is the decline in contractility,
while the biochemical sequelae show marked individual
differences. Therefore, a decline in coronary flow is only one
of many factors determining the fall in contractility.

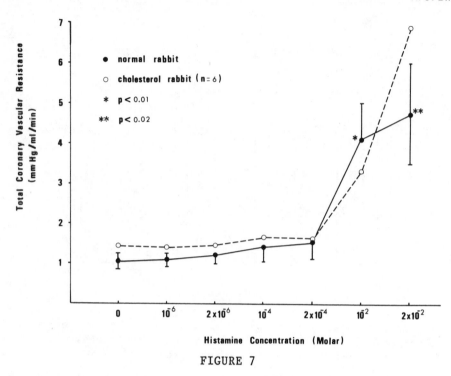

FIGURE 7

Dose response curve after intaatrial injection of histamine
(histamine concentrations plotted against total coronary
vascular resistance). At concentrations of histamine of 10^{-2}
M and 2 x 10^{-2} M total coronary resistance increases
significantly. No statistical change between hearts with normal
and atherosclerotic coronary arteries is noted.

Coronary Vascular Spasm

This subject is included because of the causal relationship
between coronary spasm and myocardial ischemia and necrosis.
Figure 7 shows the dose response curve relating total coronary
resistance to dosage of histamine injected intraatrially. It is
seen that concentrations of 10^{-2} and 2 x 10^{-2} M result in a
significant increase in total coronary vascular resistance; no
significant differences are noted between control animals and
rabbits with coronary atherosclerosis. Apparently in our
experimental conditions, coronary atherosclerosis does not
predispose to coronary spasm. This is in contrast to the
results of Yokoyama and Henry who found that in isolated
arteries the addition of cholesterol increases the
responsiveness of coronary arteries to spasm (19).

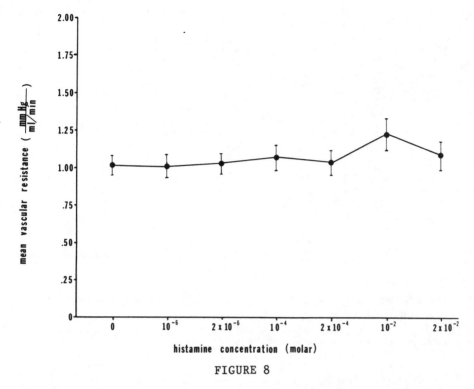

FIGURE 8

Dose response curves as in Figure 7, but histamine (2×10^{-2} M) was rapidly applied (sprayed) to the region of the l.a.d. coronary artery. Total vascular resistance is not significantly altered.

Figure 8 demonstrates that in contrast to intraatrial injection, local application of histamine (spray) in doses ranging from 10^{-6} to 2×10^{-2} M causes only a nonsignificant rise in total vascular resistance. The different effect of local versus intraatrial injection of histamine is also illustrated in Figure 9. Local applications of histamine (2 cc of a 10^{-2} M solution) do not elevate total coronary resistance, while after intraatrial injection total coronary resistance increases significantly.

On the other hand, topical spraying of histamine (2 cc of 2×10^{-2} M) significantly reduces the vascular diameter of the exposed coronary artery and increases its large vessel resistance (Figure 10). Figure 11 demonstrates similar effects of intraatrial injection of histamine (2×10^{-2} M). It is to be recalled, however, that with this type of administration

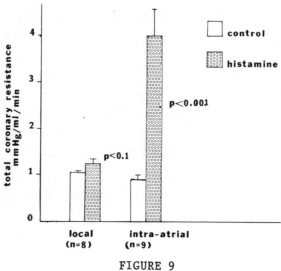

FIGURE 9

Demonstrates that total coronary vascular resistance is
increased only after intraarterial injections of histamine (2 x
10^{-2} M). Local spraying (2 cc of 10^{-2} M solution) has no
effect on total coronary vascular resistance.

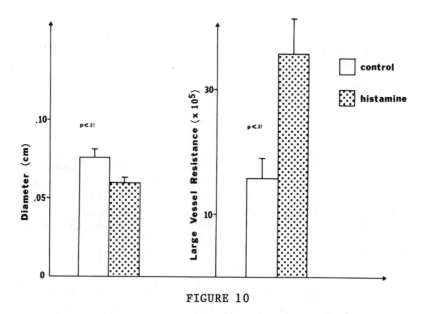

FIGURE 10

The effect of topical administration of histamine (2 x 10^{-2} M)
on vascular diameter and large vessel resistance of l.a.d. The
changes are significant.

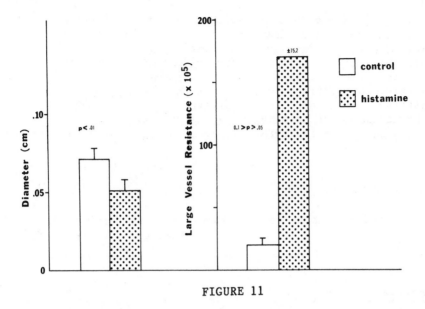

FIGURE 11

Significant increase in diameter and large vessel resistance.
Not shown is the increase in total vascular resistance.

vasoconstriction extends also to the resistance vessels, as
illustrated by the significant elevation of total coronary
resistance, illustrated in Figures 7 and 9.

Several conclusions can be drawn from these experiments.
First, there still appears to be a place in the filed of cardiac
metabolism for the study of isolated well-oxygenated perfused
hearts. The advent of perfluorochemicals as blood substitutes
together with recent developments in oxygenating devices has
made possible metabolic studies on different types of myocardial
failure produced in vitro. The finding of a wide spectrum of
hemodynamic and metabolic manifestation parallels those
described for the clinical variety of myocardial failure. This
newly developed perfusion system has also made possible the
observation and quantitation of coronary spasm in vitro, through
color arteriograms and gated high speed photography. Here the
prime lesson learned is that localized spasm of a coronary
artery with increase in large vessel resistance may not result
in changes in arteriolar coronary vascular resistance. In
clinical situations, therefore, if these conclusions are
applicable, spasm of large coronary arteries are not by
necessity accompanied by myocardial ischemia.

Our perfusion model, utilizing perfluorochemicals and bubble oxygenation has future implications. These include controlled pharmacological studies on new inotropic agents and their mode of action, such as those illustrated in this report for TA-064, and on Ca^{++} transfer in relation to deficient excitation-contraction coupling. Of particular future significance will be the availability of our model for the study of the mechanism of coronary vasoconstriction. Thus, the work of the pioneers of the 19th century is being extended to our own era.

ACKNOWLEDGEMENTS

This work was supported by grants from the Council for Tobacco Research, U.S.A., Inc., and the Margaret W. and Herbert Hoover Jr. Foundations.

REFERENCES

1. Tigerstedt, R.A. (1923): Die Physiologie des Kreislaufes, Vol. I, 2nd edition, Berlin and Wien, publisher, W. De Gruyter, p. 245.
2. Starling, E.H., & Evans, C.L. (1914): J. Physiol. 49: 67.
3. Bing, R.J. (1954): Harvey Lect. 50: 27.
4. Opie, L.H. (1969): Am. Heart J. 77: 383.
5. Neely, J.R., & Rovetto, M.J. (1975): Methods Enzymol. 39: 43.
6. Rovetto, M.J., Lambeston, W.F., & Neely, J.R. (1975): Circ. Res. 37: 742.
7. Kubler, W., & Spieckermann, P.G. (1970): J. Mol. Cell. Cardiol. 1: 351.
8. Opie, L.H. (1976): Circ. Res. 38: I-52.
9. Clark, L.C. Jr., & Gollan, F. (1966): Science 152: 1755.
10. Tomera, J.F., & Geyer, R.P. (1982): J. Mol. Cell. Cardiol. 14: 573.
11. Kino, M., Hirota, Y., Yamamoto, S., Sawada, K., Moriguchi, M., Kotaka, M., Kubo, S., & Kawamura, K. (1983): Am. J. Cardiol. 51: 802.
12. Green Cross Corp. (1976): Green Cross Tech. Info., Ser. 3, Osaka, Japan.
13. Bergmeyer, H.U. (1974): Methods in Enyzmatic Analysis, Deerfield Beach, Verlag Chemie International.
14. Wollenberger, A. (1947): Am. J. Physiol. 150: 733.
15. Lane, R.F., Hess, M.L., Gertz, E.W., & Briggs, F.N. (1968): Circ. Res. 23: 597.

16. Bing, R.J., Sugihara, J., & Metz, M. (Submitted for publication).
17. Fenton, J.C., Gudbjarnason, S., & Bing, R.J. (1962): Am. Heart Assoc., Monograph No. 1, second edition.
18. Bing, R.J. (1978): Circ. Res. 58: 965.
19. Yohoyama, M., & Henry, P.D. (1979): Circ. Res. 45: 479.

CLINICAL RELEVANCE OF FREE FATTY ACID EXCESS

L.H. Opie, M.J. Tansey, and J. de Leiris

MRC-UCT Ischemic Heart Disease Research Unit
Department of Medicine, University of Cape Town
Cape Town, South Africa

GENERAL METABOLIC RESPONSE IN MYOCARDIAL INFARCTION

A large part of this book is devoted to abnormalities of
myocardial lipid metabolism and to the possible disturbances
thereof in ischemia. This article emphasizes the importance not
only of changes in lipid but also of carbohydrate metabolism and
the interaction of these two, with special reference to clinical
situations. In acute myocardial infarction, there is a general
metabolic disturbance (1), quite apart from the changes
occurring in the myocardial muscle. There is a release of
catecholamines with increased circulating and urinary values
with an elevation of blood free fatty acids (= FFA = NEFA =
non-esterified fatty acids), and the development of glucose
intolerance. There is reasonable and increasing evidence that
each of these abnormalities may play an important role in the
evolution of myocardial ischemic injury. The fundamental change
may be the increased circulating catecholamines which probably
elevate the blood free fatty acids. The glucose tolerance
probably results both from the elevation of circulating free
fatty acids and also from the effect of catecholamines on the
release of insulin from the pancreas. The adverse effects of
catecholamines on the myocardium are complex and are probably
mediated in part by increased cylic AMP (2) and in part by
increased entry of calcium ions (3, 4). The adverse effects of
free fatty acids might be a direct detergent effect (5) or the
result of an accumulation of acyl CoA and acyl carnitine (6).

PATHWAYS IN ISCHEMIA

In broad outline, some of the relevant pathways in ischemia are as follows. In the ischemic zone there is a decreased delivery of oxygen and a decreased oxygen uptake. Because there is still some collateral flow, in most animal models there is a residual uptake of oxygen and fatty acids by the ischemic cells. The predominant pattern of metabolism remains aerobic even to very low coronary flow values; as long as there is oxygen, even a small amount of aerobic ATP will be of greater importance fot eh production of energy than the very low rates of production of anaerobic ATP. As coronary flow is reduced, glucose becomes a more important source of oxidative energy than does fatty acid oxidation; only when the flow falls to below 10% of control do glycogen and anaerobic metabolism become important energy sources (Figure 2, ref. 7). Important reservations to the model of Opie (7) are that (1) the coronary flow data were sometimes extrapolated and not measured; and (2) the model implies the existence of a hypoxic "intermediate" cell. Chance (8) has questioned the existence of such intermediate cells, suggesting instead the mitochondria respond in an "on-off way" to O_2-lack. However, patterns of mixed aerobic and anaerobic metabolism occur in dog heart infarct models (9) suggesting that hypoxia is a valid concept for the ischemic zone as a whole.

There appears to be some controversy as to whether tissue free fatty acids themselves are elevated. This question has been addressed in this book by two other investigators. Tissue triglyceride appears to be elevated in zones of modest flow impairment but not in zones of severe flow impairment. In ischemia, acyl CoA rises as does acyl carnitine (10). According to one currently favored theory, acyl CoA may inhibit the adenine nucleotide transferase to further impair ATP production by the mitochondria (11, 12). However, this theory is still controversial (13). As far as glucose metabolism is concerned, there is enhanced glucose extraction relative to that of free fatty acid. In other words, ischemia changes the oxidative metabolism from being fatty acid-dependent to carbohydrate-dependent (14). This change probably occurs in zones of moderately severe ischemia and not in zones of severest ischemia (9). In severest ischemia, products of glycolysis such as lactate, H^+ and NADH may inhibit the rate of glycolysis at the level of glyceraldehyde-3-phosphate dehydrogenase (15, 16). In zones of modest flow impairment, and also in non-ischemic tissue (17) the theory is that enhanced glucose metabolism may protect the myocardium, possibly by an enhanced rate of aerobic glycolysis or by reduction of blood free fatty acids. Such glycolysis, although accelerated, does not play any significant contribution to the myocardial energy needs (18).

PATIENT OBSERVATIONS

Arrhythmias

In patients the first and classic observations were made by Oliver and his group from Edinburgh (5, 19). Kurien and Oliver (5) reported that in a patient who had been monitored before and after the onset of myocardial infarction, the onset of infarction was associated with an increase of blood free fatty acids. They reported the data on blood samples usually taken at relatively infrequent intervals. Much later Tansey and I (20) undertook hourly measurements in patients with acute myocardial infarction. We found that if fatty acids were measured at such regular intervals, that there was a considerable hour-to-hour variation. If we allowed for this variation and looked at the effect of the mean free fatty acid value in the first hours of infarction on the incidence of arrhythmias, then like Oliver, we found a positive relation between high free fatty acid values and arrhythmias (Table 1). This does not prove that free fatty acids themselves are arrhythmogenic, which still remains a controversial issue. Rather, we propose that fatty acids are "co-arrhythmogenic" factors, providing a "last straw" situation in the presence of more powerful factors such as adrenergic stimulation and hypokalemia. Otherwise it is difficult to understand those animal studies where high free fatty acids even in the presence of hypokalemia (K^+ = 3 mM) have no apparent arrhythmogenic effect (21). The complexities of this problem are reviewed elsewhere (22).

Estimated infarct size

We also examined the relationship between free fatty acids and infarct size, estimating the infarct size in patients by creatine kinase release patterns (23). The peak free fatty acid levels were higher in patients with large estimated infarct sizes (Figure 1). Thus, as the plasma fatty acid values increase, so does the estimated infarct size. The increased infarct sizes could either be the consequence of the raised free fatty acid and catecholamine values or else the large infarct size could be indirectly associated with high free fatty acids, as a consequence of high blood catecholamine levels.

Hypothesis tested

The hypothesis presented in the Lancet is as follows (Figure 2). In the acute stage of myocardial infarction, increased ischemic damage increases infarct size. There is a relationship between estimated infarct size and its complications (24) and also between infarct size and circulating catecholamine values

TABLE 1   FFA and arrhythmias in the first 12 hours

| | Number (%) of patients with | | | | |
	Any arrhythmia	VPBs only	VF or VT	Heart block	VT, VF, or heart block
Admission FFA					
Low (n=23)	13* (57)	2 (9)	10* (23)	1 (4)	11* (48)
High (n=12)	10* (83)	2 (17)	7 (58)	1 (8)	8 (87)
P	NS	NS	NS	NS	NS
Peak FFA					
Low (n=15)	6 (40)	2 (13)	4 (27)	0	4 (27)
High (n=20)	17* (85)	2 (10)	13* (65)	2 (10)	15* (75)
P	0.05	NS	NS	NS	0.05
Mean FFA					
Low (n=23)	11* (48)	4 (17)	7* (30)	0	7* (30)
High (n=12)	12 (100)	0	10 (83)	2 (17)	12 (100)
P	0.01	NS	0.02	NS	0.002

* One patient was hypokalemic (potassium 3.4 mmol/l) at the time of VT.
VPBs = ventricular premature beats; VF = ventricular fibrillation; VT = ventricular tachycardia;
NS = not significant.

From: Tansey & Opie, (20). By permission, The Lancet.

(25). In conscious dogs with coronary artery occlusion, a
deterioration in hemodynamics was closely related to increases
in plasma catecholamine concentrations (26). Our studies on
patients have shown a relationship between estimated infarct
size and circulating free fatty acid values. Although we have
not simultaneously measured blood concentrations of
catecholamines and of free fatty acid values, that has been done
by the Edinburgh group (27). There is a close relationship
between circulating catecholamines and free fatty acids; however
within the first hour of onset of symptoms elevated blood plasma
catecholamines and not free fatty acids are detected. So too in
our study it took 4 hours for free fatty acids to rise more in
large than in small infarcts (23). Hence high free fatty acids
are more likely to be associated with large infarcts than with
ventricular arrhythmias in the first hour of myocardial
infarction.

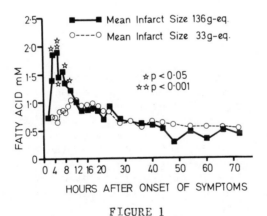

FIGURE 1

Plasma FFA concentration in eight patients with large infarcts
were significantly higher 4, 5, 6, 7 and 8 hours after onset of
symptoms than in those with small infarcts. From Opie et al.
(23) by permission, The Lancet.

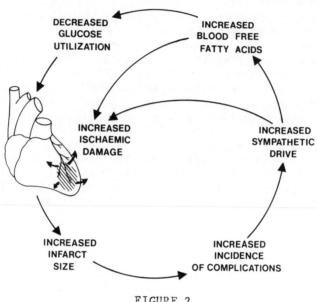

FIGURE 2

Proposed metabolic vicious circle in acute myocardial
infraction. From Opie et al. (23), by permission, The Lancet.

ANIMAL EXPERIMENTAL DATA

Ischemic damage

    Many workers have shown that gross elevations of circulating
free fatty acids can increase ischemic damage (1, 28). The
experimental system we used was the isolated rat heart model
perfused either in the Langendorff non-working mode or else in
the working mode as described by Neely et al. (29). Enzyme
release was monitored for a period of 60 minutes; the rate of
release of lactate dehydrogenase in hearts perfused with glucose
showed a very small but definite increase after coronary artery
ligation (30). When coronary ligated hearts were perfused with
physiological concentrations of free fatty acids, there was an
increased enzyme release rather similar to the increase obtained
when non-ligated hearts were perfused with unphysiologically
high fatty acid-albumin molar ratios (Figure 3). When such a
high molar ratio was combined with coronary artery ligation,
then enzyme release was greatly augmented. Similar trends were

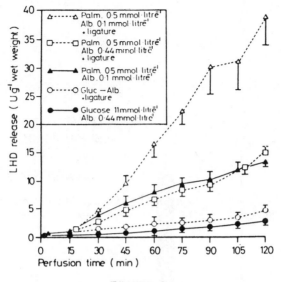

FIGURE 3

Rates of release of lactate dehydrogenase (LDH) in isolated
working rat heart with coronary ligation 15 to 105 min after the
onset of recirculation perfusion. Control hearts, without
coronary ligation, are shown in black symbols and coronary
ligated hearts in white. Note that (1) coronary ligation
doubles or trebles the rates of LDH release; (2) palmitate-
perfused hearts have higher rates than glucose-perfused hearts;
(3) an increased albumin concentration decreases LDH release in
palmitate-perfused hearts; and (4) LDH release is approximately
linear. From deLeiris and Opie (30), by permission,
Cardiovascular Research.

obtained for the release of creatine kinase. Although most
studies were with the "traditional" fatty acid palmitate,
similar data were obtained for oleate and linoleate (Figure 4).
Because the fatty acid solutions were prepared by repeated
dialysis, against a standard calcium ion concentration, it is
unlikely that alterations in perfusate calcium played any role
in the results obtained (on a few occasions calcium ion
concentration was checked by a calcium-sensitive microelectrode).

Mechanical performance

When fatty acid perfused hearts were compared with glucose
perfused hearts (Table 2), several indices of mechanical

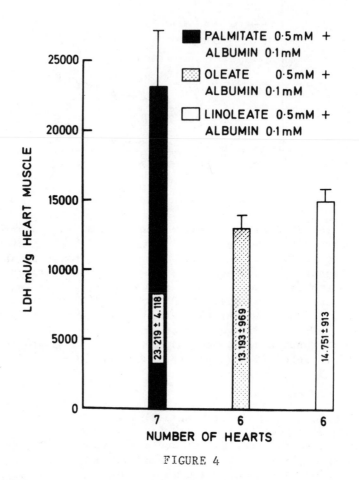

FIGURE 4

Effect of various fatty acids on release of LDH in isolated
perfused working rat heart after coronary ligation.

TABLE 2   Comparison of effects of fatty acid (palmitate 0.5 mmol/litre, albumin 0.1 mmol/litre or of glucose 11 mmol/litre) on enzyme release, mechanical performance, dP/dt_{max}, and oxygen uptake of isolated coronary ligated rat heart

Initial substrate concentration (mmol/litre)	n	Release of lactate dehydrogenase (mU/g/min)	O_2 uptake (ml/g/min)	O_2 uptake per beat per unit systolic pressure (nl/kPa)
Palmitate 0.5 Albumin 0.1	8	170 ± 16	102.2 ± 4.1	333.8 ± 11.20
Glucose 11 Albumin 0.1	7	53 ± 12	81.4 ± 4.3	356.3 ± 10.1
P		<<0.001	<0.005	<0.005

For details, see Opie & Bricknell (36).

performance such as peak systolic pressure and an index of contractility were unchanged. However, there was nevertheless a large increase in enzyme release. There was an impairment of mechanical efficiency as shown by the increased amount of oxygen required for each unit of the dP/dt measurement; the "oxygen-wasting" effect was about 25%.

Effect of glucose or glucose-insulin

The addition of either glucose or insulin reduced fatty acid-induced enzyme release (30). In further unpublished studies, the combination of the two when provided in excess had no further effect on enzyme release. Liedtke et al. (31) showed that excess glucose and insulin did not prevent ischemic damage in an isolated pig heart model. Their perfusate probably contained some glucose and insulin to start with; our recent experiments show that when excess glucose and insulin are provided, these agents do not alter the beneficial effects of a low concentration of only glucose (5 mM).

These data may suggest that excess glucose and insulin would be unlikely to modify infarct size. However, glucose-insulin-potassium is probably a very effective antilipolytic agent (18) and limits indices of infarction in dogs (32). Furthermore, controlled studies by Rackley's group in Birmingham have shown a beneficial effect of glucose-insulin-potassium in patients with acute myocardial infarction; one postulated mechanism of action is by decreasing the circulating free fatty acids (33).

ISCHEMIC CONTRACTURE

The model used was an isolated rat heart perfused by the method of Langendorff in which the perfusion pressure was abruptly decreased (34). In glucose-perfused hearts, only the peak systolic pressure decreased whereas the diastolic tension remained unchanged over 20 min. In hearts perfused with acetate, pyruvate or free fatty acids, the diastolic tension increased; this change was not due to a decreased coronary flow but to a true increase in diastolic tension.

To compare further the metabolic situations in ischemic hearts perfused with glucose in contrast to acetate, we aimed for conditions in which the myocardial level of ATP was the same in the two perfusion conditions (35). Mitochondrial production of ATP was inhibited by atractyloside which is the inhibitor of adenine nucleotide transferase, or glycolysis was inhibited by iodoacetate or deoxyglucose. In acetate-perfused hearts, when mitochondrial metabolism provided the source of ATP, there was a large degree of ischemic contracture. In glucose-perfused

hearts, when only glycolysis provided energy because of the
presence of atractyloside, there was little or no ischemic
contracture. Thus it seemed as if glycolysis was in some way
preventing the formation of ischemic contracture.

Our unpublished experiments support this proposal more
directly. The rate of glycolysis was monitored constantly by
the rate of formation of tritiated water from tritiated
glucose. All mechanical activity was stopped by a combination
of ischemia and potassium arrest; the diastolic tension fell to
zero. When glycolysis was inhibited by the addition of
iodoacetate, then the rate of glycolysis fell as the diastolic
tension rose. Thus there appeared to be a close inverse
relationship between the rate of glycolysis and the development
of diastolic tension; the difference could not simply be
explained by the ATP level in the ischemic heart.

We have developed two hypotheses to try to explain the
effect of glycolysis. First, glycolysis may provide glycolytic
ATP which in turn could be used for the calcium pump of the
sarcoplasmic reticulum. Secondly, glycolysis may act to prevent
accumulation of myocardial cyclic AMP (34).

CONCLUDING REMARKS

The model of ischemia chosen by most workers would appear to
be that of a reduction of flow frequently regional, sometimes
global, but usually not the total cessation of flow. In most
models there is still some collateral flow with some uptake of
oxygen. The oxygen uptake of the ischemic tissue is reduced.
We do not know whether in the ischemic area there are some
mitochondria working normally and some completely arrested, or
whether there are hypoxic mitochondria working at "half-speed".
The overall pattern of metabolism is hypoxic (7). Depending on
the severity of ischemia and the anatomical distribution, many
different patterns of metabolism can be found. One pattern that
can be described at least in cells of moderately ischemic
severity, is an increase of glucose metabolism relative to that
of free fatty acid (15). The question arises whether further
therapeutic modification of external glucose and fatty acid can
influence the internal cellular events. There seems to be
little doubt that an extreme modification from fatty acid to
glucose can greatly alter the severity of the ischemic process.
When trying to apply this to patients, we have to bear in mind
that in patients there are already elevated glucose levels in
acute myocardial infarction and that glucose intolerance which
in turn may impair the rate of glucose utilization by the
heart. One promising avenue of approach would be to regulate
circulating free fatty acid levels either directly by various

antilipolytic agents or indirectly by altering the balance between carbohydrate and fatty acid metabolism in the myocardium.

REFERENCES

1. Opie, L.H. (1975): Am. J. Cardiol. 36: 938.
2. Horak, A.R., Podzuweit, T., & Opie, L.H. (1980): IN Advances in Myocardiology, Vol. 1, (ed) Tajuddin, M., Dass, P.K., Tariq, R., & Dhalla, N.S., University Park Press, Baltimore, p. 367.
3. Opie, L.H., Thandroyen, F.T., Muller, C., & Bricknell, O.L. (1979): J. Mol. Cell. Cardiol. 11: 1073.
4. Horak, A.R., & Opie, L.H. (1983): IN Advances in Myocardiology, Vol. 4, (eds) Chazox, E., Saks, V., & Rona, G., Plenum Publishing Corp., New York, p. 23.
5. Kurien, V.A., & Oliver, M.F. (1970): Lancet 2: 122.
6. Feuvray, D., Idell-Wenger, J.A., & Neely, J.R. (1979): Circ. Res. 44: 322.
7. Opie, L.H. (1976): Circ. Res. 53 (Suppl. 1): 52.
8. Chance, B. (1976): Circ. Res. 38(Suppl. 1): 69.
9. Opie, L.H., Owen, P., & Riemersma, R.A. (1973): Eur. J. Clin. Invest. 3: 419.
10. Whitmer, J.T., Idell-Wenger, J.A., Rovetto, M.J., & Neely, J.R. (1978): J. Biol. Chem. 253: 4305.
11. Shug, A.L., Shrago, E., Bittar, N., Folts, J.D., & Kokes, J.R. (1975): Am. J. Physiol. 228: 689.
12. Kotaka, K., Miyazaki, Y., Ogawa, K., Satake, T., Sugiyama, S., & Ozawa, T. (1982): J. Mol. Cell. Cardiol. 14: 223.
13. Lochner, A., Van Niekerk, I., & Kotze, J.C.N. (1981): J. Mol. Cell. Cardiol. 13: 991.
14. Owen, P., Thomas, M., & Opie, L.H. (1969): Lancet 1: 1187.
15. Rovetto, M.J., Lamberton, W.F., & Neely, J.R. (1975): Circ. Res. 37: 742.
16. Mochizuki, S., & Neely, J.R. (1979): J. Mol. Cell. Cardiol. 11: 221.
17. Liedtke, A.J., Nellis, S.H., & Whitesell, L.F. (1982): J. Mol. Cell. Cardiol. 14: 195.
18. Opie, L.H., & Owen, P. (1976): Am. J. Cardiol. 38: 310.
19. Oliver, M.F., Kurien, V.A., & Greenwood, T.W. (1968): Lancet 1: 710.
20. Tansey, M.J.B., & Opie, L.H. (1983): Lancet In press.
21. Didier, J.P., Moreau, D., & Opie, L.H. (1980): J. Mol. Cell. Cardiol. 12: 1191.
22. Opie, L.H. (1975): Am. J. Cardiol. 36: 938.
23. Opie, L.H., Tansey, M., & Kennelly, B.M. (1977): Lancet 2: 890.
24. Grande, P., Christiansen, C., & Pedersen, A. (1983): Eur. Heart J. 4: 20.

25. Karlsberg, R.P., Cryer, P.E., & Roberts, R. (1981): Am. Heart J. 102: 24.
26. Karlsberg, R.P., Penkoske, P.A., Cryer, P.E., Corr, P.B., & Roberts, R. (1979): Cardiovasc. Res. 13: 523.
27. Vetter, N.J., Strange, R.C., Adams, W., & Oliver, M.F. (1974): Lancet 1: 284.
28. Liedtke, A.J., Nellis, S., & Neely, J.R. (1978): Circ. Res. 43: 652.
29. Neely, J.R., Liebermeister, H., Battersby, E.J., & Morgan, H.E. (1967): Am. J. Physiol. 212: 804.
30. De Leiris, J., & Opie, L.H. (1978): Cardiovasc. Res. 10: 585.
31. Liedtke, A.J., Hughes, H.C., & Neely, J.R. (1976): Am. J. Cardiol. 38: 17.
32. Dalby, A.J., Bricknell, O.L., & Opie, L.H. (1981): Cardiovasc. Res. 15: 588.
33. Rogers, W.J., Segall, P.H., McDaniel, H.G., Mantle, J.A., Russell, R.O., & Rackley, C.E. (1979): Am. J. Cardiol. 43: 801.
34. Bricknell, O.L., & Opie, L.H. (1978): Circ. Res. 43: 102.
35. Bricknell, O.L., Daries, P., & Opie, L.H. (1981): J. Mol. Cell. Cardiol. 13: 941.
36. Opie, L.H., & Bricknell, O.L. (1979): Cardiovasc. Res. 12: 693.

IODINE-123 PHENYLPENTADECANOIC ACID: DETECTION OF ACUTE MYOCARDIAL INFARCTION IN ANESTHETIZED DOGS

J. S. Rellas, J. R. Corbett, P. Kulkarni, C. Morgan,
M. Devous, L. M. Buja, R. W. Parkey, J. T. Willerson
and S. E. Lewis

Departments of Internal Medicine (Cardiovascular
Division), Radiology (Nuclear Medicine), and Pathology
The University of Texas Health Science Center and
Parkland Memorial Hospital
5323 Harry Hines Boulevard
Dallas, TX   75235

Long-chain fatty acids are the preferred substrate of
cardiac muscle. Therefore, radiolabeled free fatty acids are a
natural choice for the non- invasive evaluation of myocardial
metabolism and extensive research has focused on the development
of radiolabeled free fatty acids for myocardial imaging (1-5).
Evans et al. in 1965 successfully radioiodinated (I-131) oleic
acid across a double bond and produced crude images of the
myocardium in dogs, thus demonstrating the potential of
radiolabeled free fatty acids for external, noninvasive
myocardial imaging (1). Subsequently, heptadecanoic acid and
hexadecanoic acid have been studied extensively in experimental
animals and have shown promise in preliminary clinical
assessments (2-5). However, for myocardial imaging, the
terminally iodinated straight-chain free-fatty acids have two
major problems, including (a) they are metabolized rapidly by
the myocardium and (b) significant blood pool radioactivity
results from free iodide released along with beta oxidation of
the fatty acid in the myocardium and liver.

Recently, Machulla et al. (3) have proposed a means to

stabilize chemically the carbon-iodine bond by replacing the
alkyl carbon-iodine bond by an aryl carbon-iodine bond. The
by-product of beta-oxidation of the iodophenyl free-fatty acid
is benzoic acid which is rapidly excreted with the iodine moiety
still attached. Kulkarni et al. have recently developed simple,
convenient, reproducible, and efficient (> 90%) labeling of
phenylpentadecanoic acid (PPA) using an organothallium
intermediate (6-8). Preliminary studies by Kulkarni et al.
(6-8) and Chien et al. (9) using serial myocardial biopsies have
demonstrated rapid extraction by normal myocardium and a
bi-exponential clearance with a fast component half-time of 3.5
minutes and a slow component half-time of approximately 130
minutes. Blood clearance was also rapid being approximately 2.5
minutes. Thus, IPPA appears similar in its myocardial uptake
and blood clearance to carbon-11 palmitate (9, 10). Indeed,
work by Chien et al. (9) suggests that there is no discernible
difference in the myocardial localization of the two agents.

The hypothesis tested in the present study was that the
regional uptake and/or clearance of IPPA measured with single
photon emission computed tomography (SPECT) allows the
relatively noninvasive detection of myocardial infarction in
anesthetized, open-chest canine models.

MATERIALS AND METHODS

Mongrel dogs were fasted overnight, anesthetized with sodium
pento- barbital, intubated, and ventilated with a Harvard
respirator. The jugular vein and carotid artery were
cannulated, the heart was exposed via a left thoracotomy and
suspended in a pericardial cradle. A catheter was inserted into
the left atrium through the appendage. Technetium-99m or
thallium-201 point sources (5-15 mCi) were sewn to the left
ventricular apex and base. These markers were used to ensure
correspondence between tomographic and pathologic sections.

Five anesthetized, open-chest dogs were studied as control
animals. Following placement of the radioactive point sources,
tracer microspheres were injected into the left atrium for a
determination of regional myocardial blood flow by the reference
method (11, 12). The animal's chest was closed and myocardial
tomographic imaging performed immediately following the
injection of I-123 PPA.

Eleven anesthetized, open-chest dogs were studied following
proximal ligation of the left anterior descending (LAD) coronary
artery. In nine dogs, tracer microspheres were injected for
determination of regional myocardial blood flow prior to

coronary artery occlusion. Ten minutes later, the LAD was
ligated proximally and a second tracer microsphere species was
injected 60 minutes following LAD occlusion. The animals were
then transported to the imaging facility and imaging was begun
immediately after the intravenous injection of 2-6 mCi of I-123
PPA and approximately 90-120 minutes after LAD occlusion.

Radiopharmaceutical Preparation

PPA was radioiodinated via an organothallium intermediate
(6-8). PPA (0.5 mg) was dissolved in 0.2 ml trifluoroacetic
acid with 2 mg of thallium trifluoroacetate and incubated at
room temperature for at least one hour. The in situ formed
PPA-Tl complex was treated with 5-10 mCi Na I-123 in 0.1 N NaOH
(5-100 µl) along with the carrier (KI) (12 µg). The reaction
mixture was heated at 100° C for 15 minutes and the labeled
product purified by solvent extraction silica gel column
chromatography. After evaporation of the solvent, the product
was dissolved in 100 µl ethanol and reconstituted with 6% human
albumin solution. The final product was filtered through a 0.1
µ membrane filter to remove any aggregates.

Single Photon Tomographic Imaging (SPECT)

SPECT was performed with a rotating wide field of view gamma
camera (General Electric 400T, General Electric Medical Products
Division, Milwaukee, WI) equipped with a general purpose 200 keV
parallel hole collimator. Animals were positioned on the
imaging table right side down with the spine approximately
parallel to the axis of rotation. The position was adjusted so
that the radioactive point sources were superimposed in the
anterior projection and were within the same row in the lateral
projection. Acquisition of the first tomogram was begun within
5 minutes after the intravenous injection of 2-6 mCi I-123 PPA.
Energy discrimination was provided by a 20% window centered on
the 159 keV photopeak. Thirty-two, 64 x 64 x 16 projection
images each containing a minimum of 40,000 counts were acquired
at equally-spaced intervals from 60° right anterior oblique to
30° left posterior oblique projections. Sequential tomograms
were acquired with identical technique, approximately 20 and 40
minutes after the IPPA injection.

Postmortem Tissue Preparation

Animals were killed by an overdose of pentobarbital. Hearts
were removed and sliced carefully into 1 cm sections
perpendicular to a line connecting the radioactive point sources
sewn to the left ventricular apex and base. Slices were

incubated in a warm solution of 1% 2,3,4-triphenyl-tetrazolium chloride (TTC) for 20 minutes or until the normal myocardium was stained. Color slides were taken of each slide for permanent documentation and for direct comparison to the I-123 PPA tomographic sections.

Infarcted tissue, defined by an absence of TTC staining was dissected from normal tissue. Transmural tissue blocks were cut from the infarct and posterior left ventricular free wall, weighed, and placed in scintillation vials containing 10% formalin and counted in a Packard multichannel scintillation counter for 5 minutes per vial with appropriate window settings for each isotope. Tissue blocks were processed into paraffin, sectioned for light microscopy, and stained with hematoxylin and eosin. The extent of myocyte injury was estimated from these histologic sections.

Image Processing

Projection images were corrected for field non-uniformity (using an iodine-123 flood source) and for center of rotation. Sixteen transverse sections, each 1 pixel thick, were reconstructed by filtered backprojection (Medical Data Systems A2 computer system, Ann Arbor, MI). Coronal sections were extracted from the reconstructed volume. Coronal slices were used for quantitative analysis to minimize attenuation effects within the same plane and for comparison to pathologic sections. Planar resolution of the imaging system was measured to be 15.7 mm full width at half maximum at a depth of 20 cm in water. Voxel dimensions were determined using a volume phantom. Attenuation correction was not attempted. After masking for all non-cardiac activity, absolute I-123 PPA radioactivity was measured in each of 15, 24° radial sectors for all 16 slices and for all 3 tomograms (Figure 1). Processing was performed on a Technicare 560 computer system using the integrated array processor (Technicare Corp., Cleveland, OH). Sector radioactivity was also expressed as a percentage of maximal activity within the same slice. I-123 PPA clearance was calculated from the formula:

$$\text{Clearance} = \frac{\text{initial radioactivity (tomo set 1)} - \text{radioactivity (tomo set 2 or 3)}}{\text{initial radioactivity (tomo set 1)}} \times 10$$

Data from 5 control dogs were grouped to determine means and standard deviations of I-123 PPA uptake in similar LV regions, expressed as percentage of maximal activity within the same slice, and clearance for each of the 15 sectors in each corresponding slice.

Pathologic and tomographic sections from the dogs with permanent LAD occlusions were compared directly. The initial uptake of I-123 PPA, as a percentage of maximal activity within the same slice in sectors corresponding to infarcts as defined by TTC were analyzed to develop criteria to identify infarcted tissue from the tomograms. When infarcts were defined by: (1) initial relative uptake less than mean control uptake minus 2 standard deviations, (2) initial relative uptake less than mean control values minus 1 standard deviation and less than 60% of maximal activity within the same slice, and (3) continuity with similar areas within the same or adjacent slices, there was excellent correlation between tomography and pathology. This algorithm was applied to all of the dogs with permanent LAD occlusion to measure cumulative I-123 PPA uptake and clearance values for infarct sectors, sectors immediately adjacent to the infarct, and normal sectors.

RESULTS

Control Studies

Five dogs were studied under control conditions. Corresponding segments of normal myocardium demonstrated uniform uptake of I-123 PPA with all values within 10% of the maximal radioactivity. There was also uniform clearance of I-123 PPA from the first to second tomograms which were separated by approximately 20 minutes. The mean tolerance for all segments was approximately 40% of initial uptake between the first and second tomograms. There was little change in segmental activity from the second to third tomograms.

Dogs with Permanent LAD Occlusion

Eleven dogs were studied after 90-120 minutes of fixed LAD coronary arterial occlusion. Myocardial blood flow in regions supplied by the occluded LAD was significantly reduced in 10 of the 11 dogs immediately after LAD occlusion. One remaining dog without significant flow reduction after LAD occlusion did not show gross evidence of infarction by TTC staining and demonstrated only mild scattered necrosis in a very small percentage of the histologic sections.

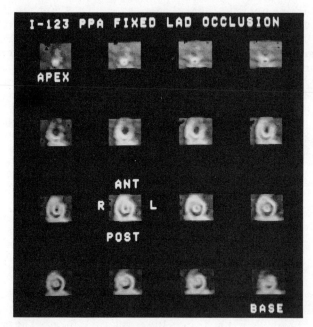

FIGURE 1

Sixteen individual slices from the apex through the base of the
left ventricle in a dog with proximal left anterior descending
coronary artery occlusion imaged with I-123 PPA are
demonstrated. Note the reduction in septal, apical and
anterolateral I-123 PPA uptake demonstrated in the last 2 slices
in the second row and all slices in the third row of images.

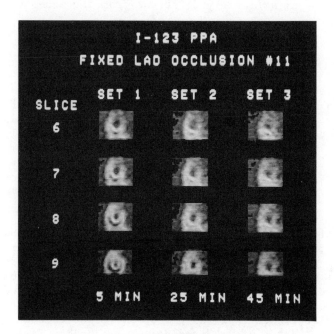

FIGURE 2

The clearance of I-123 PPA in a dog with permanent left anterior descending coronary artery occlusion and an acute anterior myocardial infarction is shown. Note the delayed clearance of I-123 PPA from the anteroapical regions in the tomograms obtained 20 minutes after the injection of I-123 PPA.

Infarct and peri-infarct regions were correlated on the TTC gross pathology specimens with the corresponding tomographic sections. Initial uptake of I-123 PPA within the infarct was 48 ± 6.2% (S.D.) of maximal radioactivity within the same slice (p < 0.001) (Figure 1). Clearance of I-123 PPA from the first to the second tomograms was reduced in the infarct and peri-infarct regions. In infarct tissues, I-123 PPA activity showed an increase of 9 ± 11.8% compared to a clearance of 3.7 ± 15.8% in peri-infarct zones and 15.4 ± 1.83 in normal LV tissue; each of these values was significantly different from the other (p < 0.05) (Figure 2).

DISCUSSION

In the present study, we used single photon emission tomography to measure the relative uptake and clearance of I-123 PPA in canine myocardium under control conditions and following permanent left anterior descending coronary artery occlusion. PPA was radiolabeled with iodine-123 via an organothallium intermediate (6, 7). This labeling technique has a significant advantage over other methods, because it is relatively simple, reproducible and efficient.

Tomograms were performed with a rotating gamma camera system with relatively limited resolution compared to state-of-the-art positron tomographs and no attempt was made to correct for attenuation. The time available for sequential tomographic imaging was limited, because of the need to acquire sufficient data to permit reasonable estimates of segmental uptake and clearance. Despite these limitations, there were consistent, significant differences in I-123 PPA uptake and clearance between infarct, peri-infarct, and normal myocardium following permanent LAD occlusion and these differences were identified within 1-2 hours of the LAD occlusion.

In dogs with fixed LAD coronary artery occlusions, myocardial infarcts identified by an absence of staining with TTC, demonstrated reduced uptake and clearance of I-123 PPA. Indeed, the infarct region could be identified from the tomogram as an area with initial uptake of I-123 PPA at least 2 standard deviations below mean control values for the same segment and no appreciable clearance of I-123 PPA approximately 20 minutes after its intravenous injection.

Thus, these data demonstrate an ability to identify acute myocardial infarction produced by LAD occlusion in canine myocardium using SPECT and I-123 PPA. The data also suggest the need to further evaluate I-123 PPA and SPECT in the study of myocardial metabolism and the detection of myocardial injury with acute and chronic heart disease in the patient.

REFERENCES

1. Evans, J.R., Gunton, R.W., Baker, R.G., Beanlands, D.S., & Spears, J.C. (1965): Circ. Res. 16: 1.
2. Poe, N.D., Robinson, G.D., & MacDonald, N.S. (1975): Proc. Soc. Exp. Biol. Med. 148: 215.
3. Machulla, H.J., Marsmann, M., & Dutschka, K. (1980): Eur. J. Nucl. Med. 5: 171.
4. Freundlieb, C., Hock, A., Vyska, K., Feinendegen, L.E., Machulla, H.J., & Stocklin, G. (1980): J. Nucl. Med. 21: 1043.
5. Van der Wall, E.E., Heidendal, G.A.K., den Hollander, W., Westera, G., & Roos, J.P. (1981): Eur. J. Nucl. Mes. 6: 391.
6. Kulkarni, P.V., & Parkey, R.W. (1982): J. Nucl. Med. 23: 105.
7. Kulkarni, P.V., Parkey, R.W., Lewis, S.E., & Willerson, J.T. (1983): Eur. J. Nucl. Med. In press.
8. Kulkarni, P.V., Buja, L.M., Willerson, J.T., Lewis, S.E., & Parkey, R.W. (1983): Eur. J. Nucl. Med. In press.
9. Chien, K., Han, A., White, J., & Kulkarni, P. (1983): Am. J. Physiol. 14: H957.
10. Schelbert, H.R., Phelps, M.E., Hoffman, E., Huang, S.C., & Kuhl, D.E. (1980): Am. J. Cardiol. 46: 1269.
11. Heyman, M.A., Payne, B.D., Hoffman, J.E., & Rudolph, A.M. (1977): Prog. Cardiovasc. Dis. 20: 55.
12. Roan, P.G., Buja, L.M., Izquierdo, C., Hashimi, H., Saffer, S., & Willerson, J.T. (1981): Circ. Res. 49: 31.

FREE FATTY ACIDS, CATECHOLAMINES AND ARRHYTHMIAS IN MAN

D. C. Russell and M. F. Oliver

Cardiovascular Research Unit
Hugh Robson Building, George Square
Edinburgh EH8 9XF Scotland

The role of free fatty acids (FFA) in the pathogenesis of malignant arrhythmias associated with myocardial ischemia or infarction remains controversial. Such an association first was suggested by Kurien and Oliver in 1970 (1) in their "FFA hypothesis" on the basis of clinical observations in patients following acute myocardial infarction. It was proposed in their hypothesis that increased substrate availability of FFA to the ischemic myocardium either alone or acting synergistically with catecholamines might exert adverse electrophysiological effects. Subsequent clinical and experimental evidence, however, has been confusing and contradictory and the concept remains neither fully confirmed nor refuted.

In the last few years, however, understanding of basic electrophysiological mechanisms of arrhythmogenesis and of their interactions with both catecholamines and alterations in cardiac metabolism has advanced considerably and necessitates a re-examination of these concepts and also re-interpretation of much earlier data. Several discrete phases of arrhythmogenesis may occur for example with respect to the time of onset of coronary occlusion, each with differing mechanisms of pathogenesis, some catecholamine related and some not. Similarly multiple electrophysiological phenomena may be involved. Furthermore, although a clear relationship certainly exists between sympathetic activation, elevated plasma catecholamines and the genesis of certain arrhythmias, it is unclear whether this is mediated by direct electrophysiological effects or more indirectly by chronotropic, inotropic or metabolic sequelae of adrenergic activation. In a clinical setting the situation is

further complicated as sympatho-adrenal activation occurs not in
isolation but as part of a broader stress response with complex
modulation of autonomic outflow to the heart and other organs,
multiple endocrine responses and peripheral metabolic changes in
carbohydrate metabolism and lipolysis.

Disentangling of possible FFA-mediated from
catecholamine-mediated arrhythmogenic effects is difficult as
enhanced adrenergic activity results in stimulation of both
peripheral and intramyocardial lipolysis with plasma elevation
pari passu of both FFA and catechols. Furthermore alterations
in intramyocardial lipolysis either in ventricular muscle or
Purkinje tissue may be of more importance than previously
recognized in initiating arrhythmias and under certain
circumstances could outweigh metabolic effects mediated by
changes in plasma FFA alone. Plasma FFA elevations may occur,
however, independent of catecholamines under certain
circumstances for example by reduction in insulin induced
inhibition of lipolysis or slower plasma clearance of FFA
relative to catecholamines following an adrenergic stimulus.

It would seem relevant, therefore, to re-appraise current
concepts of the possible interrelations between FFA, altered
lipolytic activity and arrhythmogenesis in the light of recent
advances in understanding of adrenergic activity and
electrophysiological mechanisms of arrhythmogenesis.

The FFA Hypothesis

The background of this hypothesis suggested by Kurien and
Oliver in 1970 was the clinical observation that plasma FFA are
usually elevated in the first 24 hours of acute myocardial
infarction and that those patients with very high plasma FFA
levels suffered more arrhythmic deaths (2). A significant
correlation was found between high levels of plasma FFA and
arrhythmias and deaths in a series of 200 patients with acute
myocardial infarction. Thirty-three percent of patients with
plasma FFA greater than 1200 $\mu Eq.1^{-1}$ died compared with 5% of
patients with plasma FFA levels below 380 $\mu Eq.1^{-1}$.

It was not established, however, whether the changes were
causally related to plasma FFA levels or whether both FFA
elevation and arrhythmogenesis followed an increase in
catecholamine or sympathetic activity. Furthermore, it was not
suggested that these possible effects necessarily arose as a
result of changes in plasma FFA alone but rather from
accumulation of intracellular "unbound" FFA or their derivatives
or synergistic effects with those of catecholamines.

It is perhaps worth quoting from the original publication as this has been often cited, yet suffered misinterpretation by many authors, viz: -

"Some arrhythmias which occur during acute myocardial hypoxia could be explained on a metabolic basis. Acute lipid mobilisation from adipose tissue can lead to plasma concentrations of FFA in excess of the primary binding sites of albumin. In the presence of myocardial ischaemia elevated FFA levels lead to accumulation of triglycerides. Intracellular fatty acids may increase when glucose uptake is inadequate due to insulin suppression. Accumulation of FFA in an ´unbound´ form could lead to detergent effects on the cell membrane with cation loss and resultant development of ectopic pacemaker activity."

In addition, it was not suggested that all arrhythmias have a metabolic cause but rather that the FFA hypothesis may explain how catecholamines could produce arrhythmias in the presence of myocardial ischemia by inducing lipid mobilization and glucose intolerance viz: -

"In ischaemic myocardium in which triglyceride has accumulated, catecholamines released . . . may promote high intracellular concentrations of ´unbound´ FFA . . . by activation of myocardial tissue lipase . . . and predispose to sudden and serious arrhythmias."

These concepts as originally described are illustrated in Figure 1.

One factor was considered to be acute lipid mobilization from adipose tissue by noradrenaline with elevation in plasma FFA and hence increased myocardial uptake of FFA in proportion to the concentration of "unbound" FFA in plasma. This might be expected to be increased above an FFA albumin binding ratio of 2 (plasma FFA above 1200 $\mu Eq.l^{-1}$). An additional factor to be considered was the possible effect of accumulation of triglyceride as FFA oxidation became limited. This was thought possibly to predispose to arrhythmias during further or continued ischemia.

Circumstantial evidence quoted in favor of the FFA hypothesis relates to effects of increasing plasma FFA on enhancing oxygen consumption (3, 4); to the association between high metabolic rate and elevated FFA in conditions such as thyrotoxicosis or diabetic ketosis (5); and to known detergent effects of unbound FFA on cell membranes which might have

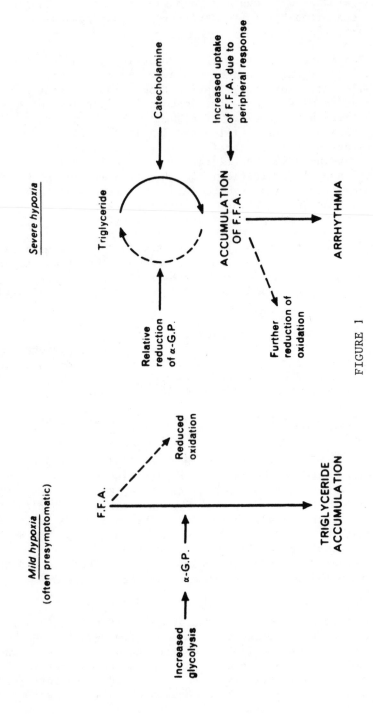

FIGURE 1

Suggested interactions between FFA metabolism, catecholamines
and arrhythmias in the "FFA hypothesis" of Kurien and Oliver (1).

electrophysiological sequelae (6). Initial experimental studies
performed in the dog appeared to support this concept in that
infusions of triglyceride-heparin following acute circumflex
coronary occlusion were followed after 20 minutes by bursts of
ectopic activity including ventricular tachycardia and this
effect was reversed by administration of protamine (7, 8).
These studies, however, were inadequately controlled and in
retrospect difficult to interpret in the light of current
knowledge of the phasic nature of early ventricular
arrhythmias. Findings were not confirmed in a parallel series
of experiments by Opie et al. (9), although these were not
comparable, with occlusion of different vessels at different
durations of ischemia and different FFA-albumin binding ratios.

Subsequent clinical studies similarly have proved
confusing. In retrospect these seem largely empirical, do not
assess electrophysiological phenomena, are performed at variable
durations following onset of myocardial ischemia and are clouded
by gross methodological errors. An association between elevated
plasma FFA and arrhythmias was confirmed in some clinical
studies (10-12) yet other studies failed to do so (13, 14).
Rutenberg et al. (15) showed no correlation in 73 patients
between initial fasting FFA and development of arrhythmias,
cardiogenic shock or late death, although there was a tendency
for FFA to be elevated at the time of any complication such as
heart block, junctional rhythm or VPB's. Nelson (13) found no
increase in arrhythmias in 24 patients treated with heparin
(which stimulates lipolysis by release of lipoprotein lipase and
hence results in elevation of plasma FFA) within the first 24
hours of myocardial infarction. A definite correlation was
shown between arrhythmias and plasma noradrenaline. We have
demonstrated recently, however, that gross overestimations of
plasma FFA may result after clinical administration of heparin
due to continuing in vitro lipolysis prior to plasma
extraction. Thus in Nelson's study although a mean elevation in
plasma FFA from around 1100 to 1800 µEq/l was reported following
administration of heparin within the first 6 hours of acute
myocardial infarction, the true increment may well have been
one-third of this value. Our own studies suggest the "true"
elevation in plasma FFA after heparin in man during acute
myocardial infarction is no more than 300 µEq/l and may not
increase levels above the binding capacity of albumin for FFA
said to be obtained when plasma FFA levels exceed around 1200
µEq/l (17). The proportion of "unbound" FFA therefore may not
be disproportionately in excess of the physiological range.

Apart from these methodological considerations some
re-examination of the concepts suggested in the original

hypothesis is required. That greater importance should be attached to the role of catecholamine-mediated intramyocardial lipolysis has been suggested in clinical studies by Simonsen and Kjekshus (18) examining the effects of antilipolytic therapy on myocardial oxygen consumption during isoprenaline infusions and also in experimental studies (19). Forty-five percent of increased myocardial oxygen consumption in the catecholamine-stimulated human heart is accounted for by the associated elevation in peripheral plasma free fatty acids compared with 29% from an increase in contractility and 23% from an increase in heart rate, although the relationship with elevated plasma FFA could be coincidental and the main effect mediated through intramyocardial lipolysis. In addition absolute levels of "unbound" FFA may not rise to such an extent during ischemia as considered previously although their derivatives do accumulate (20).

Perhaps more importantly regarding possible links between FFA metabolism and arrhythmogenesis is a consideration of the discrete phases of arrhythmias associated with myocardial ischemia and their varied electrophysiological mechanisms, not all of which may be modulated by metabolic factors. These phases will be considered therefore and their possible interactions with FFA and catecholamine metabolism discussed.

Natural History of Malignant Ventricular Arrhythmias During Acute Myocardial Ischemia

Natural history studies have revealed distinct periods of genesis of malignant ventricular arrhythmias and ventricular fibrillation (VF) with respect to the duration after onset of symptoms of acute myocardial ischemia or infarction (21). These may roughly be divided into very early or "pre-hospital" arrhythmias within the first 2 or 3 hours, later "in-hospital" arrhythmias between 4 and 72 hours, and "chronic" arrhythmias from 3 to 30 days of infarction. Experimental studies suggest each period of arrhythmogenesis involves differing pathogenetic and electrophysiological mechanisms and may include two or more discrete "sub-phases" of arrhythmogenesis.

Superimposed on this complex picture are the possibilities of "early arrhythmias" generated by extension of the area of coronary occlusion and of "reperfusion arrhythmias" which might result following sudden release of a coronary occlusion. Furthermore, immediate and delayed types of reperfusion arrhythmias have been described each with differing mechanisms of pathogenesis (22).

A hypothetical scheme of the interrelationships of these phases of arrhythmogenesis following onset of symptoms of acute myocardial ischemia or infarction is illustrated in Figure 2. By necessity this is based upon experimental studies although supported by a large body of clinical evidence. It can be seen that at any point in time several types of arrhythmia may be initiated, the origin of which may not be evident to the clinician.

A very early or "pre-hospital" phase of arrhythmias appears to occur within the first 2-3 hours after onset of symptoms of myocardial ischemia. This is associated with very high incidence of VF, particularly in the first 30 minutes and often within seconds or minutes after onset of the initiating event. An experimental parallel is found in the Harris phase I arrhythmias which may be induced within the first 30 minutes of coronary occlusion in a variety of animal models. These early arrhythmias may be sub-divided into immediate (or phase Ia) and delayed (or phase Ib) types (23), each with differing electrophysiological mechanisms of pathogenesis and differing susceptibility to pharmacological intervention. Thus, the immediate early arrhythmias appear associated with re-entrant circus movements within an ischemic area of myocardium demonstrating marked regional inhomogeneities in metabolic activity including glycolytic activity and FFA oxidation. The later early arrhythmias however, may involve adrenergic mediated or autonomic mechanisms although this is uncertain. Differentiation of these various subgroups in man has not been possible and is made difficult by the superimposition of reperfusion phenomena, which themselves could induce VF.

Following a period of 4 to 6 hours a further "in-hospital" arrhythmic phase arises (21), with much higher incidence of idioventricular rhythms and ventricular tachycardias but lower incidence of VF. Enhanced automatic activity predominates and may reflect delayed ischemic injury to more hypoxia-resistant specialized conducting tissue. Re-entrant arrhythmias can also occur, however. These arrhythmias in general subside by 48 or 72 hours of ischemia.

From 3 or 4 days onwards with organization of the infarct and preservation of areas of "chronic" ischemic injury, further arrhythmias may result, probably in association with formation of stable anatomical re- entrant circuits into and within the ischemic zone. Experimentally, such arrhythmias are easily induced by programmed stimulation techniques. Exact mechanisms of their origin are uncertain. Certain late arrhythmias appear catechol-mediated and others associated with fixed delayed depolarizations or "late potentials" conducive to re-entry.

Table 1:   CATEGORIES OF ARRHYTHMIAS DURING MYOCARDIAL
             INFARCTION AND THEIR POSSIBLE MODULATION BY FFA

Duration of Ischaemia	Phase of Arrhythmias	Probable Mechanism	Possible FFA Modulation
0-3 hrs.	Early: 1a	Re-entry	Yes
	1b	Unknown	Unknown
	Reperfusion:		
	Immediate	Re-entry	Yes
	Delayed	Automatic	? Yes
4-72 hrs	"In-hospital"	Automatic	Yes
3-30 days	"Chronic"	Re-entry	Unknown

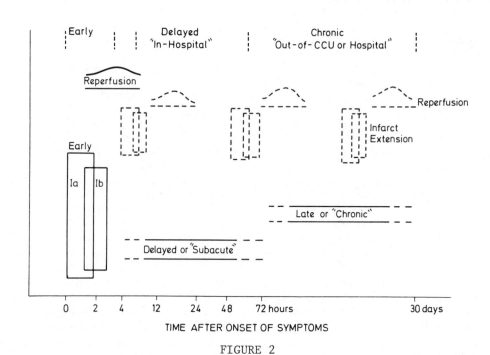

TIME AFTER ONSET OF SYMPTOMS

FIGURE 2

Multiple electrophysiological mechanisms either singly or in combination, affecting ventricular muscle, specialized conducting tissue or both may therefore be operative in the same heart at varying durations of ischemia. A variety of phenomena may be implicated including re-entrant excitation, focal excitation, enhanced automaticity and triggered early and late after-depolarizations (24). The extent to which metabolic factors may modulate these effects is largely unknown. The variety of these arrhythmias, their postulated mechanisms and possible modulation by changes in intracellular FFA are outlined in Table 1.

The failure of clinical studies to contribute to our understanding of possible interrelationships between FFA metabolism, catecholamine and arrhythmias, may have been due partly to a failure to relate data to known pathophysiological mechanisms of arrhythmogenesis, and to particular discrete phases of arrhythmogenesis. The various types of ischemia related arrhythmias will be briefly described therefore with reference to man and fragmentary clinical evidence interrelating and implicating FFA and catecholamines in their pathogenesis.

FFA and Early Ischemic Arrhythmias

VF may result within a few minutes of onset of a presumed coronary occlusive event. Clinical evidence implicating elevations in either plasma FFA or catecholamines in the pathogenesis of this early VF or of "pre-hospital" ventricular arrhythmias is therefore fragmentary and indirect. Studies in Edinburgh have demonstrated that plasma catecholamines may be elevated certainly within 15 minutes of onset of symptoms of a coronary occlusive event and probably sooner (25). This is likely to be associated with rapid activation of a peripheral metabolic response either from activation of cardio-sympathetic reflexes or a more general stress response. The nature of these responses have been more carefully studied under the more controlled circumstances of stress such as following exercise, psychological stress, trauma, burns or acute painful conditions.

That such stress responses may be associated with early ischemic arrhythmias is supported by epidemiological evidence. On the basis of retrospective studies of sudden cardiac death victims, Lown et al. (16) have suggested that the vulnerability of ischemic myocardium to VF may be profoundly influenced by psychological "trigger factors" which mediate stress responses and hence autonomic effects. Furthermore, the influence of these "trigger factors" seems more important the less marked is the coronary arterial disease in sudden cardiac death victims. Immediate antecedent events to sudden cardiac death have been

examined in several other clinical studies which conclude that
acute emotional arousal may precede the event in between 20 and
40% of the cases (27, 28).

Such stimuli are likely to induce release of catecholamines
from both adrenal glands and sympathetic nerve terminals and
hence stimulate both peripheral and intramyocardial lipolysis
which is cyclic AMP mediated. A net efflux of plasma FFA and
glycerol from adipose tissue thus ensues and plasma levels may
be elevated to three or four times normal levels. Plasma FFA
are elevated to around twice basal levels within the first 30
minutes of onset of symptoms of a coronary occlusive event (25)
indicating significant activation of lipolysis. Maximum levels,
in excess of 1200 μEq.1^{-1} were only observed after 1 to 2
hours of ischemia after the period of early arrhythmias. Only
at this level when the FFA:albumin binding ratio exceeds 3:1 are
the two main binding sites of albumin for FFA saturated and
myocardial FFA uptake expected to be greatly increased (17).
Irrespective of plasma FFA levels, however, early activation of
intramyocardial lipolysis may occur within minutes of onset of a
coronary occlusive event. Indeed plasma FFA levels may reflect
poorly overall tissue lipolysis since the lipolytic response to
sympathetic stimulation may be modulated by additional
concomitant endocrine effects. Cortisol release enhances
lipolysis as does release of thyroxine and growth hormone.

Of further importance may be the early complex interactions
between FFA, catecholamine and glucose metabolism. An early
change in man, within 15 minutes of onset of symptoms of
infarction is hypoinsulinaemia leading to mild or overt
hyperglycaemia as a result of either reduced glucose uptake or
reduction of insulin sensitivity. This may be initiated by an
inhibitory effect of adrenaline on the pancreatic β-cell insulin
response (29). At this time plasma FFA levels are elevated when
plasma glucose levels are normal and insulin levels are low.
The later elevation in glucose levels is influenced by the
glycogenolytic effect of adrenaline on the liver and by release
of glucagon, throxine and growth hormone. Adrenaline in
contrast to noradrenaline has a weaker effect on beta$_1$-
mediated adipose tissue lipolysis than on glycogenolysis which
is largely beta$_2$-mediated (30).

The net intramyocardial and peripheral metabolic response to
acute ischemia with mobilization of FFA, glucose and
catecholamines, although appropriate for increased energy
requirements in the normal heart may be inappropriate in many
respects to the ischemic cell. Experimental studies strongly
suggest that the vulnerability to VF within the first 30 minutes
of ischemia relates in part to both the severity of myocardial

ischemia injury and to its rate of development. An increase in heart rate for example may greatly increase both ischemic injury and the incidence of malignant ventricular arrhythmias or VF (31).

The importance in terms of electrophysiological effects of direct adrenergic responses with respect to indirect responses resulting from hemodynamic metabolic effects is unclear. Marked effects on conduction, refractoriness, diastolic depolarization, autonomic activity and a variety of electrophysiological phenomena may follow sympathetic stimulation or elevations in plasma catecholamines during acute myocardial ischemia and ventricular vulnerability to VF may be greatly reduced (32).

A critical factor at least in the very early malignant ventricular arrhythmias appears to be regional inhomogeneity of electrophysiological activity within the ischemic zone, leading to multiple re-entrant circus movements and hence VF. Evidence from our own laboratory suggests that regional inhomogeneities in adrenergic responsiveness also may exist within the ischemic zone relating to regional severity of ischemic injury (unpublished). This may be influenced by chronotropic and inotropic effects of catecholamines, with increased heart rate and myocardial oxygen consumption, and also by their direct or indirect myocardial metabolic effects.

Further studies in our laboratory have demonstrated that manipulation of metabolic responses to ischemia may have significant anti-arrhythmic effects. Thus, infusion of glucose sufficient to double arterial levels in the dog is effective in reducing the arrhythmia threshold and ameliorating conduction and repolarization abnormalities, although not under conditions of very severe ischemia (34). Similar beneficial effects of antilipolytic therapy on conduction and refractoriness are found using nicotinic acid to suppress lipolysis induced by infusion of isoprenaline, during 15 minute periods of acute myocardial ischemia (35). Effects, however, are small and confined to small reductions in divergence of refractoriness, action potential duration shortening and epicardial activation delays but nevertheless, potentially antiarrhythmic. The role of elevation in plasma FFA per se in the absence of catecholamine stimulated intramyocardial lipolysis is less clear. Using a differential cell separation centrifuge to administer oleic acid at plasma concentrations of 1200-1800 μEq.1^{-1} the incidence of VF during 15 minute periods of myocardial ischemia was not affected (36).

An electrophysiological effect of antilipolytic therapy has been demonstrated during acute ischemia in man using a nicotinic

acid analogue (5-fluoronicotinic acid) in patients with stable
angina of effort. Pretreatment with the antilipolytic agent was
found to be effective in significantly reducing the degree of
ST-segment depression during exercise although not the degree of
effort intolerance (37). This effect was independent of
hemodynamic factors. The corollary of this is that stimulation
of lipolysis during the first hour after onset of symptoms of
myocardial infarction may have adverse electrophysiological
effects against a background of adrenergic stimulation.

A further possibility is that the composition rather than
the absolute level of free fatty acids may be of importance.
Ravens and Ravens (14) for example found an elevation of plasma
free fatty acids in patients following myocardial infarction but
relatively lower levels of oleic acid and higher levels of
linoleic acid in the arrhythmic compared with the non-arrhythmic
groups. Elevated levels of docosahexanoic acid are found in
myocardial biopsies in hearts of sudden cardiac death victims
(38). Differential electrophysiological effects of different
chain length fatty acids are therefore a possibility. Effects
in addition could relate to diet in different subjects.
Retardation of myocardial metabolism with brassica based fatty
acids such as erucic or cetoleic acid is described for example.
Beyond the scope of this review is the potential importance of
differences in dietary fatty acid intake on platelet aggregation
and coronary thrombosis which may determine the presence or
absence of a coronary occlusive event.

FFA and Reperfusion Arrhythmias

Sudden reperfusion of an occluded coronary vessel either by
spontaneous thrombolysis of an occlusive thrombus or by release
of coronary vasospasm may induce VF often within a few seconds
of reperfusion. The clinical importance of this phenomenon is
unclear although it could be of major importance in sudden
cardiac death perhaps following a transient coronary occlusion.
Limited experimental data would suggest that the incidence of
reperfusion arrhythmias relates to both duration and severity of
the ischemia. It is possible, therefore, that FFA mediated
enhancement of ischemic injury prior to reperfusion might
increase the likelihood of serious reperfusion arrhythmias.
Furthermore, delayed metabolic recovery of the myocardium
following short periods of myocardial ischemia relates to
delayed recovery in fatty acid oxidation, and could be a factor
in the genesis of later delayed reperfusion arrhythmias.

Delayed "In-Hospital" Arrhythmias

The early studies of Oliver et al. (2) demonstrated a crude but positive relationship between incidence of serious ventricular arrhythmias and elevated plasma free fatty acids within the first few hours after onset of symptoms of myocardial infarction. More recently Tansey and Opie (39) made similar observations and have shown a better correlation between mean levels of FFA than peak levels within the first 12 hours of myocardial infarction although plasma catecholamine levels were not determined nor distinction made between differing etiologies of ventricular arrhythmias. These arrhythmias may be categorized as being largely of the delayed "in-hospital" phase with differing mechanisms of pathogenesis to arrhythmias occurring during early ischemia. These "in- hospital" arrhythmias often arise against a background of established infarction of "chronic" ischemia and may involve generation of abnormal automatic activity in ischemic Purkinje tissue rather than electro- physiological abnormalities confined to ischemic ventricular myocardium.

As in the case of early arrhythmias both plasma catecholamines and FFA may be elevated. Catecholamines, in particular noradrenaline, are elevated in plasma and urine for 36 hours or more after onset of symptoms of myocardial ischemia. FFA and glycerol may remain elevated for up to 48 hours. The relative role of catecholamines, FFA and other factors such as electrolyte shifts, ischemic injury, autonomic tone etc. in the genesis of these arrhythmias is controversial.

In favor of an arrhythmogenic effect of stimulation of lipolysis independent of plasma catecholamine levels are clinical studies by Rowe et al. within the first 5 hours of acute myocardial infarction using the nicotinic acid analogue 5-fluoronicotinic acid (40). A significant reduction in the incidence of ventricular tachycardia was obtained with effects confined to a sub-group of patients in whom rapid normalization of plasma FFA levels was achieved (see Table 2).

Effects were not associated with significant hemodynamic changes nor alterations in plasma catecholamine levels. Confirmatory evidence of a significant metabolic effect of antilipolytic therapy during the early hours of acute myocardial infarction was obtained in a similar study examining the evolution of ST-segment changes within the first 8 hours following onset of symptoms of myocardial infarction (41). A small but significant amelioration of ST-segment elevation was observed in association with a reduction in plasma free fatty acid levels. This effect was attributed to a reduction in

Table 2. Incidence of V.T. During Acute Myocardial Infarction

	Placebo (71) 3-12 hrs.	Nicotinic Acid (32) Within 5 hrs.	Analogue (36) 5-12 hrs.
Delay from onset			
FFA Levels			
>50% fall in 4 hrs. <800 µEq/1 (20 hrs)	42%	0%[**]	70%
<50% fall in 4 hrs. >800 µEq/1	70%	29%	77%

*P<0.01   **P<0.003

From Rowe, Neilson, and Oliver, 1975 (40).

ischemic injury in surviving ischemic tissue. Any potentially arrhythmogenic effects of FFA might be expected, however, to differ from patient to patient. At least four different myocardial metabolic patterns have been described during acute infarction by Mueller et al. (42). Of their 173 patients 41% exhibited a pattern of predominant myocardial free fatty acid uptake and metabolism whereas 18% showed predominantly carbohydrate metabolism and 20% demonstrated high plasma substrate levels but low myocardial substrate uptake suggestive of generalized metabolic breakdown. Plasma levels of adrenaline and noradrenaline also vary greatly from patient to patient. In addition, the relative role of enhancement of fatty acid metabolism versus inhibition of glucose metabolism is unclear.

Antiarrhythmic effects of glucose or glucose-insulin-potassium regimes have been suggested since the early studies of Sodi-Pollares with "polarising" solutions (43). Attempts to reproduce these findings have not been uniformly successful largely due to gross differences in dosage and time of administration. More recently, Rogers et al. have demonstrated a 50% reduction in "in-hospital" ventricular tachycardias using a high concentration glucose-insulin-potassium regime (44). Interestingly, antiarrhythmic effects only occur in those patients in whom adequate suppression of lipolysis and marked reduction in plasma FFA is achieved. Undoubtedly, a variety of different mechanisms may generate ventricular arrhythmias during this period only some of which may relate to FFA or catecholamines. Antiarrhythmic effects of antilipolytic therapy can be demonstrated at this time, however, and could be mediated

by metabolic actions on "chronically" ischemic myocardial cells
or perhaps more likely on ischemic Purkinje fibres which may
exhibit ischemic automatic activity.

Late Ventricular Arrhythmias

Ventricular arrhythmias or VF may occur following patient
transfer from CCU to the ward or subsequently "out-of-hospital"
within the first few weeks of infarction. Similar arrhythmias
may be easily elicited by ventricular extrastimulation between 3
and 30 days following experimental infarction, and may derive
either from continued automatic activity within the specialized
conducting tissue or from generation of fixed re-entry pathways
within ventricular aneurysms or areas of patchy myocardial
fibrosis. The role of metabolic factors in genesis of these
arrhythmias is obscure, although some appear mediated by
adrenergic mechanisms. Clinical trials have demonstrated
significant reductions in mortality within the first few months
of infarction using a variety of beta-blocking agents. The role
of the antilipolytic action of beta-blockade in these
circumstances is unknown.

Are FFA Arrhythmogenic?

Despite over a decade of research since the formulation of
the "FFA hypothesis" by Kurien and Oliver no simple answer to
this question has emerged. What has become clearer, however, is
that cellular electro- physiological events may be profoundly
influenced by the state of energy metabolism particularly in
ischemic tissue and that this in turn may be modulated by
alterations in substrate availability of FFA or an alteration in
the rate of intramyocardial lipolysis. In the clinical setting
it is evident that changes in FFA metabolism may be merely a part
of a more generalized stress reaction involving altered autonomic
outflow, elevated plasma catecholamines and other endocrine
effects from which it may be difficult to dissociate the isolated
effect of alterations in intracellular FFA. Finally, potential
arrhythmogenic effects of FFA must be viewed against the
background of a variety of discrete phases or types of
arrhythmias occurring during acute myocardial infarction each
with quite different and as yet incompletely understood
mechanisms of pathogenesis, and susceptible to differing degrees
of severity of ischemic damage, adrenergic stimulation or
metabolic factors.

Nevertheless, with these provisos, sufficient evidence has
been presented to implicate a likely role of FFA in the
pathogenesis of serious ventricular arrhythmias in man. A
hypothetical scheme of possible relevant interactions between

FFA, catecholamines and arrhythmogenesis is shown in Figure 3. This is by necessity highly speculative, applicable to varying degrees to early compared with later ischemic arrhythmias and based largely on experimental studies.

It can be seen that FFA associated electrophysiological effects might be mediated by effects on energy dependent processes in turn regulating conduction or ionic channel activity or by direct toxic effects on the cell membrane perhaps with structural changes to the ionic channels themselves induced by accumulation of amphiphilic derivatives such as fatty acyl carnitines or lysophosphatides or by peroxide formation. These effects must be to an extent interdependent, and occur in association with direct adrenergic cyclic AMP-mediated electrophysiological phenomena.

Cellular effects of adrenergic stimulation are many and include enhanced diastolic depolarization of specialized conduction tissue, initiation of abnormal automatic activity or triggered after-depolarization amelioration of slowed conduction or conduction block and accelerated repolarization with shortened periods of refractoriness (45). Several effects are mediated by an increase in slow inward current, largely carried by Ca ions. This slow inward current is also, however, energy dependent and can be shown to be altered by changes in production of cytosolic ATP largely derived from the anaerobic phase of glycolysis.

In addition to modulating slow channel activity cytosolic ATP is necessary for ionic pumping, Na^+-K^+ ATPase activity, maintenance of the electrogenic Na pump and a variety of functions, including nexus junction conduction (46) which may influence several cellular electrophysiological properties.

Such ATP availability for electrophysiological processes could be limited during ischemia (47) by (a) reduced glucose and increased FFA utilization, (b) "futile" energy cycling of re-esterification - lipolysis, accelerated by catecholamine-induced intramyocardial lipolysis or fatty acyl CoA synthesis and hydrolysis, (c) ATP entrapment within mitochondria resulting from accumulation of fatty acyl CoA derivatives and inhibition of mitochondrial adenine nucleotide translocase activity, (d) depletion of glycogen reserves, (e) uncoupling of oxidative phosphorylation. Requiring particular attention, we believe, are the metabolic effects of catecholamines or sympathetic stimulation. Elevations of plasma FFA may compound the effects of catechol induced activation of intramyocardial lipolysis by leading to a further increase in intracellular levels of FFA or their acyl CoA or carnitine derivatives which in turn may have direct or indirect electrophysiological effects. Indeed, it has

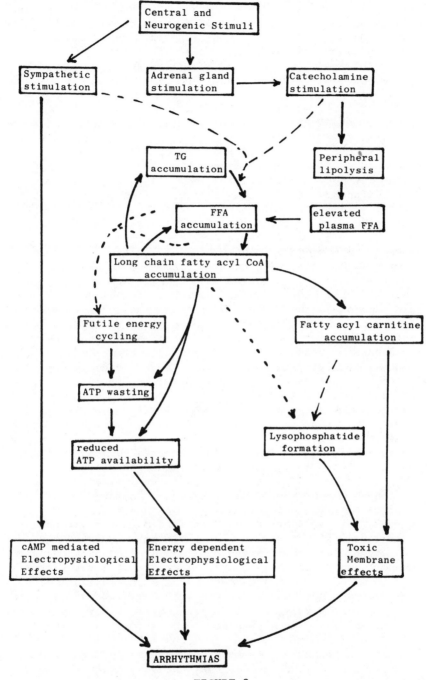

FIGURE 3

Hypothetical scheme of possible interactions
between FFA, catecholamines and arrhythmogenesis
during myocardial ischaemia.

been suggested that a vicious circle of events may exist whereby enhanced sympathetic drive may lead to stimulation of peripheral and intramyocardial lipolysis with resulting inhibition of glucose metabolism and further increase in severity of ischemia. Thus, both catecholamine release and elevated plasma FFA would increase myocardial ischemic injury and hence vulnerability to arrhythmias.

Lipid accumulation within the myocardium may be an additional factor. That this may be arrhythmogenic is by no means a new concept. In the nineteenth century it was held that the fatty heart was linked to sudden cardiac death (48). Although reflecting previous myocardial ischemia and the phenomenon of triglyceride accumulation within ischemic tissue, the possibility exists that lipid accumulation could be the substrate for profound activation of intramyocardial lipolysis following adrenergic stimulation and hence further accumulation of intracellular FFA or derivatives. These effects are accompanied by the complex biochemical changes of ischemic injury, including H^+ ion accumulation, K^+ leakage and accumulation of a variety of potentially toxic metabolites which may have direct effects on the cell membrane. Both "unbound" FFA and their derivatives in high enough concentrations could have "detergent" effects on the membrane although intracellular concentrations in practice may not reach these levels (20). Experimentally striking electrophysiological effects have been demonstrated in superfused Purkinje fibres not by FFA but by amphiphilic FFA derivatives such as long chain fatty acid carnitine and lysophosphatides derived from membrane phospholipid (49, 50). These effects are similar in many respects to those observed in vivo during acute ischemia and are observed at much lower concentrations possibly within the physiological range. Thus, marked loss of transmembrane potential, slow conducting action potentials, alternating electrical activity and post-repolarization refractoriness may be simulated in vitro by low concentrations of palmitoyl carnitine, concentrations of which are known to increase progressively during ischemia and more rapidly when substrate levels of FFA are increased. Similar phenomena occur with the lysophosphatide lysophosphatidyl choline particularly under conditions of acidosis. Initial studies suggest tissue concentrations of these substances approach levels shown to have adverse electrophysiological effects within minutes of onset of ischemia. Alternatively, toxic membrane effects may result from accumulation of fatty acid peroxides or free oxygen radicals.

Translation of these phenomena into genesis of ventricular arrhythmias in a clinical setting is unproven, however. Potential mechanisms clearly exist but require further evaluation.

Clinical Prospects for the Future

A strong case may be made for the existence of clinically important interactions between FFA metabolism, catecholamines and genesis of serious ventricular arrhythmias during acute myocardial ischemia or infarction. Undoubtedly, understanding of the relative importance of these phenomena will parallel advances in understanding of electrophysiological mechanisms of arrhythmogenesis. The original somewhat simplistic "FFA hypothesis" would appear therefore still tenable and worthy of active research. Areas demanding particular clarification in man include the role of accumulation of toxic FFA metabolites and amphiphiles, metabolic effects of adrenergic stimulation, effects of triglyceride accumulation in myocardium and the possible influence of diet on FFA composition and metabolism and arrhythmogenicity.

In addition, several therapeutic avenues are open which could hold promise for the future. Antilipolytic therapy may be used to limit intramyocardial FFA accumulation, drugs devised to limit accumulation of toxic metabolites and dietary modification evaluated. Furthermore, conventional anti-arrhythmic therapy including beta-blockade under a variety of circumstances requires re-evaluation in terms of effects on cardiac metabolism.

REFERENCES

1. Kurien, V.A., & Oliver, M.F. (1970): Lancet 1: 813.
2. Oliver, M.F., Kurien, V.A., & Greenwood, T.W. (1968): Lancet 1: 710.
3. Challoner, D.R., & Steinberg, D. (1966): Am. J. Physiol. 210: 280.
4. Mjos, O.D. (1971): J. Clin. Invest. 50: 1386.
5. Carlson, L.A., & Liljedahl, S.O. (1963): Trauma. Acta Med. Scand. 173: 25.
6. Pande, S.V., & Mead, J.F. (1968): J. Biol. Chem. 243: 6130.
7. Kurien, V.A., Yates, P.A., & Oliver, M.F. (1969): Lancet ii: 185.
8. Kurien, V.A., Yates, P.A., & Oliver, M.F. (1971): Eur. J. Clin. Invest. 1: 225.
9. Opie, L.H., Norris, R.M., Thomas, M., Holland, J.A., Own, P., & Van Norden, A. (1971): Lancet 1: 818.
10. Gupta, D.K., Young, R., & Jewitt, D.E. (1969): Lancet 2: 1209.
11. Reimann, R., & Schwandt, O. (1971): D. Med. Wochenschr. 96: 93.
12. Prakash, R., Parmley, W., Horvat, M., & Swan, H.J.C. (1972): Circulation 45: 736.

13. Nelson, P.G. (1970): Lancet 1: 733.

14. Ravens, K.G., & Jipp, P. (1972): Arzneim.-Forschung 22: 1831.

15. Rutenberg, H.L., Panintuan, J.L., & Soloff, L.A. (1969): Lancet ii: 559.

16. Riemersma, R.A., Logan, R., Russell, D.C., Smith, H.J., Simpson, J., & Oliver, M.F. (1982): Br. Heart J. 48: 134.

17. Spector, A.A. (1968): Ann. N.Y. Acad. Sci. 149: 768.

18. Simonsen, S., & Kjekshus, J.K. (1978): Circulation 58: 484.

19. Vik-Mo, H., Mjos, O.D., Riemersma, R.A., & Oliver, M.F. (1980): Adv. Physiol. SC 8: 121.

20. Van der Vusse, G.J., Rueman, T.H., Prinzen, F.W., Coumons, W.A., & Reneman, R.S. (1982): Circ. Res. 50: 538.

21. Bigger, J.J., Dresdale, R.J., Heissenbuttel, R., Weld, F.M., & Wit, A.L. (1977): Prog. Cardiovasc. Dis. 19: 255.

22. Kaplinsky, E., Ogawa, S., Michelson, E.C., & Dreifus, L.S. (1980): Circulation 63: 333.

23. Kaplinsky, E., Ogawa, S., Balke, C.W., & Dreifus, L.S. (1979): Circulation 60: 391.

24. Wit, A.L., Rosen, M.R., & Hoffman, B.F. (1974): Am. Heart J. 88: 664.

25. Vetter, N.J., Adams, W., Strange, R.C., & Oliver, M.F. (1974): Lancet 1: 248.

26. Lown, B., & de Silva, R.A. (1978): Am. J. Cardiol. 41: 979.

27. Bruhn, J.G., Paredes, A., Adsett, C.A., & Wolf, S. (1978): J. Psychosom. Res. 18: 187.

28. Hinkle, L.E. (1981): Acta Med. Scand. (Supp. 51) 210: 207.

29. Porte, D., Graber, A.C., Kazuya, T., & Williams, R.H. (1966): J. Clin. Invest. 45: 228.

30. McLeod, A.A., Brown, J.E., Kahn, C., Kitchell, B.B., Sedor, F.A., Williams, R.S., & Shand, D.G. (1983): Circulation 67: 1065.

31. Kent, K.M., Smith, E.R., Redwood, D.R., & Epstein, S.E. (1975): Circulation 42: 291.

32. Verrier, R.L., Thompson, P., & Lown, B. (1974): Cardiovasc. Res. 8: 602.

33. Russell, D.C., Riemersma, R.A., Lawrie, J.S., & Oliver, M.F. (1982): Cardiovasc. Res. 41: 613.

34. Russell, D.C., Lawrie, J.S., Riemersma, R.A., & Oliver, M.F. (1981): Acta Med. Scand. (Supp. ii) 230: 71.

35. Russell, D.C., & Oliver, M.F. (1983): J. Mol. Cell. Cardiol. 15(Suppl 3): 18.

36. Riemersma, R.A., Michorowski, B., & Oliver, M.F. (1983): J. Mol. Cell. Cardiol. 15(Suppl 3): 17.

37. Luxton, M.R., Miller, N.E., & Oliver, M.F. (1976): Br. Heart J. 38: 1204.

38. Gudbjarnason, S., Oskarsdottir, G., Doell, B., & Hallgrimsson, J. (1978): Adv. Cardiol. 25: 130.

39. Tansey, M.J.B., & Opie, L.H. (1983): S. Afr. Heart J. In press.

40. Rowe, M.J., Neilson, J.M.M., & Oliver, M.F. (1975): Lancet 1: 295.

41. Russell, D.C., & Oliver, M.F. (1978): Brit. Heart J. 40: 117.

42. Mueller, H.S., & Ayres, S.M. (1973): Am. J. Cardiol. 42: 363.

43. Sodi-Pallares, D., Ponce de Leon, J., Bisteri, A., & Medrano, G. (1969): Lancet 1: 1315 (Letter).

44. Rogers, W.J., Stanley, A.W., Breinig, J.B., Prather, J.W., McDaniel, A.G., Maraski, R.E., Mantle, J.A., Russell, R.O., & Ruckley, L.E. (1976): Am. Heart J. 92: 441.

45. Carmeliet, E. (1982): IN Catecholamines in the Non-Ischaemic and Ischaemic Myocardium (eds) R.A. Riemersma & M.F. Oliver, Elsevier Biomedical Press, Amsterdam, p. 77.

46. Carmeliet, E. (1978): Circ. Res. 42: 577.

47. Vik-Mo, H., & Mjos, O.D. (1981): Am. J. Cardiol. 48: 361.

48. Broadbent, W.H., & Broadbent, J.F.H. (1897): Heart Disease, p. 282, London.

49. Sobel, B.E., Corr, P.B., Robisan, A.K., Goldstein, R.A., Witkowski, F.X., & Klein, M.S. (1978): J. Clin. Invest. 62: 546.

50. Corr, P.B., & Sobel, B.E. IN Early Arrhythmias Resulting from Myocardial Ischaemia (eds) J.R. Parratt, Macmillan Press, New York, p. 199.

CONCLUSIONS

Lipids are essential for normal myocardial function; free
fatty acids, for example, represent the major substrate for
cardiac energy production, and a variety of complex lipids play
essential structural and functional roles in the heart. Under
certain circumstances, however, abnormalities in lipid metabolism
can be harmful to the heart. A large body of recent experimental
findings has shown that the abnormal accumulation of certain
classes of lipid can impair myocardial function and, at high concentrations, may lead to cell death. Over the past decade, these
detrimental effects of lipids have attracted the attention of basic
scientists who study the response of the heart to disease, and
physicians charged with the care of the cardiac patient. Major
advances in both the medical and surgical therapy of cardiac
diseases, notably the wide use of open-heart surgery and a growing number of interventions for the therapy of coronary occlusion
and myocardial infarction, have brought this subject to the fore-
front of research in Cardiology.

In July 1983, a group of investigators assembled in Rome for
what we believe to have been the first International Meeting on
the role of lipid abnormalities in the pathogenesis of arrythmias,
the loss of contractile function, and cell death in the ischemic
myocardium. For three days, brief lectures on these subjects were
followed by heated, though congenial, discussions of these subjects.
The broad scope of this meeting is presented in Supplement 3
(August, 1983) to Volume 15 of the Journal of Molecular and Cellular
Cardiology, which contains the abstracts of both the formal lectures and more than 50 posters that were presented and discussed
at this meeting. The present text, which contains a series of
chapters written by the speakers at this meeting, provides an over-
view of this field as it is understood at the present time.

This book is divided into 5 sections that consider normal lipid
metabolism, lipid-induced membrane abnormalities, lipid-induced
changes in myocardial function in the ischemic heart, interventions
that can modify these abnormalities in the ischemic heart, and clinical aspects of these lipid abnormalities. These divisions, however,

329

are more or less arbitrary as it proved impossible to separate these aspects of this important subject.

Although our current understanding of the normal role of lipids in myocardial function is clear in its broad outline, a number of important details are still lacking. These are discussed in the Chapters by Siliprandi et al., Bremer et al., and Hulsmann et al. Powerful techniques now exist to localize lipids in membranes, as discussed by Severs, but it remains impossible to localize the lipids that accumulate in the ischemic heart. Thus, values for such substances as free fatty acids, fatty acyl CoA, and fatty acyl carnitine continue to be expressed as content (moles per unit of weight) rather than as concentration (moles per unit of a particular volume in the heart). As these lipid are highly soluble in the membrane bilayer, it is probable that they find their way into such membranes as the sarcolemma and sarcoplasmic reticulum, but it is not now possible to determine where these lipids are located in the membranes of the ischemic heart.

One of the major mechanisms by which abnormal concentrations of lipids can alter myocardial function is through their ability to modify membrane function. In addition, lipases can damage cells by hydrolysing membrane phospholipids, which both alters membrane function and leads to the release of fatty acids and lysophospholipids. Shaikh et al., who point out that it is essential to distinguish between the effects of membrane damage per se and those produced by the hydrolytic products, present evidence that membrane hydrolysis rather than the accumulation of hydrolytic products is of greatest importance in producing functional alterations in ischemia. On the other hand, studies in vitro indicate that free fatty acids and lyosphosphatides, at least in high concentrations, can have important effects on membrane function. These include modification of ion channel function, postulated by Pappano and Inoue to be due in part to a modification of surface charge, and effects on membrane permeability and the various ion transport systems localized in membranes that are discussed by Lamers et al. An effect of palmitic acid to trap calcium inside the sarcoplasmic reticulum is discussed by Messineo et al., while Ferrari et al, and Paulson and Shug describe the relationship between mitochondrial and contractile abnormalities in terms of the lipid abnormalities seen in the ischemic heart, and after reperfusion. Chien et al., who use the appearance of arachidonic acid as a marker for membrane degradation, suggest that impaired reincorporation of fatty acids into membrane lipids may represent a novel consequence of ATP depletion in the ischemic heart. Neely and McDonough, and van der Vusse et al., examine the amounts of lipid that accumulate in the ischemic heart, as well as their potential role in the pathogenesis of ischemic damage. The latter group reviews the measurements of fatty acids in the ischemic heart and notes that improved methodology has led to 1000-fold decrease in the amounts estimated to

appear in these injured hearts. This parallels a similar downward
revision in the amount of lysophospholipid that appears in the
ischemic heart, first pointed out by Shaikh.

Effects of carnitine on these lipid-induced abnormalities are
discussed by Shug and Paulson, and the ability of carnitine and
oxfenicine, which can reduce the amounts of fatty acid that accumulate in the ischemic heart, to improve function in the ischemic
heart are discussed by Liedtke and Miller. Chiariello et al.,
describe the ability of quinacrine, a phospholipase inhibitor, to
reduce the extent of ischemic myocardial damage while Bing presents
important data regarding coronary spasm. Opie et al., and Russell
and Oliver highlight the clinical significance of the many experimental studies described in this text while Rellas et al. point out
an important application of this approach in the non-invasive imaging of acute myocardial infarction.

Several conclusions emerged as a consensus at the end of this
meeting. The first is that this is a dynamic subject in which the
number of important questions far exceeds the answers that are currently available. Secondly, several discussants highlighted the
problems in methodology that have plagued this field. Accurate
measurements of various lipids are often difficult, and a number of
errors have appeared because of problems in the quantification of
such lipids as free fatty acids and lysophosphatides in the ischemic
heart. Finally, it was agreed that the role of lipid abnormalities
in the pathogenesis of ischemic damage remains an unsolved question
that is of intense interest and considerable practical importance
to Cardiology. Further interactions between basic scientists and
clinical investigators in this field clearly hold promise for the
development of clinically important information regarding means to
reduce the detrimental effects of cardiac ischemia in man.

                                             Arnold M. Katz

CONTRIBUTORS

Albertini, A.
  Institute of Chemistry
  School of Medicine
  University of Brescia
  Brescia, Italy

Ambrosio, G.
  Department of Medicine
  2nd School of Medicine
  University of Naples, Italy

Angelino, P.F.
  Cardiological Department
  Hospital Molinette
  Torino, Italy

Bigoli, M.C.
  Chair of Cardiology
  University of Brescia
  Brescia, Italy

Bing, R.J.
  Huntington Medical Research
  Institutes and Huntington
  Memorial Hospital
  Pasadena, California, U.S.A.

Borrebaek, B.
  University of Medical Biochemistry
  University of Oslo
  Oslo, Norway

Bremer, J.
  Institute of Medical Biochemistry
  University of Oslo
  Oslo, Norway

Brusca, A.
  Chair of Cardiology
  University of Torino
  Torino, Italy

Buja, L.M
  Departments of Internal
  Medicine, The University of
  Texas Health Science Center
  Dallas, Texas, U.S.A.

Caldarera, C.M.
  Institute of Biochemistry
  University of Bologna
  Bologna, Italy

Cappelli - Bigazzi, M.
  Department of Internal Medicine
  2nd School of Medicine
  University of Naples
  Naples, Italy

Ceconi, C.
  Chair of Cardiology
  University of Brescia
  Brescia, Italy

Cherchi, A.
  Chair of Cardiology
  University of Cagliari
  Cagliari, Italy

Chiariello, M.
  Dept. of Internal Medicine, 2nd
  School of Medicine, Univisity of
  Naples, Italy

333

Chien, K.R.
  Departments of Internal Medicine
  The University of Texas Health
  Science Center
  Dallas, Texas, U.S.A.

Condorelli, M.
  Department of Internal Medicine
  2nd School of Medicine
  University of Naples
  Naples, Italy

Corbett, J.R.
  Departments of Internal Medicine
  The University of Texas Health
  Science Center
  Dallas, Texas, U.S.A.

Curello, S.
  Chair of Cardiology
  University of Brescia
  Brescia, Italy

Dagianti, A.
  Chair of Cardiology
  University of Rome
  Rome, Italy

Davis, E.J.
  University School of Medicine
  University of Indianapolis
  Indianapolis, Indiana, U.S.A.

Devous, M.
  Departments of Internal Medicine
  The University of Texas
  Health Science Center
  Dallas, Texas, U.S.A.

Di Lisa, F.
  Institute of Biochemistry
  University of Padova
  Padova, Italy

Downar, E.
  Clinical Science Division
  University of Toronto
  Toronto, Canada

Ferrari, R.
  Chair of Cardiology
  University of Brescia
  Brescia, Italy

Harris, P.
  Cardiothoracic Institute
  London, England, UK

Hülsmann, W.C.
  Department of Biochemistry
  Erasmus University
  Rotterdam, The Netherlands

Inoue, D.
  Division of Cardiology
  2nd Department of Internal
  Medicine, Kyoto Prefectural
  University of Medicine
  Kyoto, Japan

Katz, A.M.
  Department of Medicine
  Division of Cardiology
  University of Connecticut
  Health Center
  Farmington, Connecticut, U.S.A.

Kulkarni, P.
  Departments of Internal
  Medicine, The University of
  Texas Health Science Center
  Dallas, Texas, U.S.A.

Lamers, J.M.J.
  Department of Biochemistry
  Erasmus University
  Rotterdam, The Netherlands

De Leiris, M.J.
  Université Scientifique et
  Medicale de Grenoble, Labora-
  toire de Physiologie Animale
  Grenoble, France

Lewis, S.E.
  Department of Internal Medicine
  The University of Texas Health
  Science Center
  Dallas, Texas, U.S.A.

Liedtke, A.J.
  Cardiological Department
  University of Wisconsin
  Madison, Wisconsin, U.S.A.

Magnani, B.
  Chair of Cardiology
  University of Bologna
  Bologna, Italy

Manzoli, U.
  Chair of Cardiology
  University of Rome
  Rome, Italy

Marone, G.
  Department of Internal Medicine
  2nd School of Medicine
  University of Naples
  Naples, Italy

Mattioli, G.
  Chair of Cardiology
  University of Modena
  Modena, Italy

Mc Donough, K.H.
  Department of Physiology
  Louisiana State University
  Medical Center
  New Orleans, Louisiana, U.S.A.

Messineo, F.C.
  Department of Medicine
  Division of Cardiology
  University of Connecticut
  Health Center
  Farmington, Connecticut, U.S.A.

Montfoort, A.
  Department of Biochemistry I
  Erasmus University
  Rotterdam, The Netherlands

Moret, K.R.
  Centre de Cardiologie
  Hospital Cantonal Genève
  Genève, Switzerland

Morgan, C.
  Departments of Internal
  Medicine, The University of
  Texas Health Science Center
  Dallas, Texas, U.S.A.

Muiesan, C.
  Clinic of General Medicine
  and Medical Therapy
  University of Brescia
  Brescia, Italy

Neely, J.R.
  Department of Physiology
  The Milton S. Hershey Medical
  Center, Penn. State University
  Hershey, Pennsylvania, U.S.A.

Oliver, M.
  Cardiovascular Research Unit
  Edinburgh, Scotland

Opie, L.H.
  Health Unit, Department of
  Medicine, University of
  Cape Town
  Cape Town, South Africa

Paoletti, R.
  Pharmacology Institute
  University of Milano
  Milano, Italy

Pappano, A.J.
  Department of Pharmacology
  University of Connecticut
  Health Center
  Farmington, Connecticut, U.S.A.

Parkey, R.W.
  Departments of Internal Medicine
  The University of Texas
  Health Science Center
  Dallas, Texas, U.S.A.

Parson, J.
  Clinical Science Division
  University of Toronto
  Toronto, Canada

Paulson, D.J.
  Metabolic Research Laboratory
  William S. Middleton Memorial
  Veteran Hospital and Dept. of
  Neurology, University of Wisconsin
  Madison, Wisconsin, U.S.A.

Pocchiari, F.
  High Institute of Health
  Rome, Italy

Preti, A.
  Institute of Biological Chemistry
  University of Brescia
  Brescia, Italy

Prinzen, F.W.
  Department of Physiology
  University of Limburg
  Maastricht, The Netherlands

Raddino, R.
  Chair of Cardiology
  University of Brescia
  Brescia, Italy

Rathier, M.
  Department of Medicine
  Division of Cardiology
  University of Connecticut
  Farmington, Connecticut, U.S.A.

Reale, A.
  Chair of Cardiology
  University of Rome
  Rome, Italy

Rellas, J.S.
  Departments of Internal
  Medicine, The University of
  Texas, Health Science Center
  Dallas, Texas, U.S.A.

Reneman, S.R.
  Department of Physiology
  University of Limburg
  Maastricht, The Netherlands

Rizzon, P.
  Chair of Cardiology
  University of Bari
  Bari, Italy

Rossi, C.R.
  Institute of Biochemistry
  University of Padova
  Padova, Italy

Russel, D.C.
  Cardiovascular Research Unit
  University of Edinburgh
  Edinburgh, Scotalnd

Severs, N.J.
  Department of Cardiac Medicine
  Cardiothoracic Institute
  University of London
  London, England

Shaikh, N.A.
  Clinical Science Division
  University of Toronto
  Toronto, Canada

Shug, A.
  Metabolic Research Laboratory
  William S. Middleton Memorial
  Veterans Hospital and Dept.
  of Neurology
  University of Wisconsin
  Madison, Wisconsin, U.S.A.

Siliprandi, N.
  Institute of Biochemistry
  University of Padova
  Padova, Italy

Stam, H.
  Department of Biochemistry I
  Erasmus University
  Rotterdam, The Netherlands

Stinis, H.T.
  Department of Pathological
  Anatomy I, Erasmus University
  Rotterdam, The Netherlands

Strano, A.
  Clinic of General Medicine
  University of Palermo
  Palermo, Italy

Takenaka, H.
  Department of Medicine
  Division of Cardiology
  University of Connecticut
  Farmington, Connecticut, U.S.A.

Tansey, M.J.
  Department of Medicine
  University of Cape Town
  Cape Town, South Africa

Toniniello, A.
  Institute of Biochemistry
  University of Padova
  Padova, Italy

Van Der Vusse, G.J.
  Department of Physiology
  University of Limburg
  Maastricht, The Netherlands

Visioli, O.
  Chair of Cardiology
  University of Brescia
  Brescia, Italy

Watras, J.M.
  Department of Medicine
  Division of Cardiology
  University of Connecticut
  Farmington, Connecticut, U.S.A.

Willerson, J.T.
  Department of Internal Medicine
  The University of Texas
  Health Science Center
  Dallas, Texas, U.S.A.